ATLAS OF
OPHTHALMIC
SURGERY

The **Slide Atlas of Ophthalmic Surgery,** based on the material in this book, is also available. The Slide Atlas is organized into 12 topic-based units, each consisting of superbly illustrated text, with 35 mm color slides corresponding to the photographs in the next text. In this unique format, all of the slides are labeled and numbered for easy reference. In addition, each unit is presented in a durable vinyl binder, and the complete collection comes in an attractive and sturdy presentation slip case.

Units 1 to 5	Cataract Surgery and Intraocular Lens Implantation
Unit 6	Techniques in Corneal Transplantation
Unit 7	Surgery for Glaucoma and Related Conditions
Unit 8	Surgery of the Retina and Vitreous
Unit 9	Techniques in Strabismus Surgery
Unit 10	Surgery of Acquired Lid Malpositions
Unit 11	Refractive Surgery
Unit 12	Laser Surgery of Chorioretinal Diseases

For further information, please contact:
Gower Medical Publishing
101 Fifth Avenue
New York, NY 10003

ATLAS OF
OPHTHALMIC
SURGERY

EDITOR

NORMAN S. JAFFE, MD

Clinical Professor of Ophthalmology
Bascom Palmer Eye Institute
University of Miami School of Medicine
Miami, Florida

With Original Illustrations by Alan Landau

J.B. LIPPINCOTT • PHILADELPHIA
GOWER MEDICAL PUBLISHING • NEW YORK

Distributed in USA and
Canada by:
J.B. Lippincott Company
East Washington Square
Philadelphia, PA 19105
USA

Distributed in UK and
Continental Europe by:
Harper & Row Ltd.
Middlesex House
34-42 Cleveland Street
London W1P 5FB
UK

Distributed in Australia
and New Zealand by:
**Harper & Row
(Australasia) Pty, Ltd.**
P.O. Box 226
Artarmon, N.S.W. 2064
Australia

Distributed in Southeast
Asia, Hong Kong, India
and Pakistan by:
**Harper & Row Publishers
(Asia) Pte, Ltd.**
37 Jalan Pemimpin 02-01
Singapore 2057

Distributed in Japan by:
Igaku-Shoin Ltd.
Tokyo International
P.O. Box 5063
Tokyo
Japan

Library of Congress Cataloging-in-Publication Data

Atlas of ophthalmic surgery / editor, Norman S. Jaffe.
   p. cm.
  Bibliography: p.
  Includes index.
  ISBN 0-397-44664-0
  1. Eye—Surgery—Atlases.   I. Jaffe, Norman S., 1924–
  [DNLM: 1. Eye—surgery—atlases.   WW 17 A8813]
RE80.A86 1990
617.7′1′0222—dc20
DNLM/DLC   89-11915
for Library of Congress   CIP

Editors: Meryl R. G. Muskin, Joy Noel Travalino
Illustrator: Alan Landau
Art Director: Jill Feltham
Interior Design: Judy Morgan
Layout and Cover Design: Maura Burke

10 9 8 7 6 5 4 3 2 1

Printed in Singapore by Imago Productions (FE) PTE, Ltd.

PREFACE

The goal of *Atlas of Ophthalmic Surgery* is to provide a comprehensive visual reference combined with an integrated text of the important surgical subspecialties of ophthalmology. I have enlisted the aid of authors and teachers who are recognized as experts both in the United States and abroad. It is inevitable that style will vary from chapter to chapter but it is hoped that quality will be consistent because of the expertise of the authors.

I have long been aware of the "how-to-do-it" preference of ophthalmologists for learning surgical techniques. Most of us appreciate the value of carefully designed illustrations and action photography in the art of communication. Visual stimuli are more effective than auditory stimuli in teaching surgical techniques. When necessary, drawings have been used to clarify details not easily seen in photographs.

We have attempted to be highly selective in describing those methods in each subspecialty that are most universally accepted. It is impossible to include the seemingly endless number of new ideas presented in ophthalmic surgery. The authors have attempted to describe those techniques that ophthalmologists will find most useful.

This book is intended for the experienced ophthalmologist as well as for those in training. It is hoped that it will be sufficiently comprehensive to aid the ophthalmic surgeon in performing competent surgery and in the management of complications.

No attempt was made to provide an exhaustive bibliography. The suggested reading list includes textbooks, classic papers, review articles, and pertinent up-to-date references to supplement the material presented in this book.

The *Slide Atlas of Ophthalmic Surgery*, which serves as a source for all the illustrations in the text, is useful for reviewing the techniques presented. It can also be used for teaching and course presentation. A unique feature is the separate availability of the text and slide collection. Individual chapters are also available for those surgeons interested in one or more of the subspecialties.

Ophthalmology is a dynamic specialty of medicine. Old concepts change and new ideas are plentiful. Most of the techniques described have been accepted and form the background of modern ophthalmic surgery.

I would like to acknowledge the expert artistic support of Alan Landau and the superb editorial assistance of Meryl Muskin, a tireless worker. I am grateful to Abe Krieger of Gower Medical Publishing for inviting me to prepare this atlas.

Norman S. Jaffe

CONTENTS

CHAPTER 2   TECHNIQUES IN CORNEAL TRANSPLANTATION

Roger H. S. Langston, MD, CM, FACS

CHAPTER 3   SURGERY FOR GLAUCOMA AND RELATED CONDITIONS

George Nardin, MD
Thom J. Zimmerman, MD, PhD

CHAPTER 4   SURGERY OF THE RETINA AND VITREOUS
H. M. Freeman, MD

CHAPTER 5   TECHNIQUES IN STRABISMUS SURGERY
Robert W. Lingua, MD

CHAPTER 6   SURGERY OF ACQUIRED LID MALPOSITIONS
Richard R. Tenzel, MD

CHAPTER 7 REFRACTIVE SURGERY

Lee T. Nordan, MD
W. Andrew Maxwell, MD, PhD

CHAPTER 8 LASER SURGERY OF CHORIORETINAL DISEASES

Peter H. Judson, MD
Lawrence A. Yannuzzi, MD

CONTRIBUTORS

H. MacKenzie Freeman
Associate Clinical Professor
   of Ophthalmology
Harvard Medical School
Surgeon in Ophthalmology
Massachusetts Eye and Ear Infirmary
Clinical Senior Scientist
Eye Research Institute of
   Retina Foundation
Boston, Massachusetts

Norman S. Jaffe, MD
Clinical Professor of Ophthalmology
Bascom Palmer Eye Institute
University of Miami School
   of Medicine
Miami, Florida

Peter H. Judson, MD
Clinical Instructor in
   Vitreoretinal Diseases
University of Connecticut
   Health Sciences Center
Farmington, Connecticut

Roger H. S. Langston, MD, CM, FACS
The Cleveland Clinic Foundation
Department of Ophthalmology
Cornea Service
Cleveland, Ohio

Robert Lingua, MD
Assistant Professor
Department of Ophthalmology
Bascom Palmer Eye Institute
University of Miami School
   of Medicine
Miami, Florida

W. Andrew Maxwell, MD, PhD
Department of Ophthalmology
University of California
at San Francisco
San Francisco, California

George F. Nardin, MD
Assistant Professor
Department of Ophthalmology and
   Visual Sciences
University of Louisville
Louisville, Kentucky

Lee T. Nordan, MD
Assistant Clinical Professor
Jules Stein Eye Institute
University of California
   at Los Angeles
Los Angeles, California

Richard R. Tenzel, MD
Clinical Professor of Ophthalmology
University of Miami School
   of Medicine
Chief of the Plastic Surgical Service
Bascom Palmer Eye Institute
Miami, Florida

Lawrence A. Yannuzzi, MD, FACS
Vice Chairman, Academic Affairs
Department of Ophthalmology
Manhattan Eye, Ear and
   Throat Hospital
New York, New York

Thom J. Zimmerman, MD, PhD
Professor and Chairman
Department of Ophthalmology and
   Visual Sciences
University of Louisville
Louisville, Kentucky

CATARACT SURGERY AND INTRAOCULAR LENS IMPLANTATION

1

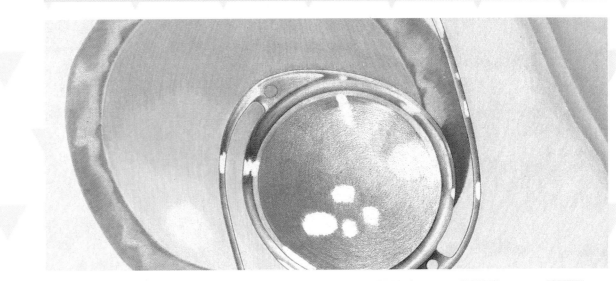

Norman S. Jaffe, MD

Cataract surgery and intraocular lens implantation is a dynamic subject filled with changing concepts and new ideas. Complications associated with it are numerous. An effort is made in this chapter to include standard surgical techniques and their complications. Some new procedures and concepts are not included since they have not yet fulfilled their promise of survival.

PHACOEMULSIFICATION

Since most phacoemulsifications include the implantation of an intraocular lens, the following technique is that used in conjunction with the placement of a posterior chamber lens.

After the preparation of a fornix-based conjunctival flap, calipers are used to mark on the sclera the intended length of the incision (Fig. 1.1). A groove incision, in this case 6.5 mm in length, is made with a diamond knife posterior to the posterior limbal border, in preparation for posterior chamber lens implantation (Fig. 1.2). An ab externo incision is made at the anterior limbal border at 1:30 o'clock (Fig. 1.3). An ab externo incision is made through the groove at its right side (Fig. 1.4). A viscoelastic material is injected into the anterior chamber (Fig. 1.5). A "can-opener" anterior capsulectomy is performed in this case with a bent-tipped, 1-in, 22-gauge disposable needle. The tip is bent at a right angle away from the bevel. Small punctures are made in the anterior capsule without stressing the zonules. The initial cuts are made at the 6 o'clock border. They are made parallel to the iris margin (Fig. 1.6). The remaining cuts are made to complete an oval-shaped capsulectomy. The oval is wider horizontally than vertically. Approximately 50 punctures are made (Fig. 1.7). The oval portion of the incised anterior capsule is then freed with the capsulectomy needle (Fig. 1.8). There is a wide variation in

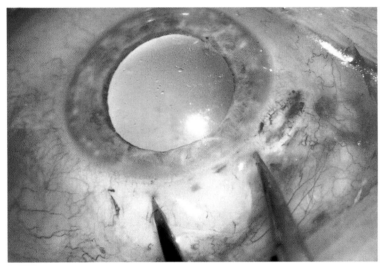
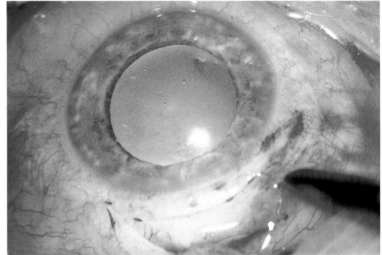

FIG. 1.1   FIG. 1.2

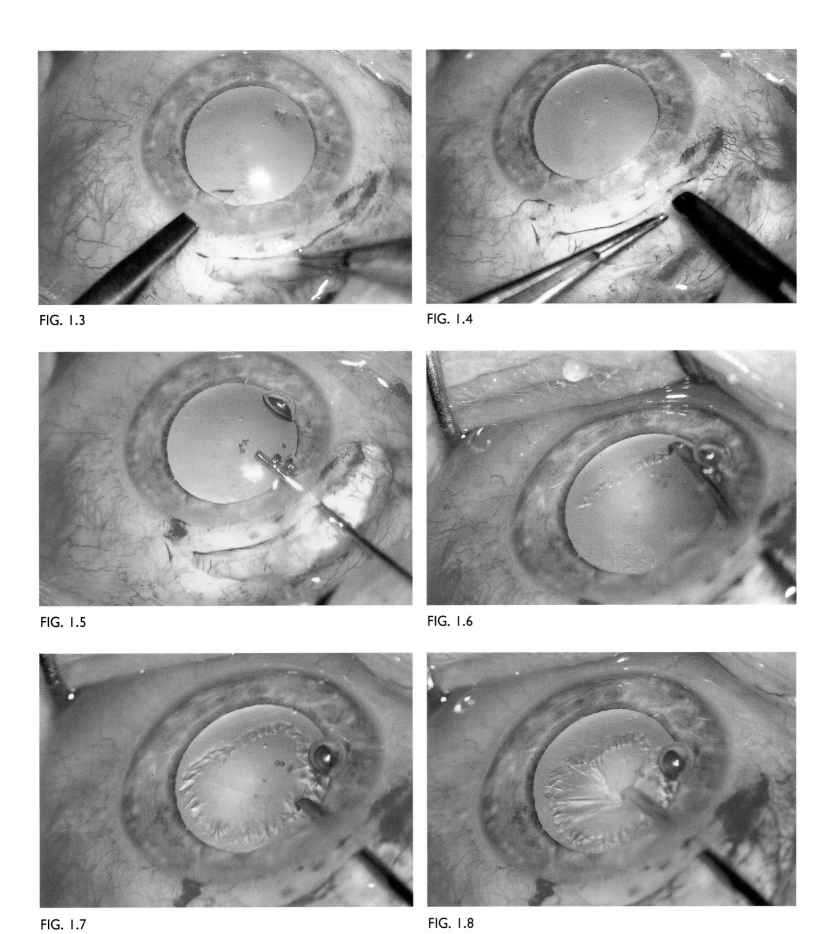

FIG. 1.3

FIG. 1.4

FIG. 1.5

FIG. 1.6

FIG. 1.7

FIG. 1.8

preference among ophthalmic surgeons as to the shape and size of the anterior capsulectomy. Most surgeons ensure that anterior margins of the capsule are available for capsular bag fixation of the posterior chamber lens. The ab externo incision is enlarged to slightly greater than 3.0 mm with a No. 55 Beaver blade or some other similar instrument (Fig. 1.9).

POSTERIOR CHAMBER PHACOEMULSIFICATION

To begin this procedure, the ultrasonic handpiece is passed into the anterior chamber. An oval, 60° bevel tip is used here. Sculpting of the anterior surface of the nucleus begins (Fig. 1.10). At least one-half of the nucleus is sculpted and a sharp border is left at the inferior margin of the sculpted area (Fig. 1.11). A Jaffe-Bechert nucleus rotator is then passed into the anterior chamber through the 1:30 o'clock incision (Fig. 1.12). The nucleus rotator displaces the nucleus toward 6 o'clock by engaging it at the inferior sculpted margin. The nucleus is allowed to rise anteriorly by assuming a foot-switch position of zero. The ultrasonic tip then passes behind the superior equator of the nucleus (Fig. 1.13). The nucleus rotator assists in rotating the nucleus so that emulsification is always performed at the equator of the nucleus (Fig. 1.14). It also keeps the nucleus away from the back of the cornea (Fig. 1.15). It feeds large pieces of nucleus into the ultrasonic tip (Figs. 1.16 and 1.17). The nucleus is finally emulsified and aspirated (Fig.

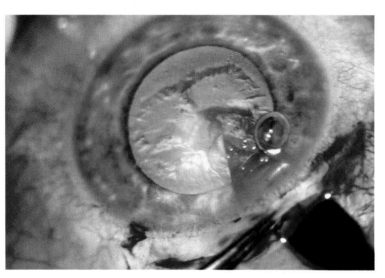

FIG. 1.9

Posterior Chamber Phacoemulsification

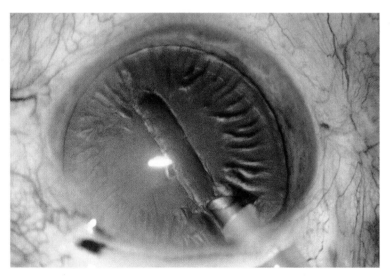

FIG. 1.10

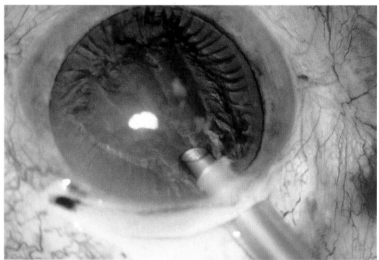

FIG. 1.11

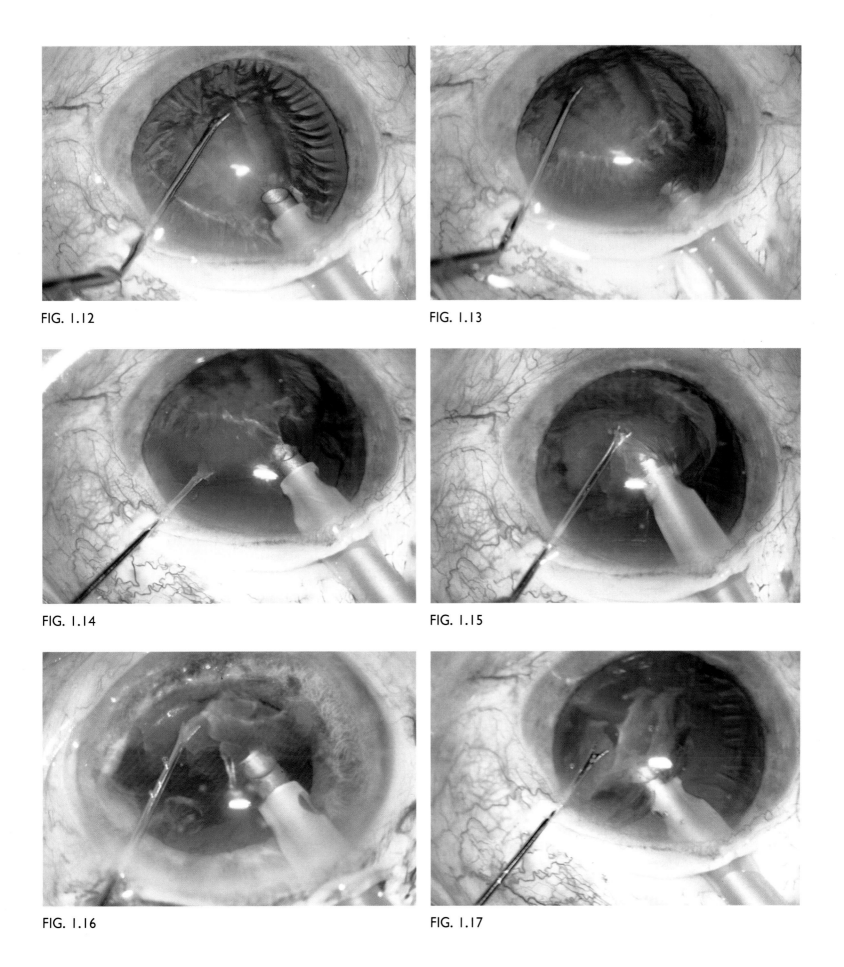

FIG. 1.12

FIG. 1.13

FIG. 1.14

FIG. 1.15

FIG. 1.16

FIG. 1.17

1.18). Aspiration of the residual cortical material is performed using the irrigation–aspiration handpiece with a 0.3-mm aspiration port. The port should face the cortex or face slightly anteriorly. A purchase is made peripherally (Fig. 1.19). The cortex is stripped toward the center of the pupil where it is aspirated (Fig. 1.20). A purchase should never be made in the center of the pupil since rupture of the posterior capsule is more likely. The posterior capsule is polished using the same handpiece with the port facing the posterior capsule. Minimal aspiration pressure is used during this process (Fig. 1.21). If the posterior capsule becomes engaged by the aspiration port, the surgeon must be quick to release it. This is done by pinching the reflux bulb of the aspiration line. The incision is then enlarged along the previously prepared groove for a distance of 6.5 mm if a 6-mm-diameter posterior chamber lens is used.

ANTERIOR CHAMBER PHACOEMULSIFICATION

This was the favored method of phacoemulsification after its introduction by Kelman. It has the advantage of less risk of rupturing the posterior capsule but it has two significant disadvantages: it causes more corneal endothelial cell loss than posterior chamber phacoemulsification, and nuclear prolapse into the anterior chamber may be a difficult technique.

The anterior capsulectomy is performed by the can-opener technique described above. The nucleus is grasped with a dull-tipped irrigating cystotome at 6 o'clock just under the incised margin of the anterior capsule, approximately 2 mm from its equator. The nucleus is pulled toward 12 o'clock until the inferior equator reaches the 3 and 9 o'clock meridian (Fig. 1.22A). The 3 and 9 o'clock equators of the nucleus are alternately rotated anteriorly to free them from the surrounding cortex. The 6 o'clock equator is then lifted anteriorly as the nucleus is slowly slid back toward 6 o'clock (Fig. 1.22B). During this movement the nucleus is rotated to the left and to the right so that it is prolapsed into the anterior chamber (Figs. 1.22C and 1.22D). The nucleus is then emulsified and aspirated as described above. However, since the nucleus is closer to the back of the cornea than with posterior chamber pha-coemulsification, the nucleus rotator is used to prevent corneal touch.

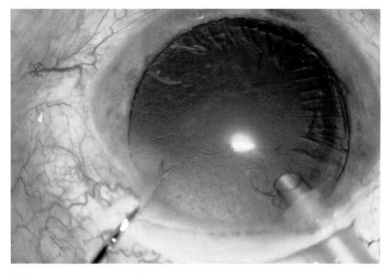

FIG. 1.18

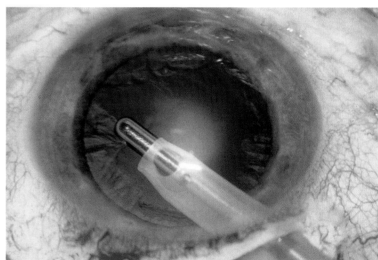

FIG. 1.19

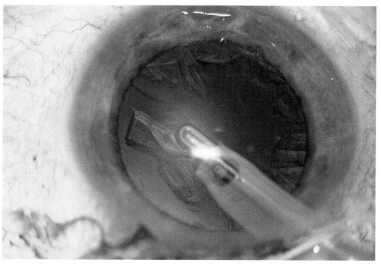

FIG. 1.20

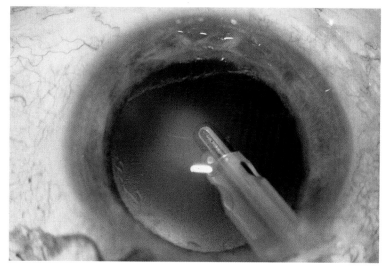

FIG. 1.21

▽ Anterior Chamber Phacoemulsification

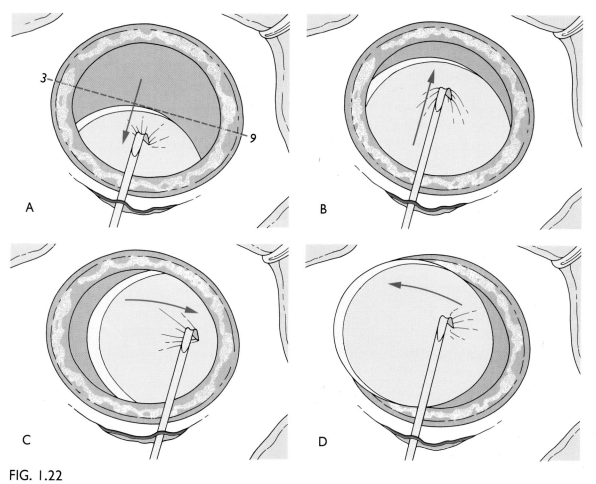

FIG. 1.22

PLANNED EXTRACAPSULAR CATARACT EXTRACTION

Following the preparation of a fornix-based conjunctival flap, a groove incision is made in the sclera behind the posterior limbal margin using a diamond knife. The incision length is approximately 11 to 12 mm. The can-opener anterior capsulectomy is performed using a bent-tipped 1-in, 22-gauge disposable needle (Fig. 1.23). The nucleus is displaced inferiorly to separate it slightly from the surrounding cortex (Fig. 1.24). The incision is then enlarged along the entire length of the previously prepared groove (Fig. 1.25).

The most popular method of nucleus delivery is by scleral expression. Pressure is exerted at the inferior limbal border with an instrument such as forceps or a muscle hook. At the same time, pressure is exerted against the sclera 2 mm posterior to the incision using a loop (e.g., Sheets irrigating vectis, Fig. 1.26). Pressure against the globe is alternated between the two instruments until the 12 o'clock border of the nucleus begins to pass through the incision (Fig. 1.27). The nucleus is delivered slowly (Figs. 1.28 and 1.29). The forceps used at 6 o'clock may then be used to draw the final portion of the nucleus out of the eye (Figs. 1.30 and 1.31). The incision is closed with three sutures. The irrigation–

Planned Extracapsular Cataract Extraction

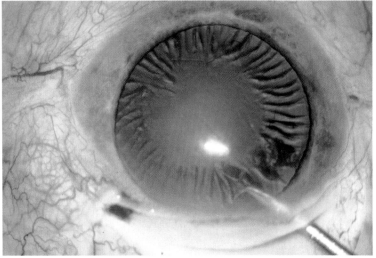

FIG. 1.23

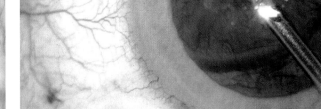

FIG. 1.24

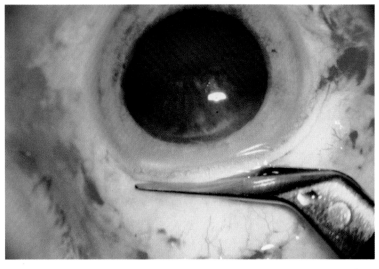

FIG. 1.25

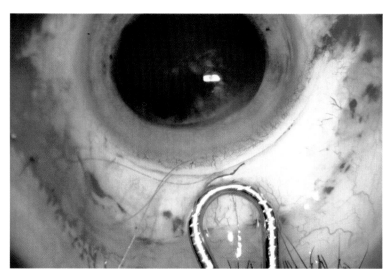

FIG. 1.26

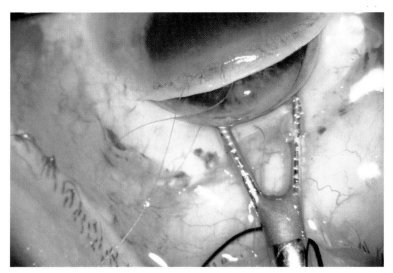

FIG. 1.27

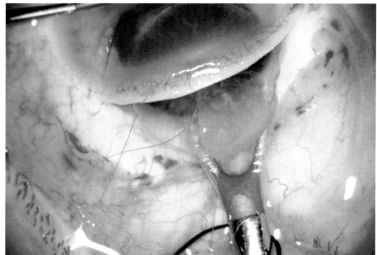

FIG. 1.28

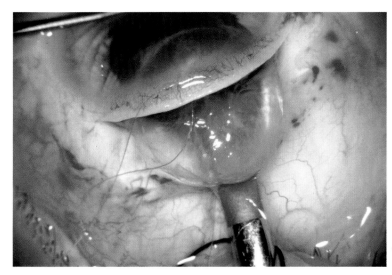

FIG. 1.29

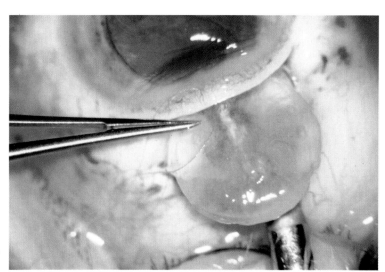

FIG. 1.30

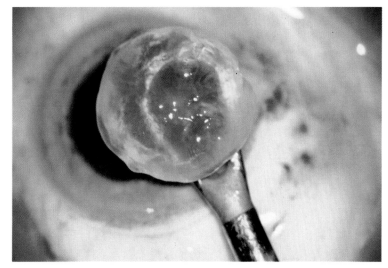

FIG. 1.31

aspiration handpiece with a 0.3-mm aspiration port is then passed between the middle and the right sutures into the anterior chamber. The orifice is directed laterally or medially to engage the cortex in the periphery. It is drawn toward the center of the pupil where it is aspirated (Figs. 1.32 to 1.36). The purchase is always made at the periphery. The posterior capsule is then polished with low aspiration pressure and with the port directed against the posterior capsule. If the posterior capsule becomes engaged inadvertently, it is imperative that the surgeon quickly cease aspiration by having a surgical assistant pinch the reflux bulb of the aspiration tubing (Fig. 1.37). The central suture is removed to permit implantation of a posterior chamber lens.

ENDOCAPSULAR–EXTRACAPSULAR CATARACT EXTRACTION

Galand and Anis, along with others, have described a method in which the procedure is performed within the capsular bag. This method may be more protective of the cornea and ensures capsular bag fixation of a posterior chamber lens. The following technique is a modification of their methods.

Several punctures are made horizontally in the anterior capsule at 6 o'clock (Fig. 1.38). A puncture is made in the anterior capsule at 10 o'clock (Fig. 1.39). The incision is enlarged to the right along a previously prepared groove (Fig. 1.40). The posterior blade of a Stern-Gills forceps (Katena) is passed through the 10 o'clock opening and the anterior capsule is incised to 2 o'clock (Fig. 1.41). The inci-

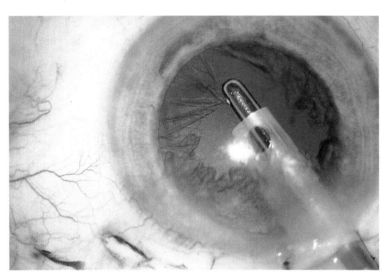

FIG. 1.32

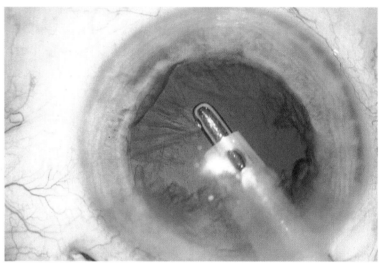

FIG. 1.33

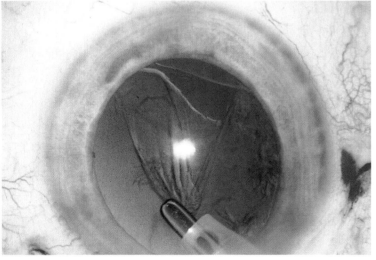

FIG. 1.34

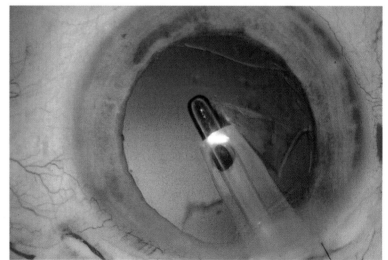

FIG. 1.35

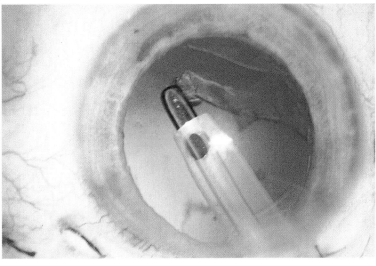

FIG. 1.36

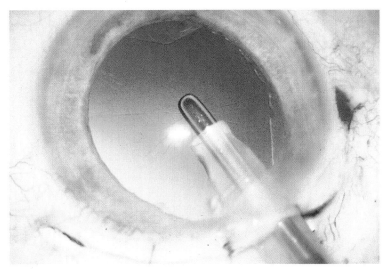

FIG. 1.37

Endocapsular–Extracapsular Cataract Extraction

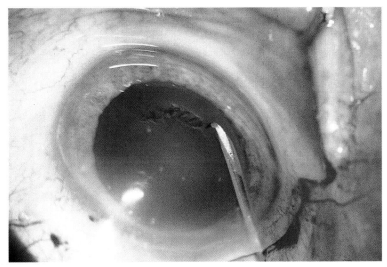

FIG. 1.38

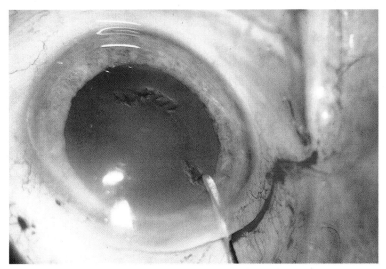

FIG. 1.39

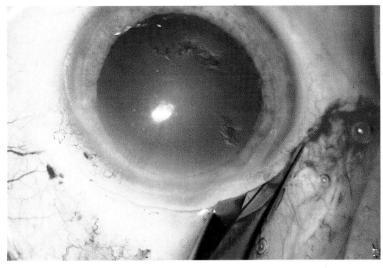

FIG. 1.40

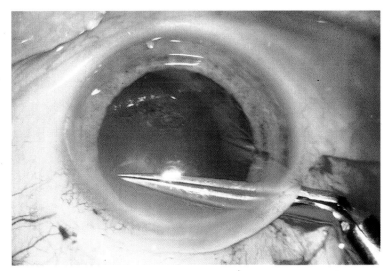

FIG. 1.41

sion in the anterior capsule is shown in Fig. 1.42. The nucleus is displaced toward 6 o'clock with the bent-tipped needle. This is performed inside the capsular bag (Fig. 1.43). The nucleus is expressed as described for a routine planned extracapsular cataract extraction (Figs. 1.44 to 1.46). Irrigation–aspiration of residual cortex is performed inside the capsular bag (Figs. 1.47 and 1.48). The posterior capsule is polished (Fig. 1.49). The opening in the anterior capsule is shown in Fig. 1.50. A viscoelastic material is injected inside the capsular bag (Fig. 1.51). The leading

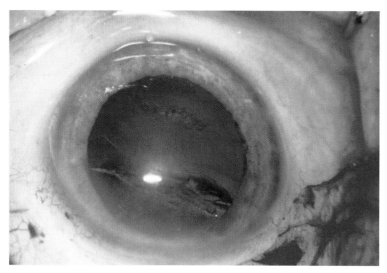

FIG. 1.42

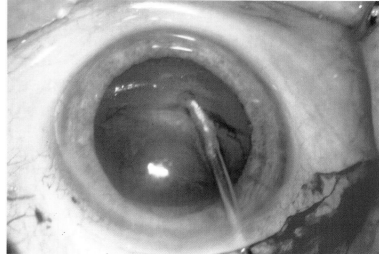

FIG. 1.43

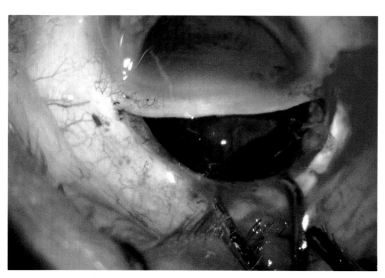

FIG. 1.44

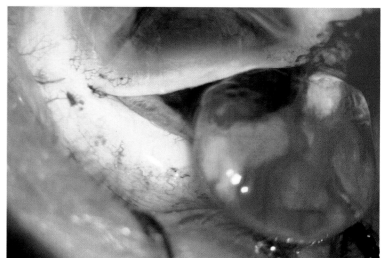

FIG. 1.45

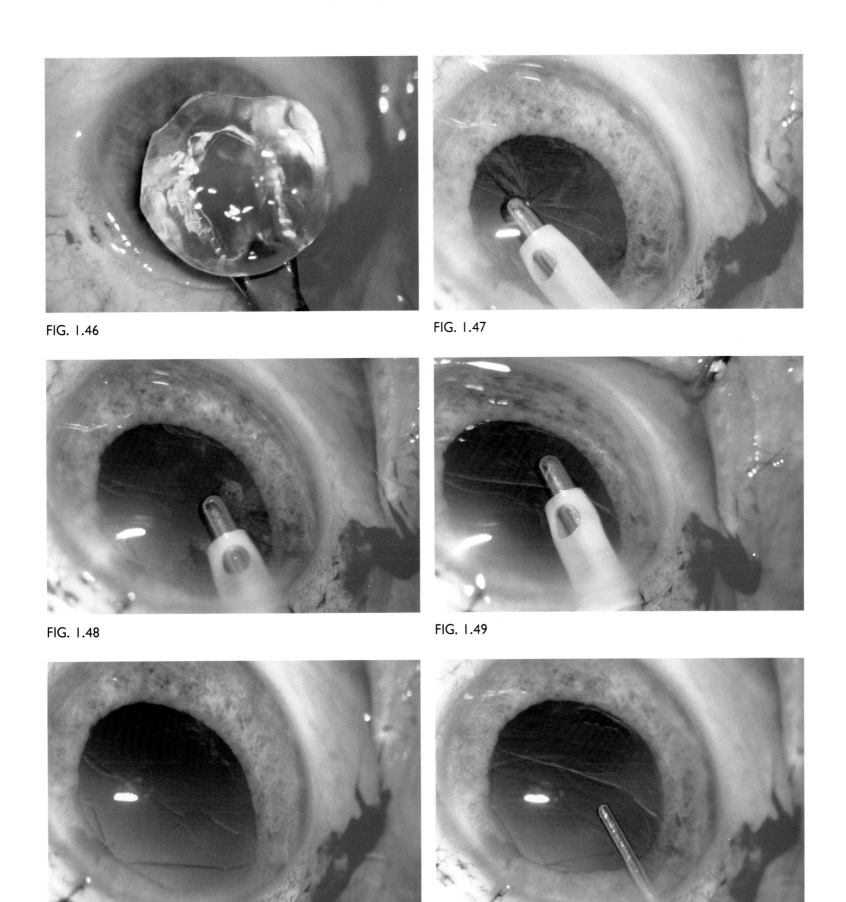

FIG. 1.46

FIG. 1.47

FIG. 1.48

FIG. 1.49

FIG. 1.50

FIG. 1.51

loop of a Jaffe 3 posterior chamber lens is passed into the capsule bag at 6 o'clock (Fig. 1.52). The hole in the convexity of the trailing loop is engaged with Jaffe-Maltzman forceps (Katena) (Fig. 1.53). The loop is flexed into the eye (Fig. 1.54). With a pronation of the wrist, the loop is passed under the superior capsular flap (Fig. 1.55). The lens is now completely within the capsular bag. The opening in the anterior capsule is shown (Fig. 1.56). A diagonal incision of the anterior capsule is made on the right. This connects the incision with the end of the previously made can-opener incision at 6 o'clock (Fig. 1.57). A similar incision is made on the left (Fig. 1.58). The anterior capsule is grasped with smooth forceps and torn free to the left (Fig. 1.59). The freed piece of anterior capsule is removed from the eye (Fig. 1.60). The lens is shown in the capsular bag (Fig. 1.61).

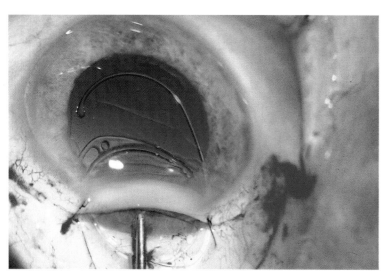

FIG. 1.52

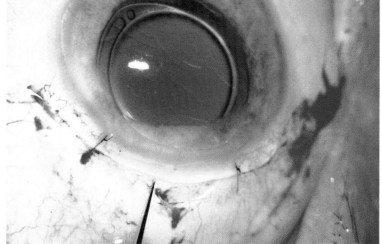

FIG. 1.53

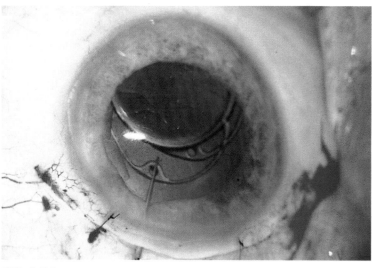

FIG. 1.54

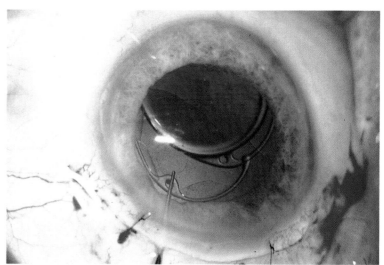

FIG. 1.55

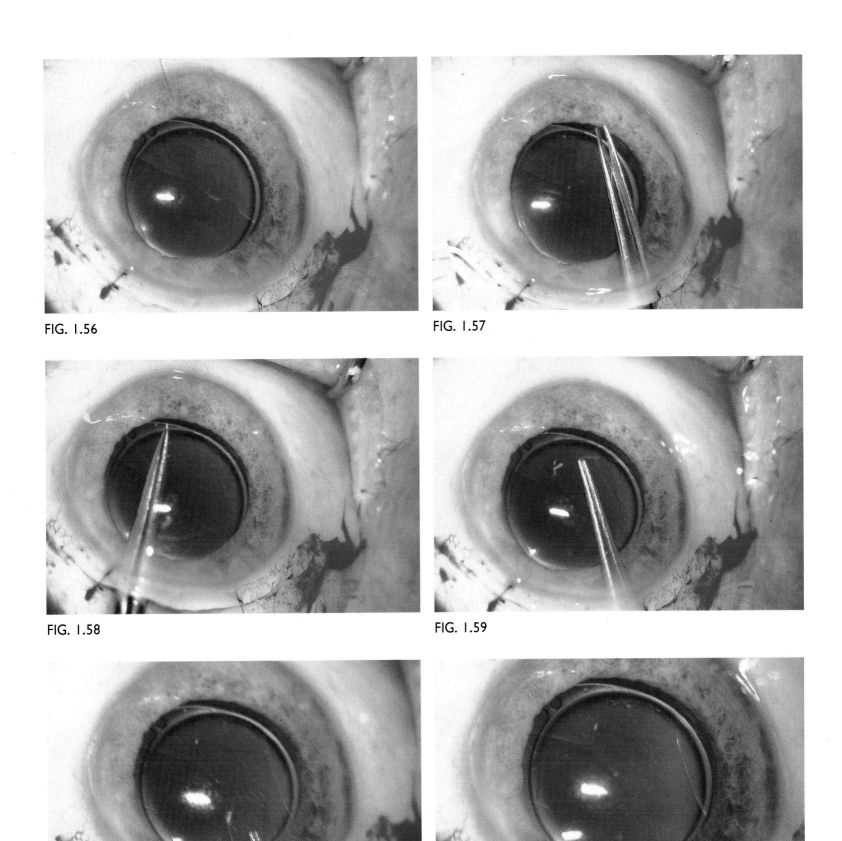

FIG. 1.56

FIG. 1.57

FIG. 1.58

FIG. 1.59

FIG. 1.60

FIG. 1.61

DELIVERY OF THE NUCLEUS

There are a variety of methods available to deliver the nucleus in a planned extracapsular cataract extraction. They fall into three categories. Nucleus 1 involves a prolapse of the nucleus into the anterior chamber and removal from the eye with a thin vectis. Nucleus 2 involves removal of the nucleus from the posterior chamber with a thin vectis. Nucleus 3 involves expression of the nucleus by scleral pressure.

Nucleus 1

The can-opener anterior capsulectomy is performed (Fig. 1.62). A vertical see-saw movement is performed as follows. The nucleus is engaged with a dull cystotome 2 to 3 mm from its inferior edge and displaced superiorly until its inferior edge reaches the horizontal meridian (Fig. 1.63). The nucleus is then engaged 2 to 3 mm from its superior edge

and displaced inferiorly until its inferior edge passes over the iris (Figs. 1.64 and 1.65). The entire nucleus is now in the anterior chamber (Fig. 1.66). A Knolle-Pearce irrigating vectis is passed through the incision (Fig. 1.67) and under the entire nucleus (Fig. 1.68). The nucleus is removed from the eye (Figs. 1.69 to 1.71).

A variation of Nucleus 1 using a combination of vertical and horizontal see-saw movements follows. The anterior capsulectomy is performed and the nucleus is engaged with a dull cystotome 2 to 3 mm from its inferior edge (Fig. 1.72). The nucleus is displaced superiorly until its inferior edge reaches the horizontal meridian (Figs. 1.73 and 1.74). The nucleus is then engaged 2 to 3 mm from one horizontal edge and rotated in the opposite direction until the entire nucleus is in the anterior chamber (Figs. 1.75 to 1.78). The nucleus is then delivered from the anterior chamber using the Knolle-Pearce irrigating vectis (Figs. 1.79 to 1.83).

Extracapsular Cataract Extraction: Nucleus 1

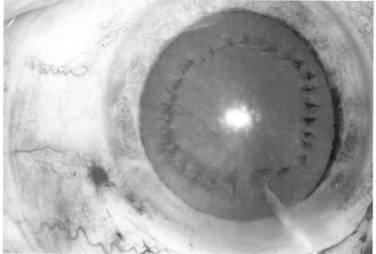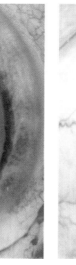

FIG. 1.62

FIG. 1.63

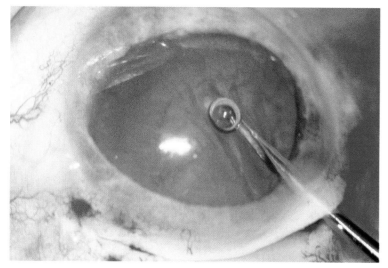

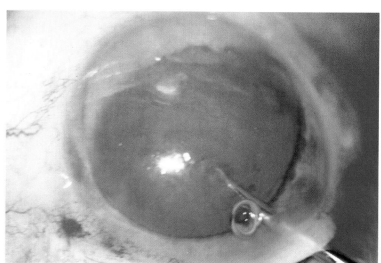

FIG. 1.64

FIG. 1.65

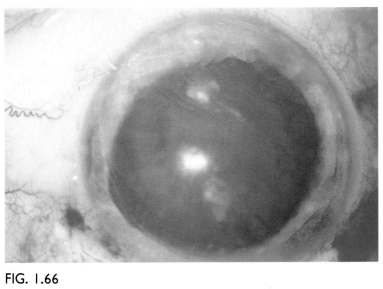

FIG. 1.66

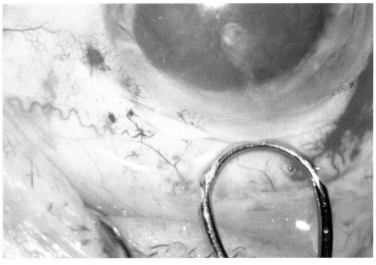

FIG. 1.67

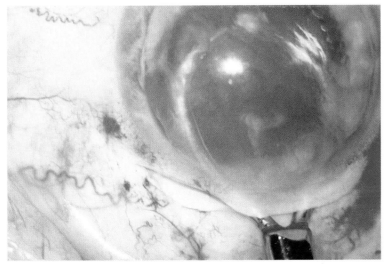

FIG. 1.68

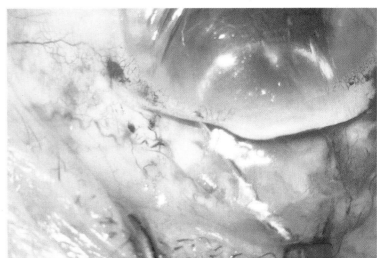

FIG. 1.69

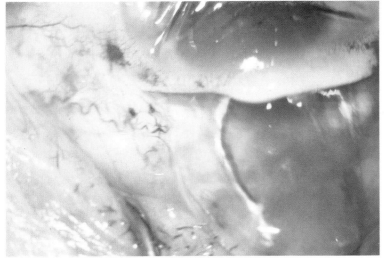

FIG. 1.70

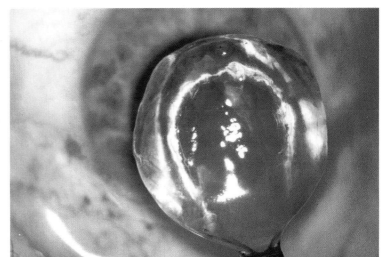

FIG. 1.71

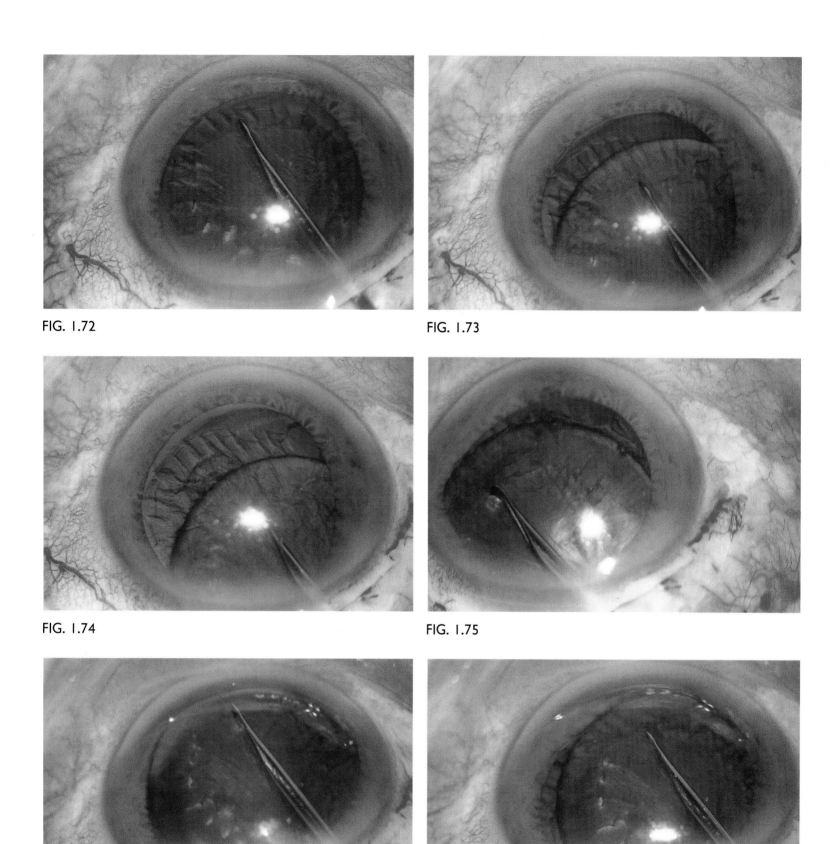

FIG. 1.72

FIG. 1.73

FIG. 1.74

FIG. 1.75

FIG. 1.76

FIG. 1.77

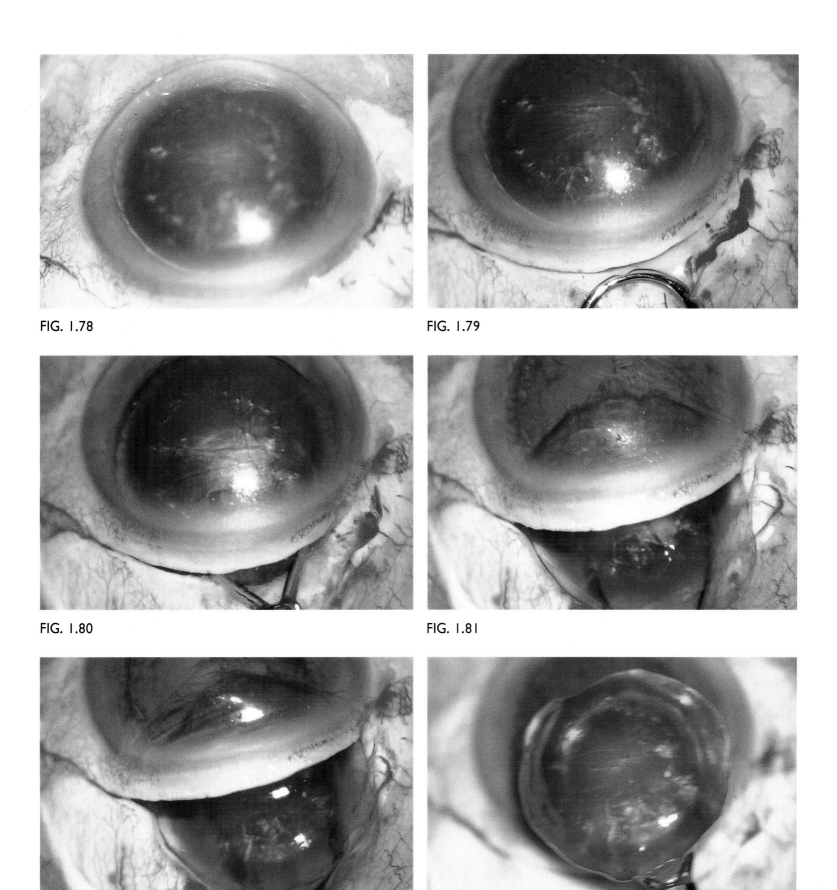

FIG. 1.78

FIG. 1.79

FIG. 1.80

FIG. 1.81

FIG. 1.82

FIG. 1.83

This method was first recommended by Kelman, who still uses it. It is probably the most difficult of the three methods to learn and the least-used today.

Nucleus 2

The can-opener anterior capsulectomy is performed and the nucleus is freed from its surrounding cortex by displacing it slightly inferiorly until the nucleus is seen to cleave from the cortex. Some use a spatula under the superior edge of the nucleus and sweep it horizontally between the nucleus and cortex. A Knolle-Pearce vectis is passed under the superior edge of the nucleus so that the edge of the vectis is clearly visible under the edge of the nucleus (Figs. 1.84 and 1.85). The vectis is then passed inferiorly until it is under the entire nucleus (Figs. 1.86 and 1.87). The nucleus is then removed from the eye (Figs. 1.88 to 1.90).

This is a very popular method and is used by many surgeons with a variety of modifications and a variety of instruments.

Nucleus 3

This is the most popular method of nucleus delivery. It involves the use of pressure exerted against the sclera superiorly and counterpressure at the inferior limbus. It has been described above (Figs. 1.26 to 1.31).

MIOTIC PUPIL TECHNIQUE

Occasionally, cataract surgery must be performed on an eye with a miotic pupil. This condition may be due to senile miosis, long-term miotic therapy for glaucoma, or a peripheral iridectomy in an eye treated with miotics. A variation in the technique of extracapsular cataract extraction is used here.

Figure 1.91 shows an eye that had a previous peripheral iridectomy for angle closure glaucoma. The pupil could not be dilated more than shown. A groove incision is made along the limbus and an ab externo incision is made at the right extremity of the groove (Fig. 1.92). The incision is

▽ Extracapsular Cataract Extraction: Nucleus 2

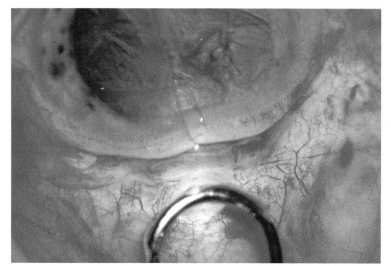

FIG. 1.84

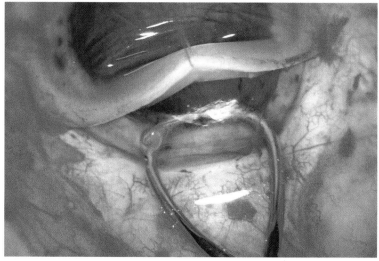

FIG. 1.85

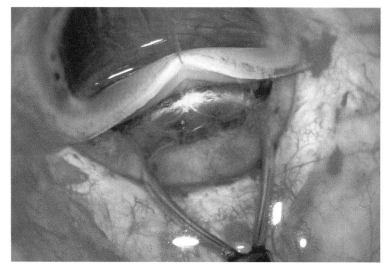

FIG. 1.86

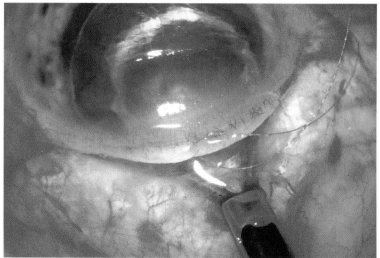

FIG. 1.87

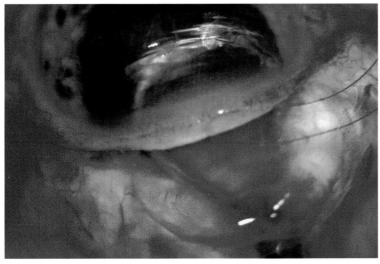

FIG. 1.88

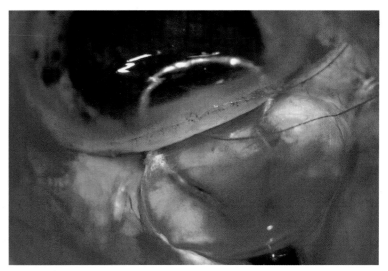

FIG. 1.89

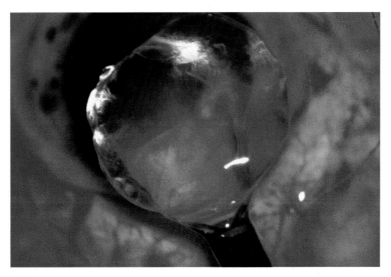

FIG. 1.90

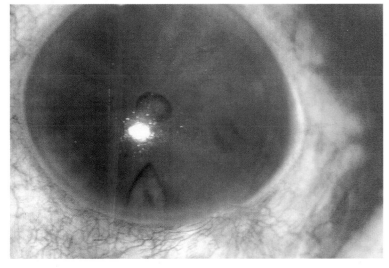

FIG. 1.91

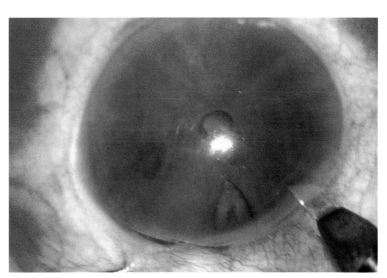

FIG. 1.92

extended to the left with scissors along the entire length of the groove (Fig. 1.93). The iris is incised with scissors between the iridectomy and the pupil (Figs. 1.94 and 1.95). A viscoelastic material is injected into the anterior chamber (Fig. 1.96). Because of the extreme miosis, an inferior iri-dotomy is performed (Figs. 1.97 and 1.98). The nucleus is expressed by the Nucleus 3 method described above (Figs. 1.99 to 1.101). The incision is closed with three sutures and irrigation–aspiration of the residual cortex is performed (Fig. 1.102). The anterior capsular margins are shown in

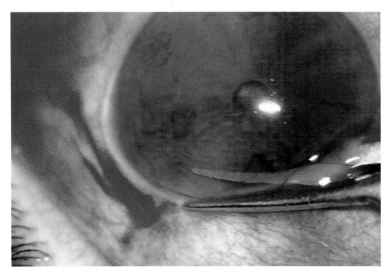

FIG. 1.93

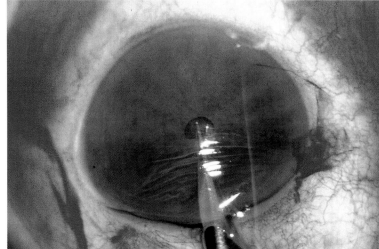

FIG. 1.94

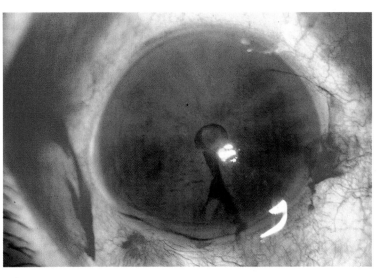

FIG. 1.95

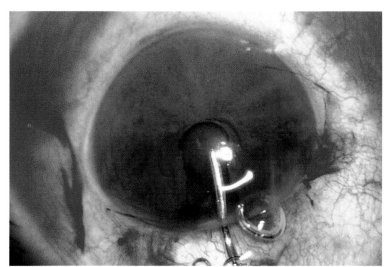

FIG. 1.96

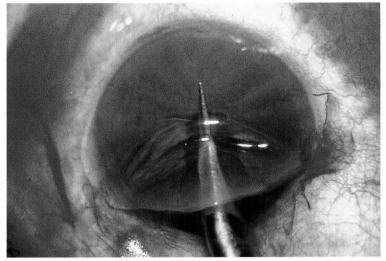

FIG. 1.97

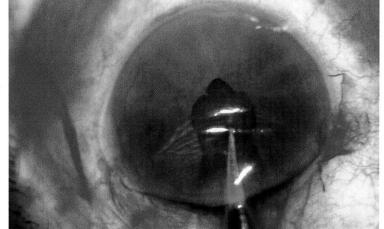

FIG. 1.98

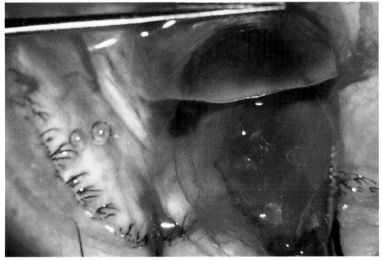

FIG. 1.99

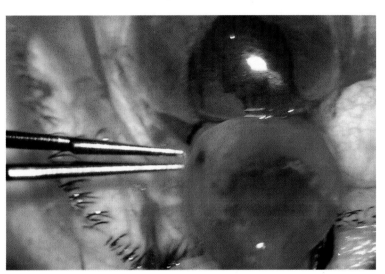

FIG. 1.100

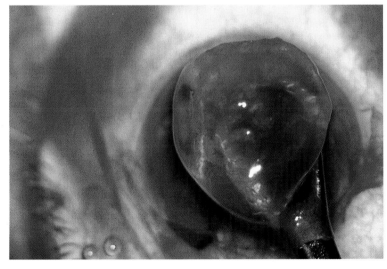

FIG. 1.101

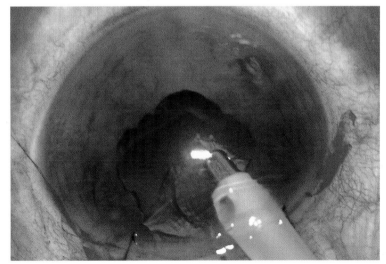

FIG. 1.102

Fig. 1.103. The capsule bag is filled with the viscoelastic material (Fig. 1.04). The Jaffe 3 posterior chamber lens is held in Blaydes forceps (Fig. 1.105). It is introduced into the eye (Fig. 1.106) and the leading loop is passed under the inferior capsular flap (Fig. 1.107). A Jaffe-Maltzman hook engages the hole in the convexity of the trailing loop

(Fig. 1.108) and flexes it into the eye (Fig. 1.109). With a pronation of the wrist, the loop is passed behind the margin of the superior capsular flap (Fig. 1.110). The viscoelastic material is aspirated (Fig. 1.111). The implant is in the capsule bag and the incision is closed (Fig. 1.112).

If the eye has a miotic pupil without a previous periph-

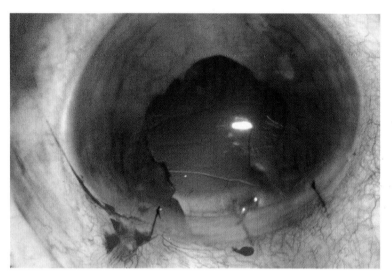

FIG. 1.103

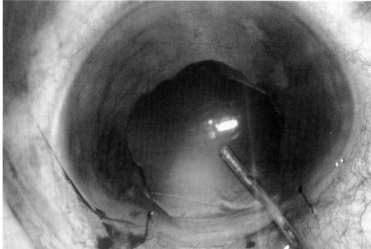

FIG. 1.104

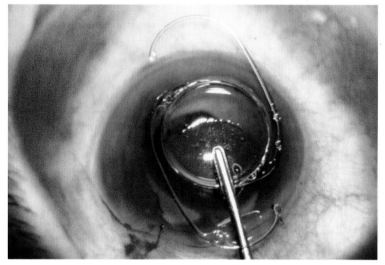

FIG. 1.105

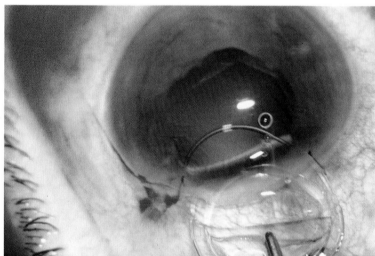

FIG. 1.106

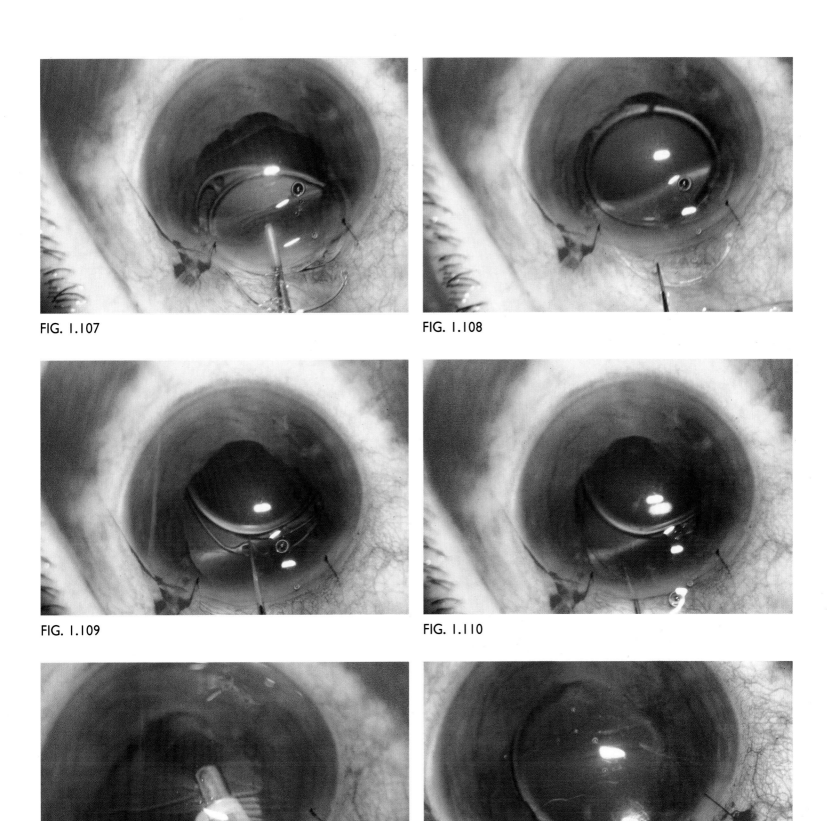

FIG. 1.107

FIG. 1.108

FIG. 1.109

FIG. 1.110

FIG. 1.111

FIG. 1.112

eral iridectomy, as in Fig. 1.113, an iridectomy is performed (Fig. 1.114). It is then made continuous with the pupil (Figs. 1.115 and 1.116). Fig. 1.117 shows an eye with two laser iridotomies and pigment over the anterior capsule of the lens. A peripheral iridectomy is again performed (Fig. 1.118) and made continuous with the pupil (Fig. 1.119). The pupil widens as the viscoelastic material is injected into the anterior chamber (Fig. 1.120). The remainder of the procedure then follows, as described above.

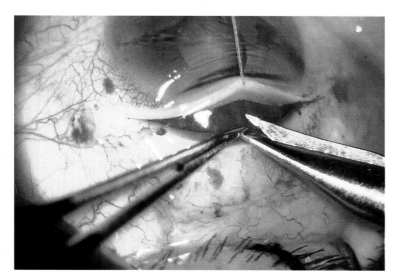

FIG. 1.113

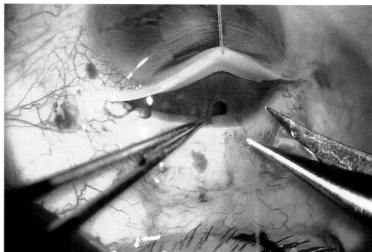

FIG. 1.114

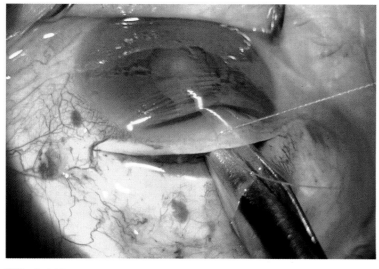

FIG. 1.115

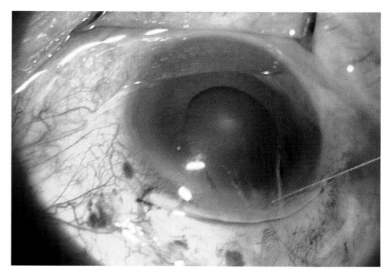

FIG. 1.116

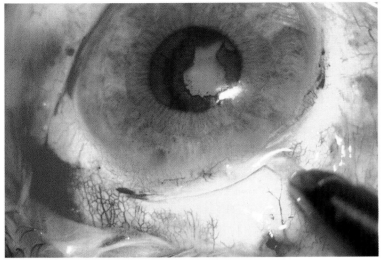

FIG. 1.117

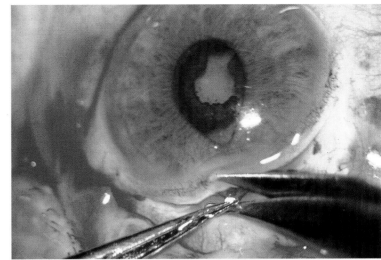

FIG. 1.118

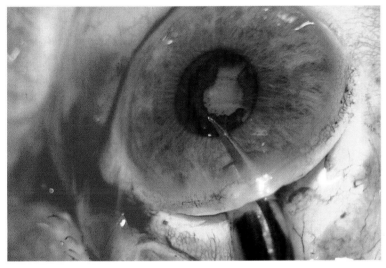

FIG. 1.119

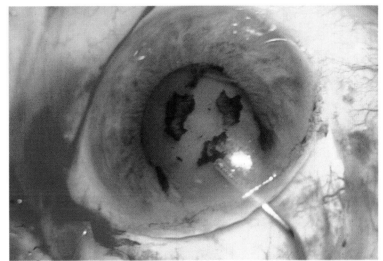

FIG. 1.120

PARS PLANA LENSECTOMY AND VITRECTOMY BY ULTRASONIC FRAGMENTATION AND IMPLANTATION OF POSTERIOR CHAMBER LENS

Louis J. Girard, MD

INTRODUCTION

Pars plana lensectomy and vitrectomy by ultrasonic fragmentation (USF) is a bimanual, two-needle technique of cataract surgery that can be performed at any age and in any type of cataract: senile, congenital, traumatic, subluxated, dislocated, retrolental fibroplasia (RLF), persistent hyperplastic primary vitreous (PHPV), cataract and glaucoma, cataract and healed retinal detachment, and hypermature cataract. The technique can also be combined with implan-

tation of any type of intraocular implant. A posterior chamber lens implant is preferred.

SURGICAL TECHNIQUE

Incisions are made through the sclera and pars plana and into the lens at 10 and 2 o'clock (Fig. 1.121). The irrigating needle is inserted at the 2 o'clock incision. This needle is connected to an overhead bottle of BSS plus containing epinephrine 1:100,000. The ultrasonic fragmentation (USF) needle is inserted at 10 o'clock and both needles brought into the soft anterior cortex just under the anterior lens capsule (Figs. 1.122 and 1.123). Fragmentation and aspiration along with irrigation are begun and removal of the anterior cortex is begun. The fragmenting needle is then moved across the lens, removing more and more of the anterior cortex (Figs. 1.124 and 1.125). The procedure is continued with deeper removal of the lens nucleus (Figs. 1.126 and 1.127). All of the nucleus is removed before removal of the

---

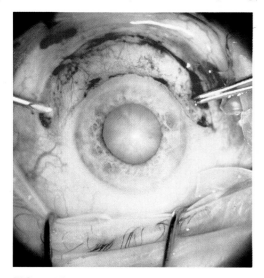

FIG. 1.121

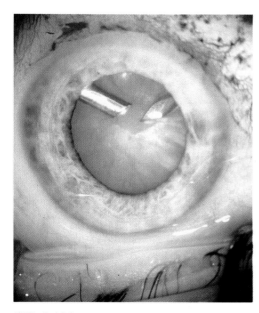

FIG. 1.122

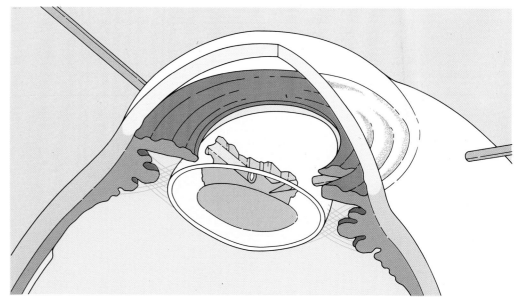

FIG. 1.123

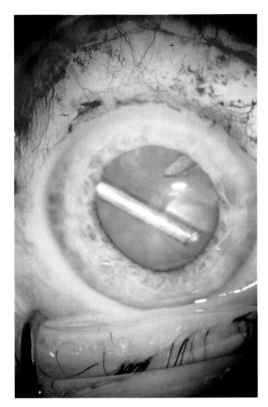

FIG. 1.124

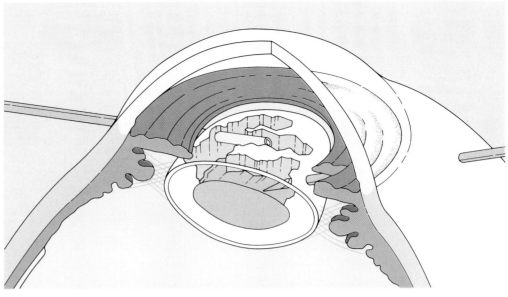

FIG. 1.125

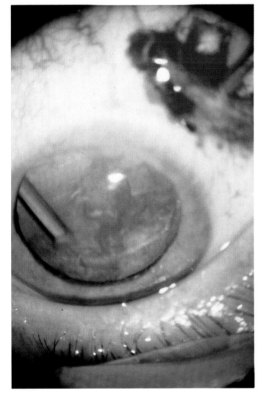

FIG. 1.126

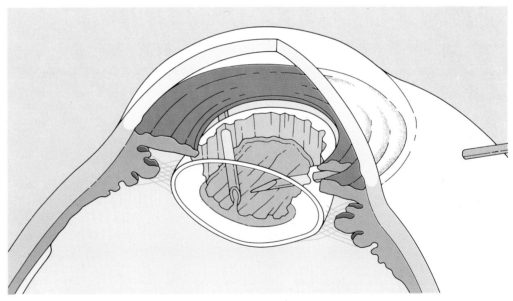

FIG. 1.127

posterior and peripheral cortices. The posterior and peripheral cortices are removed, sometimes only with aspiration (Figs. 1.128 and 1.129). Fluorescein solution, made by dipping a Fluor-i-strip in 1½ ml of BSS, is injected into the vitreous cavity to stain the formed vitreous. Removal of the cortex continues. The posterior capsule is removed and vitrectomy begun (Figs. 1.130 and 1.131). Vitreous, remaining cortex, and remnants of the posterior capsule are removed. Vitrectomy is then carried through the central portion of the vitreous (Figs. 1.132 and 1.133). Fluorescein staining helps to make the remaining vitreous visible. Peripheral vitreous is removed with the help of scleral depression. Note how the scleral depression brings the peripheral vitreous into view (Figs. 1.134 and 1.135). The anterior lens capsule, which has been kept intact, is then fenestrated centrally (Figs. 1.136 and 1.137). The fenestrated anterior capsule will be the basis for a posterior chamber lens implant. The fundus is examined by scleral

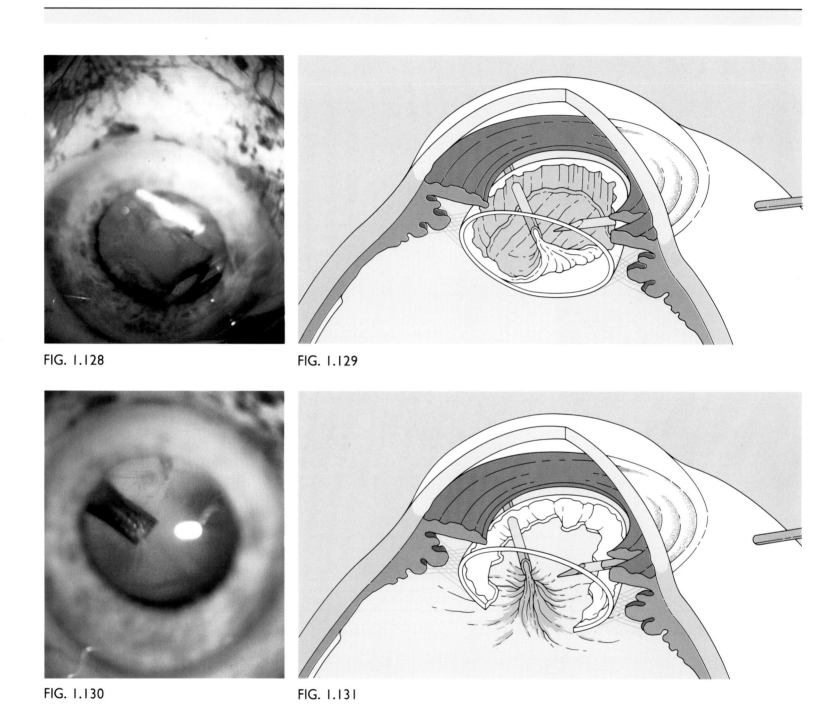

FIG. 1.128

FIG. 1.129

FIG. 1.130

FIG. 1.131

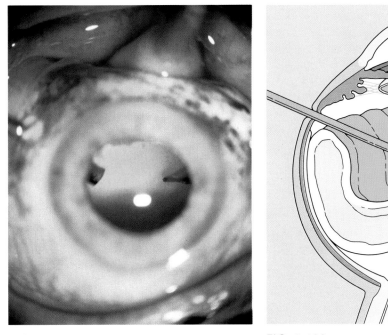

FIG. 1.132

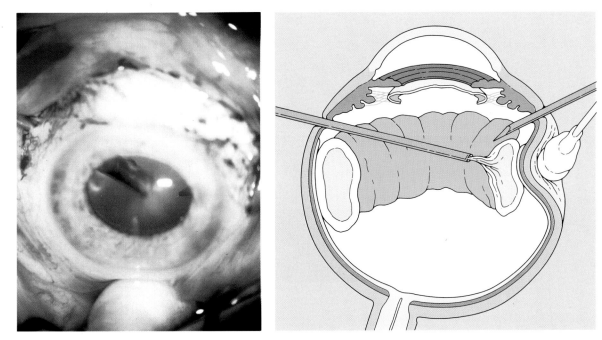

FIG. 1.133

FIG. 1.134

FIG. 1.135

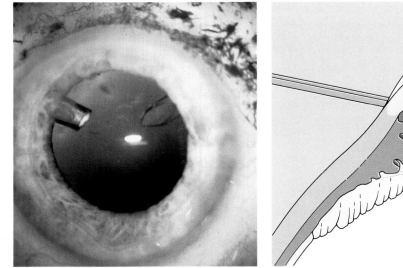

FIG. 1.136

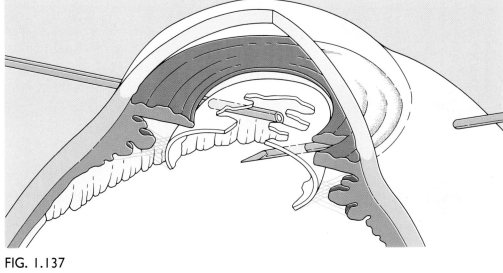

FIG. 1.137

depression and indirect ophthalmoscopy (Figs. 1.138 and 1.139). At the present time, this is the only technique of cataract surgery that allows intraocular examination at the time of surgery. While irrigation is continued with an indwelling catheter, a scleral tunnel is fashioned with a circular knife (Fig. 1.140). Dissection is carried into clear cornea (Fig. 1.141). The anterior chamber is entered just anterior to the angle meshwork (Fig. 1.142). A posterior chamber lens is inserted between the iris and anterior lens capsule (Fig. 1.143). The scleral tunnel incision is closed with interrupted 7-0 polygalactin sutures (Fig. 1.144). Conjunctiva is approximated (Fig. 1.145).

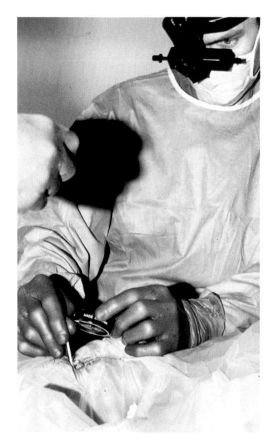

FIG. 1.138

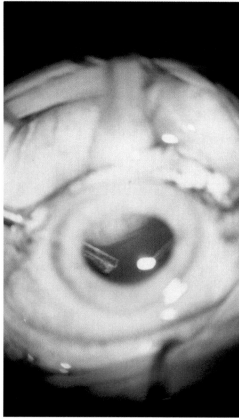

FIG. 1.139

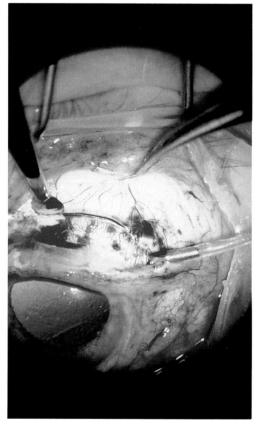

FIG. 1.140

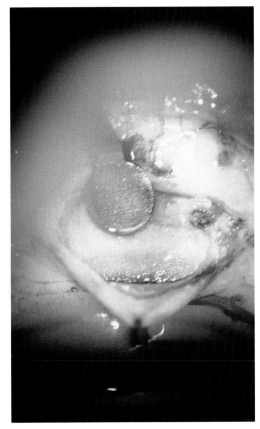

FIG. 1.141

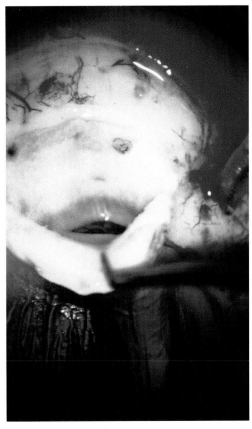

FIG. 1.142

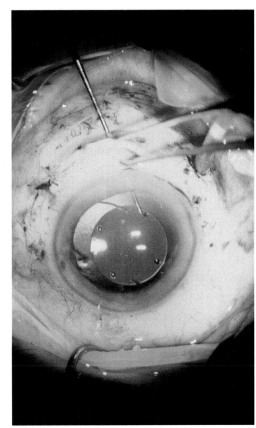

FIG. 1.143

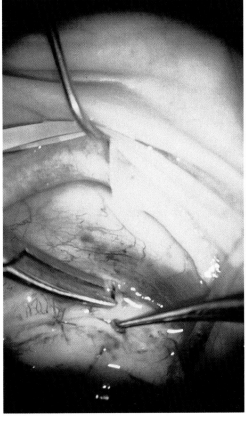

FIG. 1.144

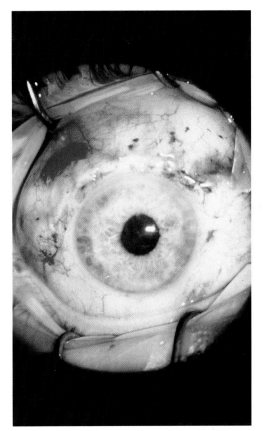

FIG. 1.145

INFANTILE CATARACT SURGERY

Robert W. Lingua, MD

Ongoing development of the anterior segment and concurrent maturation of the visual pathways in the first months of life mandate a particular philosophy, instrumentation, and technique for infant lensectomy. When one undertakes the care of the cataractous neonate, responsibility continues beyond the surgery, into optical rehabilitation, amblyopia care, and periodic evaluation for late-onset glaucoma and retinal detachment.

In the infant *under 6 months of age*, the visual pathways depend upon the transmission of formed imagery for their complete neuroanatomic development. This has been termed the "critical period" of visual maturation, and in most infants it is complete by 3 to 4 months of age. Keeping the visual axis clear and optically corrected during this early time may avoid a lifelong limitation of acuity potential. Presently, our only option with a single procedure to accomplish a clear visual axis that will remain so during these early months is the lensectomy/limited anterior vitrectomy procedure or automated lensectomy. This procedure employs a cutting and aspiration device to remove the posterior capsule along with only enough vitreous to remove a wide portion of the capsule. A generous discission is not an equivalent procedure for the following reasons:

1. It continues to provide the necessary architecture for early secondary membrane formation
2. It may predispose to secondary glaucoma due to iridocapsular adhesions
3. It often violates the vitreous face, encouraging a wick to the wound
4. It requires an iridectomy

After 6 months of age, the visual potential for the infant has been neurologically set. When the cataract has been diagnosed after 6 months of age, one must realize that the visual potential for the infant has already been established during the first several months of life. Unless other structural changes in the eye or lens exist [for example, persistent hyperplastic primary vitreous (PHPV), posterior lenticonus, rubella retinopathy suggesting early cataract onset, macular hypoplasia, anterior segment dysgenesis, or associated corneal clouding], one cannot assume that the degree of deprivation during the first several months was great, and therefore, the acuity potential is unknown. The absence of nystagmus and strabismus, however, suggest a later onset. It is my practice to treat aggressively dense *uncomplicated* cataracts, first recognized after 6 months of age, to avoid the superimposition of a dense functional amblyopia upon any existing organic limitation of acuity, with the realization and full disclosure to the parents that the final acuity result will depend on whether visual deprivation had occurred in the first 4 months of life, especially in monocular cases.

When operating on children *over 6 months of age*, opacification of the posterior capsule can still induce amblyopia ex anopsia up until visual maturity (6 to 9 years of age). This visual loss, by definition, can be reversed with elective patch therapy, after reestablishing a clear visual axis and optical correction. Any amblyopia allowed to persist through visual maturity will, of course, remain throughout life. When one decides to perform a discission, or leave the posterior capsule intact, one must be philosophically and technically prepared to regularly monitor the clarity of the capsule and manage it with surgical or laser therapy as required, as even minor degrees of opacification are amblyogenic.

In situations where an automated cutting and aspiration device is unavailable, the surgeon's preferred extracapsular technique can be performed. An irrigation–aspiration device with a 0.4-to-0.5-mm internal port diameter may be required for nuclear aspiration, after which changing to a microtip for cortical removal in the recess will minimize capsular trauma prior to its planned removal. A portable, hand-held, battery-operated vitrector of the guillotine type, with a 0.3-mm tip, is available and can remove the posterior capsule after irrigation and aspiration.

When the child *reaches visual maturity* (over 10 years of age), the planning and technique of cataract surgery proceeds as in the adult, and the reader is referred to those sections in this text.

A BRIEF NOTE ON CONTACT LENS FITTING

Prior to prepping the patient for surgery, a trial set of three silicone lenses (base curves 7.7, 7.9, and 8.1) is brought to the operating room with a Wood's light and fluorescein. Staining patterns are then used to judge the "best" base curve from this trial set. We expect the base curve to change minimally postoperatively when the bimanual 20-gauge incision technique is performed. The only calculation necessary at that time is the base curve of the preferred lens and the diameter allowed by the horizontal and vertical corneal dimensions. On the fifth to seventh postoperative day, a lens of the previously measured base curve (and, readily available, one size steeper and one size shallower) in the +20 diopter range is placed on the infant eye to reevaluate the fitting and to over-refract for the final prescription. If less than 1 year of age, 3 diopters over emmetropia are prescribed; as a toddler (1 to 3 years old), 2 diopters; over 3 years of age, 1 diopter and a reading spectacle prescribed for preschool activities. At that time, the lens can be dispensed from stock and reordered with one back-up lens for the family. I prefer to recommend daily wear for the first month for the parent and child to become accustomed to insertion and removal. Thereafter, daily wear may be continued, or in the case of silicone extended-wear lenses, weekly cleaning suffices. We have witnessed noninfective stromal opacifications when extended-wear silicone lenses were left in place for 2 or more weeks. If the child cannot be over-refracted at the time of examination, rather than lose valuable time without optical correction, it is recommended to sedate the child and try again (100 mg/kg of chloral hydrate, up to 1 g orally, or an intramuscular injection of demerol, phenergan, and thorazine in 2, 1, and 1 mg/kg respective concentrations). If corneal clarity prohibits a good retinoscopic reflex, or if the pupil is bound down despite cycloplegics, and one cannot appreciate the retinoscopic reflex within the pupil, then K readings and an A-scan axial length may be obtained under sedation to calculate the spherical equivalent for proper initial correction.

Spectacles are always dispensed even for the monocular

aphake (incorporating a balance weight plano lens for a fellow eye). When the contact lens is lost, or unable to be worn for other reasons, they are recommended for half-time wear (one-half waking hours) *only* while the phakic eye is patched. Optical correction of the operated eye, rather than binocularity, is a reasonable goal in monocular cataract care.

PREPARATION OF THE EYE

Maximum dilatation of the pupil assists in thorough removal of the cortex. However, cataracts in infancy can be associated with varying degrees of iris hypoplasia and, therefore, be somewhat refractory to dilatation. At the time the child is first evaluated, the response to mydriatic agents is assessed. One drop of 2.5% neosynephrine, 1% tropicamide, and 1% cyclopentolate, given together, is sufficient for most irides. For a darker iris, this is repeated a second time. Those children whose pupils dilate easily can be given their drops on the morning of the surgical procedure. Those responding poorly on the day of examination can be started on a regimen of daily atropinization (0.5% solution) for the days to weeks between examination and surgery. Despite this regimen, some pupils will not dilate beyond 3 or 4 mm. With the approval of the anesthetist, 0.5 mL of 1:10,000 intracardiac epinephrine (no preservatives) can be added to a 500 mL volume of irrigating solution for use intraoperatively. When the pupil will not dilate beyond 4 mm during the case, despite dilute epinephrine irrigation, sphincterotomy may be performed prior to capsular cleaning and posterior capsule management. When necessary, these are best performed in pairs, 180° apart, to prevent ectopia of the pupil. Adhesive plastic drapes can be used to isolate the lashes from the operative field.

The Bridle Suture

As the infant is often kept at a safer, "lighter" plane by the anesthetist and, therefore, the eye may elevate, a bridle suture is suggested. A single 6-0 silk suture under the superior rectus will ensure proper exposure of the superior limbus. A 0.5 forcep or larger will easily engage the tendon when the tips are rotated down onto the globe superiorly (Fig. 1.146). Care is taken to avoid dragging conjunctiva or tenons capsule anteriorly with the tendon, which will obscure the superior limbus. The suture should be gently supportive and not so taut as to raise intraocular pressure (Fig. 1.147).

PERITOMY

The bimanual technique allows complete access to the capsular recess. Moreover, the two 20-gauge incisions minimize the chance of astigmatism, and are securely closed with a single suture. In complex cases, with one port reserved for irrigation, the second port can accommodate a cutting and/or aspiration instrument, cautery, or intraocular scissors, while maintaining a full chamber throughout the case, as all are available in 20-gauge diameters. Further, the irrigating cannula can be used to manipulate tissue for proper cutting and the instruments can be interchanged from port to port as required. The 10 and 2 o'clock positions provide the maximum separation, yet keep the incision sites beneath the upper lid.

A 3-to-4-mm limbus-based peritomy is performed with a

Infantile Cataract Surgery: The Bridle Suture

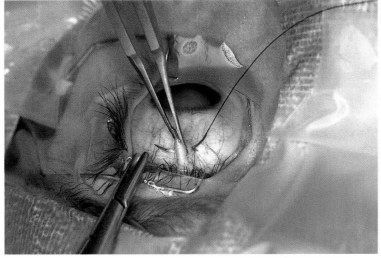

FIG. 1.146

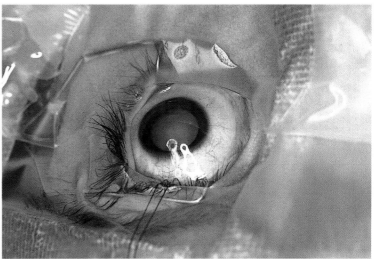

FIG. 1.147

Vannas scissor and 0.12 forcep (Figs. 1.148 and 1.149). I lightly cauterize the limbal vessels, which also assists in the removal of the limbal epithelium prior to the corneal incision. Before entering the eye, the cutting and aspiration instrument is checked for air in the line, proper port size (0.4 to 0.5 mm), and proper operation of both cutting and suction modes with saline. Only when the surgeon is satisfied with the operation of all instruments is the eye opened.

CORNEAL INCISION

The nasal incision is usually chosen for the irrigating cannula. Reserving the temporal port for the lensectomy device allows a greater range of motion than can be attained nasally when using a straight instrument. I prefer a 20-gauge "V-lance" (or House myringotomy blade), which is first oriented perpendicular to the posterior limbus (Fig. 1.150). When the initial corneal incision is vertical at the posterior limbus, no visible leukoma will occur with heal-ing. When the incision has been shelved so that the posterior entry into the anterior chamber is anterior to the anterior limbus, corneal edema may occur during the case and postoperatively a leukoma may persist. Under high magnification the blade is advanced until it is visualized to penetrate Descemet's membrane, entering the anterior chamber (Fig. 1.151). At that point the blade is turned parallel to the iris plane and advanced into the pupil (Figs. 1.152 and 1.153). The blade is then removed and the irrigating cannula introduced in order to reform the chamber prior to making the second incision (Figs. 1.154 and 1.155), minimizing iris trauma. My preferred irrigating cannula is a bent and blunted 20-gauge cannula or disposable needle (ready-made, or may be prepared so with a sandstone). A comfortable bend is 45°, made approximately 1 cm from the tip of the cannula. With the irrigating cannula in place and the chamber formed, a sufficient hold on the eye is obtained for the second corneal incision at the 10 o'clock position (Fig. 1.156).

Infantile Cataract Surgery: Peritomy

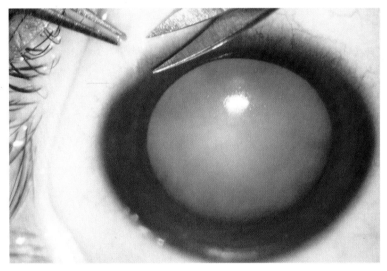

FIG. 1.148

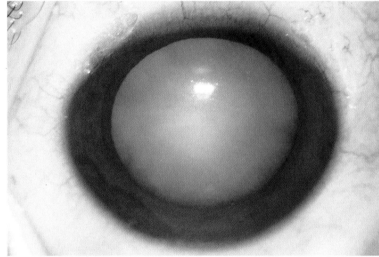

FIG. 1.149

Infantile Cataract Surgery: Corneal Incision

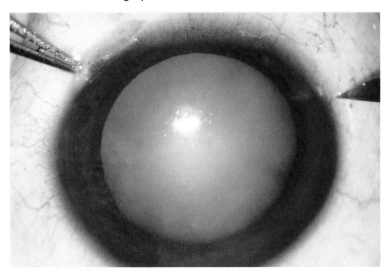

FIG. 1.150

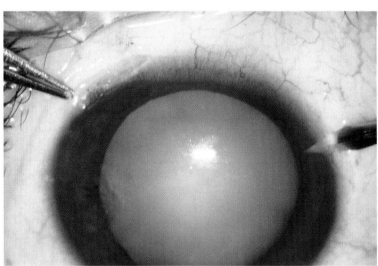

FIG. 1.151

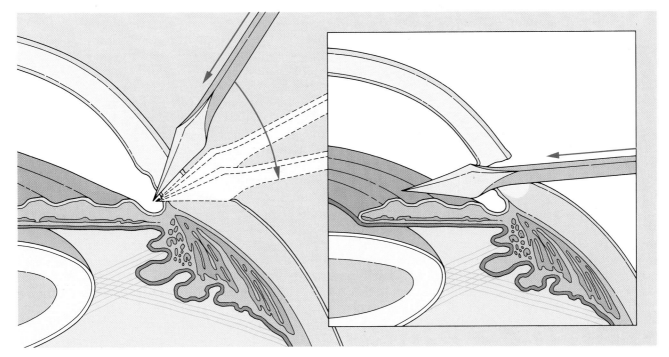

FIG. 1.152

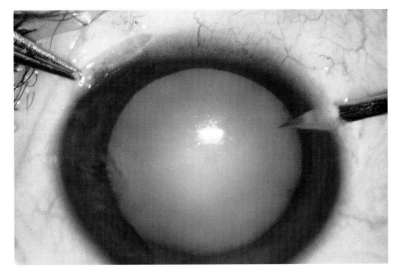

FIG. 1.153

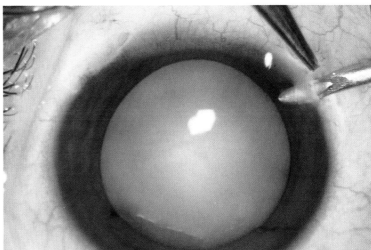

FIG. 1.154

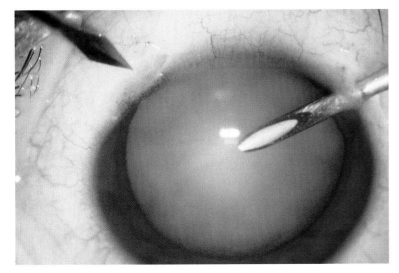

FIG. 1.155

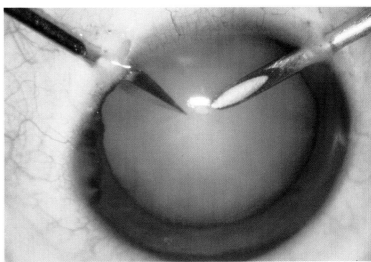

FIG. 1.156

Simultaneous anterior capsulotomy can be performed, if desired, with a rocking motion once the capsule is engaged (Figs. 1.157 and 1.158). The capsulotomy may be enlarged at this time or later performed with the cutting instrument, if it is to be used. At the conclusion of the incision the blade is exchanged for the lensectomy device (Fig. 1.159).

ANTERIOR CAPSULOTOMY

An anterior capsulotomy may be performed with the 20-gauge blade or with the cutting instrument, if one is to be used. If the cutting instrument is chosen, the port is oriented posteriorly, away from the edge of the iris, and with low suction and low cutting speed (100 cuts/minute) the capsulotomy is begun. The port is then introduced beneath the anterior capsule and, facing up, the capsulotomy is completed. Care must be exercised in some infantile cataracts, where the lens may be very thin and actually discoid. In that instance, high suction may engage the posterior capsule prematurely. One must always endeavor to remove all cortical material prior to opening the posterior capsule to avoid retained cortex in the vitreous as a mechanism for persistent inflammation.

IRRIGATION/CUTTING/ASPIRATION

When the consistency of the intracapsular contents is soft, clearing the visual axis can be accomplished with irrigation and aspiration alone. Occasionally, however, the nuclei are quite calcific and require disruption, either manually between the instrument tips or with a cutting instrument, prior to aspiration. When the surgeon prefers to use an irrigation–aspiration cannula for removal of the nucleus and cortex, he may nonetheless change to the cutting and aspiration instrument for removal of the posterior capsule/vitreous face. I find it convenient to use a cutting and aspiration instrument for the entire case, which allows me to maintain a constant chamber without having to exchange instruments and vary the intraocular pressure. In this procedure, the cutting and aspiration instrument can be used to complete the anterior capsulotomy with a low cutting mode (100 cuts/minute) and low suction. Lensectomy may then proceed with the port set to 0.4 to 0.7 mm.

The port size may be varied to accommodate the demands of the tissue. When aspiration cannot proceed at low suction, it is better to try to feed the tissue into the port or disrupt it between the two instruments rather than allow a high negative pressure to develop within the cannula, which upon release will rapidly drop the intraocular pressure and collapse the chamber. Likewise, using a much larger port size than is necessary encourages higher irrigation volumes and endothelial decompensation. The primary purpose of using the cutting and aspiration instrument for lensectomy is to allow much of the procedure to be accomplished with irrigation and aspiration alone, calling upon cutting only as is necessary to facilitate aspiration at a low suction level and small port size. Once the nucleus has been removed (Figs. 1.160 to 1.162), the anterior capsulotomy

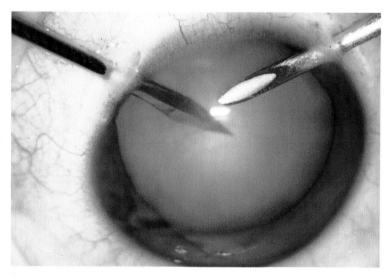

FIG. 1.157

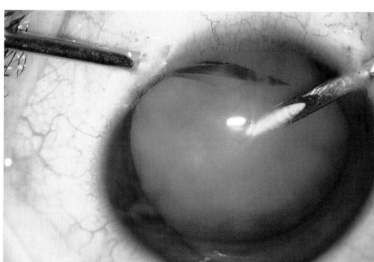

FIG. 1.158

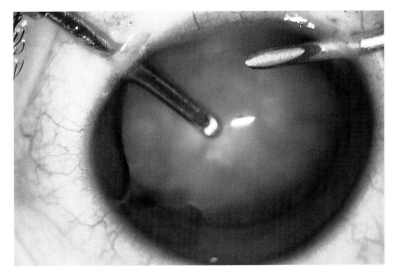

FIG. 1.159

Infantile Cataract Surgery: Irrigation/Cutting/Aspiration

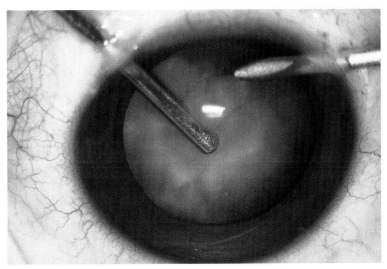

FIG. 1.160

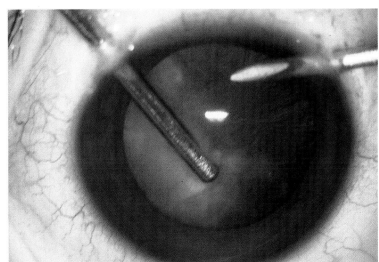

FIG. 1.161

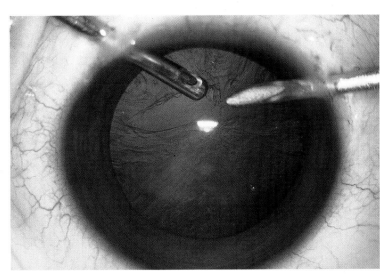

FIG. 1.162

may be enlarged (Figs. 1.163 to 1.165).

The peripheral cortex can be comfortably stripped even with a side port aspirator after reducing the port size to 0.2 to 0.3 mm. With suction off, the tip of the cannula is advanced between the leaves of the capsule into the recess, at which time low suction is used to engage the cortex. It is then pulled to the center, and only when it is in the center is the suction raised for aspiration, or cutting employed, to remove the structure without damaging the iris or posterior capsule (Figs. 1.166 and 1.167). Since both instruments are of the same caliber, they may be exchanged (Fig. 1.168) for thorough cortical removal. It is important to emphasize that use of the cutting mode, when the port is not visualized, is not recommended. Visualization is one of the primary advantages of the anterior approach.

The appearance of the posterior capsule is quite variable in these infants. It may be clear, or have varying degrees of evagination (posterior lenticonus) with or without opacifi-cation, or be variably fibrotic. In all cases, the procedure may continue without a change of instrumentation. For vitrectomy, a cutting mode of 400 cuts/minute is optimal. Occasionally, when the posterior capsule is fibrotic, it may be necessary to use a blade for incision to obtain a leading edge.

Removal of the posterior capsule with an automated device can be accomplished with minimal trauma to the capsular-zonular architecture and with minimal traction on the vitreous body (Figs. 1.169 to 1.171). It is preferable to perform a generous posterior capsulectomy (approximately 6 mm) as this obviates the need for iridectomy. Recall that the vitreous body is quite firm in these infants and, there-fore, any "stirring" maneuvers within the vitreous are to be discouraged. All attempts should be made to maintain the suction and irrigation at a low level in order to minimize traction on the vitreous and the amount of vitreous removed.

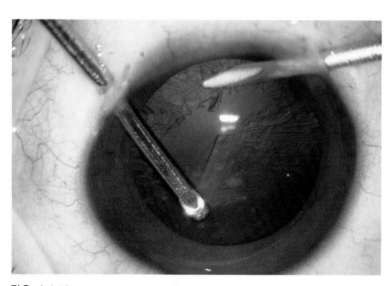

FIG. 1.163

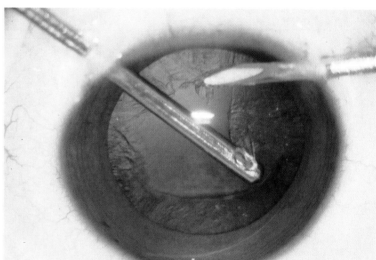

FIG. 1.164

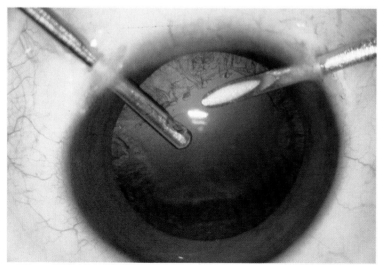

FIG. 1.165

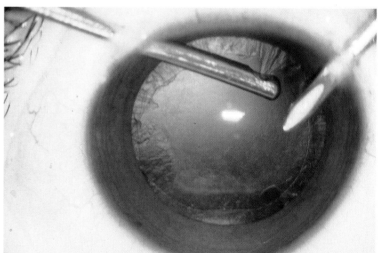

FIG. 1.166

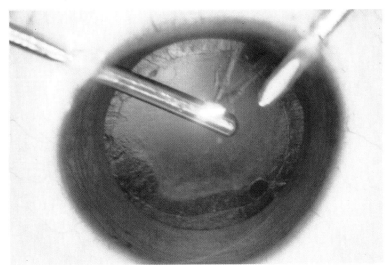

FIG. 1.167

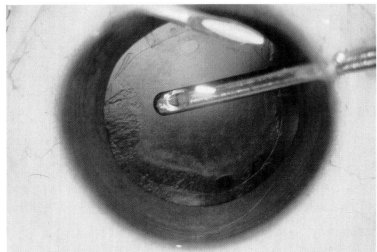

FIG. 1.168

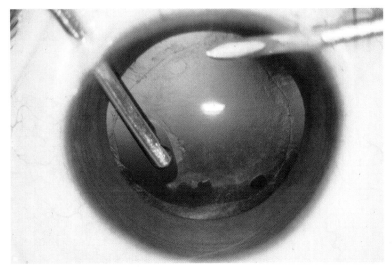

FIG. 1.169

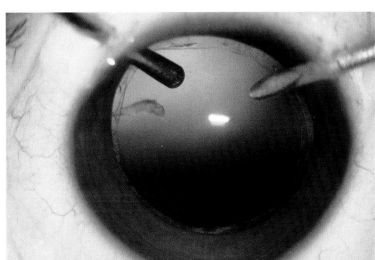

FIG. 1.170

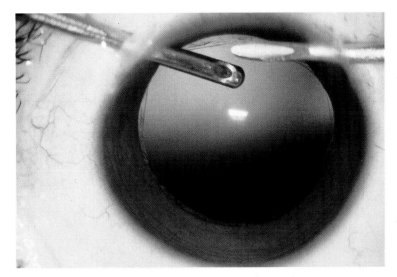

FIG. 1.171

CLOSING THE EYE

Because of firm hyaloidal capsular adherence in infancy, any violation of the posterior capsule should be considered a violation of the vitreous face. To avoid a common cause of postoperative inflammation, i.e., vitreous to the wound, I recommend closing the eye under complete air, which provides the same safety as a viscoelastic substance but is easily removed without the introduction of irrigating instruments and does not provide the risk of inflammation or transient rises in intraocular pressure associated with their use. Moreover, when air enters the anterior chamber, if the bubble is not uniformly filling the angle, the air–vitreous interface reveals vitreous in the anterior chamber, which would not be obvious with use of a viscoelastic substance (Fig. 1.172). When vitreous is present in the anterior chamber, the air will proceed posterior to the pupil, rather than fill the angle. Prior to closure, evaluate the pupil with or without Miochol for "wicks" to the wound. If necessary, continue the vitrectomy, at the pupillary margin, until symmetric. When the two 20-gauge incision technique is performed, each incision is comfortably closed with a single 10-0 nylon suture where, after four throws, the knots may be trimmed with a blade and rotated to the sclera (Fig. 1.173). At this point an air/BSS exchange can be performed with a 30-gauge cannula, removing as much air as desired from the anterior chamber. If a bridle suture was used, it is removed prior to the air/BSS exchange in order to properly reform the globe.

Rather than close the conjunctiva with a suture, the separate antibiotic and steroid injections can be performed in the episcleral space behind each incision, and balloon the conjunctiva forward to reapproximate their edges. Only 0.25 to 0.5 mL volumes are required. I prefer to use 1 mg Decadron at one port, and 10 mg Gentamycin at the other. Atropine ointment is placed between the lids along with a mild sulfa-steroid ointment. Half of an adult eye pad and infant shield protect the eye. The patient is usually discharged home as an outpatient and the dressing is changed in the morning by the surgeon. Sulfa-steroid and 0.5% Atropine ointments are continued b.i.d. until contact lens or spectacle use is begun (approximately one week), at which time the sulfa-steroid solution is reduced to q.a.m. for 2 weeks only, and the Atropine 0.5% ointment is instilled at bedtime, once weekly, for 3 months.

MANAGEMENT OF THE IRIS

The most common early complication of congenital cataract surgery, prior to the introduction of posterior capsulectomy/vitrectomy, is secondary glaucoma due to iridocapsular adhesions. Often this occurred in spite of a peripheral iridectomy. When a generous (5-to-6-mm) posterior capsulectomy is performed, an iridectomy is unnecessary. If only the central portion of the capsule is removed, or discission is performed without cutting and aspiration, an iridectomy is mandatory. Widening the incision for iridectomy is often necessary if one has begun the case with a 20-gauge incision and it is advisable to do so after the completion of the irrigation and aspiration. If enlarged prior to cortical aspiration, too great a volume of irrigating fluid is expended during this maneuver. A careful engagement of the iris will minimize intraocular bleeding and avoid dragging vitreous into the wound through the iridectomy site. Keeping the capsular-zonular architecture intact at the time of iridectomy may protect the site from vitreous plugs, after which one may return to open the posterior capsule. Should bleeding occur during the iridectomy, raising the intraocular pressure for 10 minutes "by the clock" while both ports are occluded is sufficient. Only if a large iris vessel has been cut is intraocular cautery ever required.

When the pupil cannot dilate pre- or intraoperatively beyond 4 mm, a sphincterotomy is recommended. I perform this prior to the posterior capsulectomy to avoid access of blood to the vitreous, should bleeding occur, and to improve visualization for that procedure. The cutting and aspiration device usually can be used gently to interrupt the circumferential sphincter without bleeding. To avoid a distorted pupil, two or four are performed 180° or 90° apart, respectively. If at any time iris is inadvertently caught in the cutting and aspiration device, squeezing the tubing will sufficiently reflux the system and allow it to disengage the iris prior to resuming the procedure.

PERSISTENT HYPERPLASTIC PRIMARY VITREOUS: SECONDARY MEMBRANES

In cases where the maldevelopment is mostly anterior (cataract, persistent vessels, centrally displaced elongated ciliary processes, and rudimentary stalk) with a normal posterior pole (avascular stalk, normal optic nerve, and foveal development) good acuities are feasible. When persistent vessels or ciliary processes are dragged centrally and are noted preoperatively, it is wise to prepare for the control of intraocular bleeding and the removal of dense fibrous annula from the peripheral lens. The 20-gauge intraocular cautery and intraocular scissors are sufficient. A cutting and aspiration device is indispensable in the management of persistent hyperplastic primary vitreous and the bimanual two-port approach allows for an interchange of instruments for complete access within the eye (Fig. 1.174), to feed resistant tissue into the port (Fig. 1.175), and to maintain the chamber while one employs the cautery (Fig. 1.176),

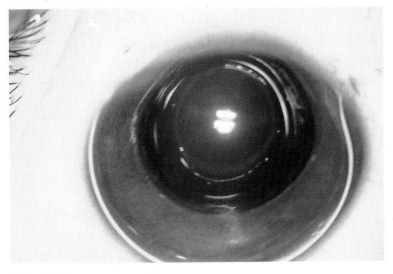

FIG. 1.172

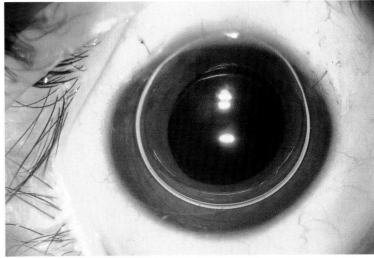

FIG. 1.173

Infantile Cataract Surgery: PHPV: Secondary Membranes

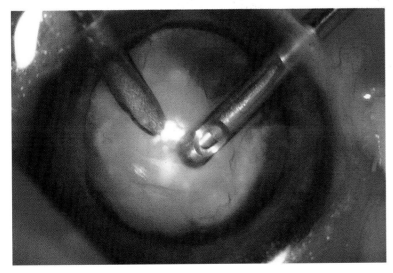

FIG. 1.174

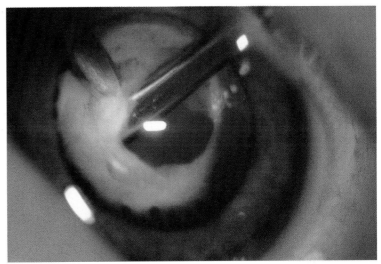

FIG. 1.175

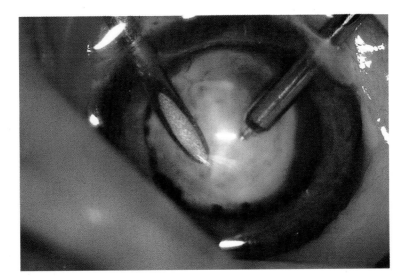

FIG. 1.176

scissors (Figs. 1.177 and 1.178), or blade to interrupt these circular fibrotic structures. Often the intraocular knife or scissor can "start the edge" when the cutting and aspiration instrument is unable to do so with modest suction. It is better to use one of these instruments than to labor too long with the cutting and aspiration device and irrigate the endothelium excessively. Removal of secondary membranes follows the same approach as described for lensectomy (Figs. 1.179 to 1.181). Two incisions are made. The anterior chamber volume is maintained with an irrigating cannula. A cutting instrument is used to remove the entire secondary membrane.

POSTERIOR CHAMBER LENS IMPLANTATION

JAFFE 3 POSTERIOR CHAMBER LENS: CAPSULAR BAG FIXATION

The cataract is extracted by phacoemulsification or planned extracapsular cataract extraction. A cannula attached to a syringe containing a viscoelastic material is passed into the anterior chamber (Fig. 1.182). The capsule bag is inflated with the viscoelastic material (Fig. 1.183). The Jaffe 3 posterior chamber lens is held in Blaydes forceps (Fig. 1.184). The implant is passed into the eye without retracting or lifting the cornea (Fig. 1.185). The leading loop of the lens is

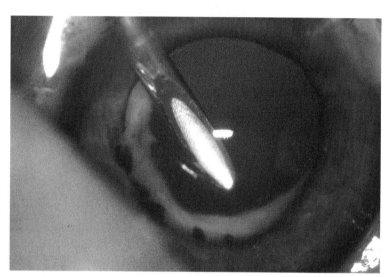

FIG. 1.177

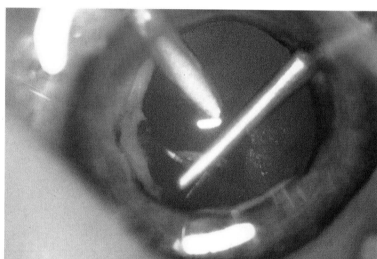

FIG. 1.178

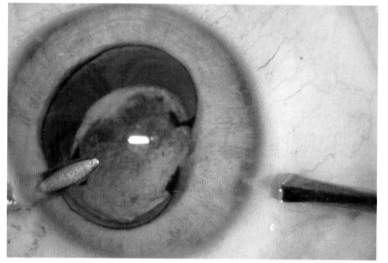

FIG. 1.179

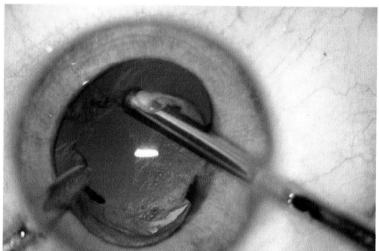

FIG. 1.180

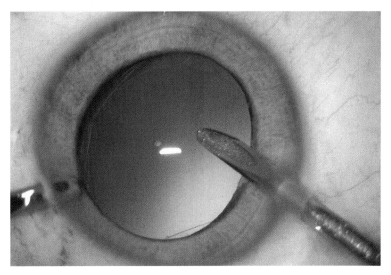

FIG. 1.181

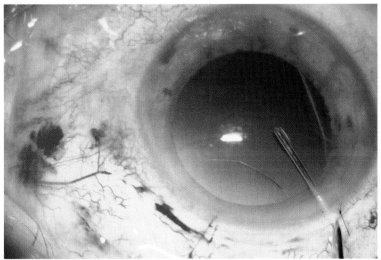

Jaffe 3 Posterior Chamber Lens Implantation: Capsular Bag Fixation

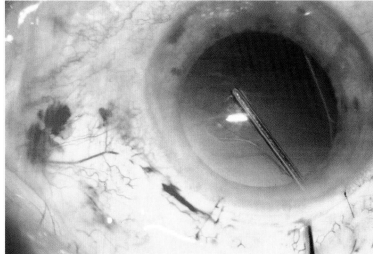

FIG. 1.182

FIG. 1.183

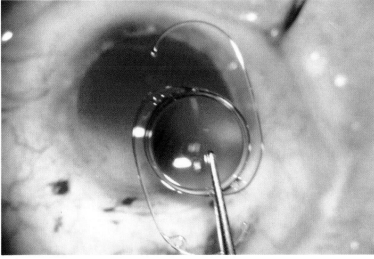

FIG. 1.184

FIG. 1.185

placed in the inferior portion of the capsule bag (Fig. 1.186). A one-handed technique is used for the trailing loop. A Jaffe-Maltzman hook engages the hole in the center of the trailing loop. The loop is flexed toward the optic (Fig. 1.187). With a slight pronation of the wrist, the loop is displaced slightly posteriorly into the capsule bag (Fig. 1.188). The lens is now in the capsule bag and it is usually not rotated (Fig. 1.189).

JAFFE I POSTERIOR CHAMBER LENS: CAPSULAR BAG FIXATION

A two-handed method is used for the trailing loop of the lens. The same method may be used for other posterior chamber lenses. The capsule bag is inflated with a visco-elastic material (Figs. 1.190 and 1.191). The Jaffe 1 posterior chamber lens is held in Blaydes forceps (Fig. 1.192). The implant is passed into the eye without lifting or retracting the cornea (Fig. 1.193). The leading loop of the lens is placed in the inferior position of the capsule bag (Fig. 1.194). Two instruments are used for the trailing loop. The iris and incised margin of the anterior capsule are retracted with a dull iris hook held in the left hand. The trailing loop is flexed into the eye with Kelman-McPherson forceps held in the right hand. The loop is then placed into the superior portion of the capsule bag with a slight pronation of the wrist (Fig. 1.195). Rotation of the lens may be performed using a hook (Jaffe or Sinskey) placed in the drill hole of the

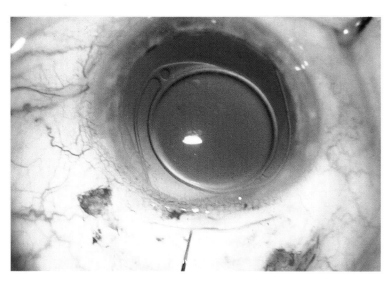

FIG. 1.186

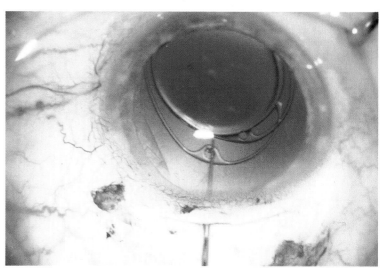

FIG. 1.187

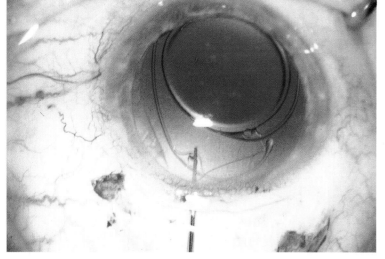

FIG. 1.188

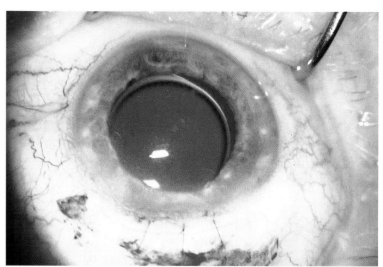

FIG. 1.189

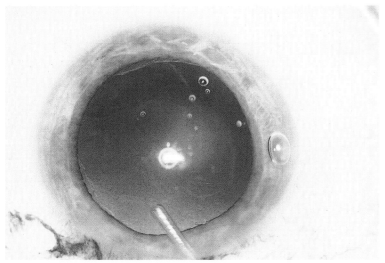

FIG. 1.190

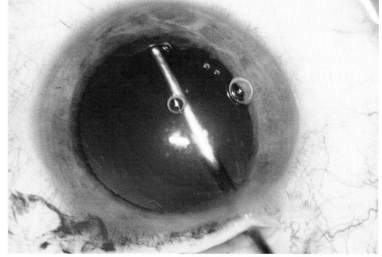

FIG. 1.191

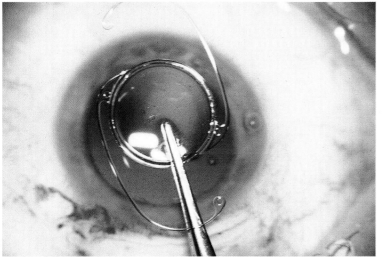

FIG. 1.192

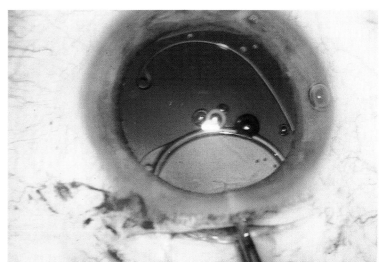

FIG. 1.193

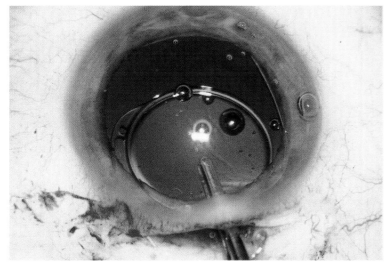

FIG. 1.194

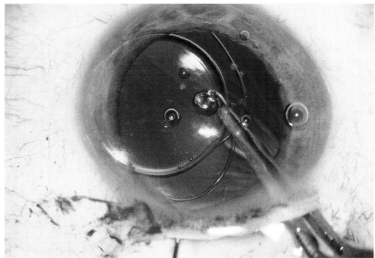

FIG. 1.195

lens outside the optic portion (Fig. 1.196). The lens is now in the capsule bag (Fig. 1.197). An alternate technique involves dialing the trailing loop into the eye after the leading loop is in the capsule bag. This is a good technique with posterior chamber lenses with polypropylene loops.

SINSKEY POSTERIOR CHAMBER LENS: SULCUS FIXATION

This lens may be placed in the ciliary sulcus or in the capsule bag. Sulcus fixation is described. The Sinskey lens is held in Blaydes forceps (Fig. 1.198). The lens is passed into the eye without lifting or retracting the cornea (Fig. 1.199). The leading loop passes anterior to the incised margin of the anterior capsule (Fig. 1.200) and then further inferiorly to the ciliary sulcus (Fig. 1.201). Two instruments are used for the trailing loop. A dull iris hook is held in the left hand and a Kelman-McPherson forceps in the right hand (Fig. 1.202). The iris is retracted with the iris hook and the loop of the lens is flexed into the eye with the Kelman-McPherson forceps (Fig. 1.203). The trailing loop is passed behind the superior portion of the iris (Fig. 1.204). The iris retraction

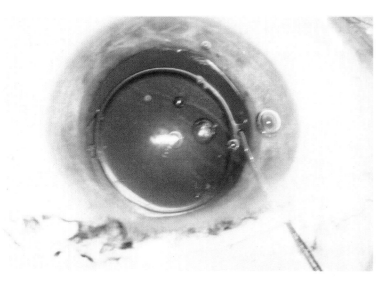

FIG. 1.196

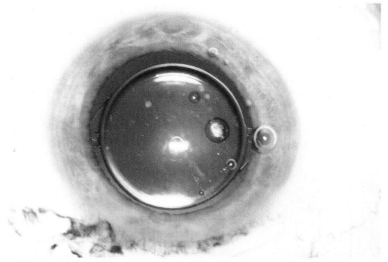

FIG. 1.197

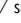 Sinskey Posterior Chamber Lens Implantation: Sulcus Fixation

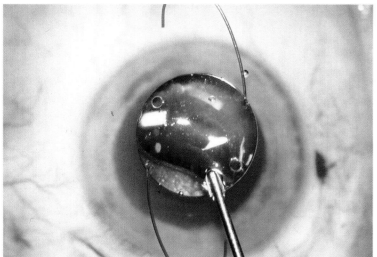

FIG. 1.198

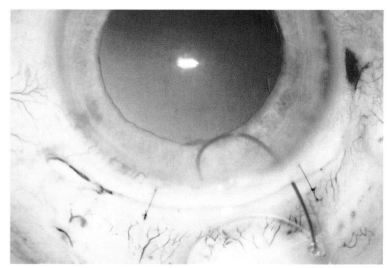

FIG. 1.199

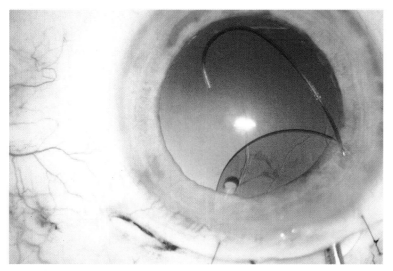

FIG. 1.200

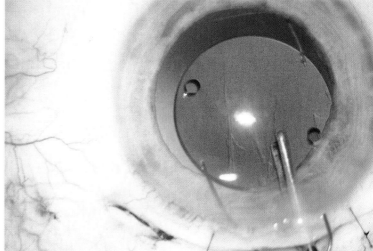

FIG. 1.201

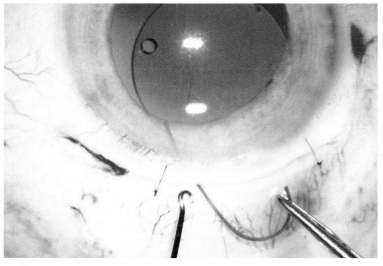

FIG. 1.202

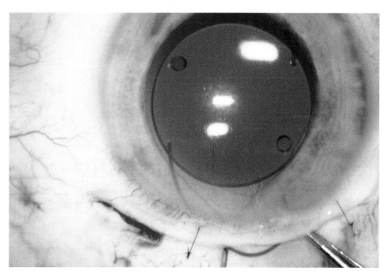

FIG. 1.203

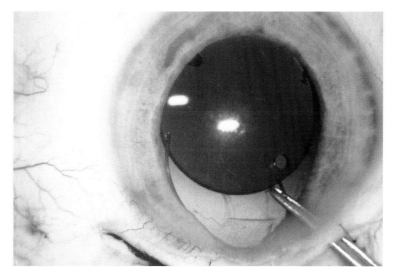

FIG. 1.204

is then released (Fig. 1.205). The lens may be rotated, if desired, to the horizontal position (Figs. 1.206 to 1.208).

SILICONE LENSES

A recent development is the introduction of foldable lenses made entirely of silicone or a combination of a silicone optic with haptics made of a different material, such as polypropylene or polyimide. The main impetus for these lenses is their ability to be inserted into the eye through a small incision since they can be folded during their insertion. Thus they enable the surgeon to use a standard phacoemulsification incision with enlargement to 3.75 to 4.25 mm. Long-term results with these lenses are not yet available.

A Staar Surgical silicone lens is shown being introduced into the eye with an injector and unfolded in the posterior chamber. It is positioned with two instruments (Figs. 1.209 to 1.213). In Figs. 1.214 to 1.221, an AMO silicone lens with polypropylene haptics is placed within the capsule bag. A Soflex silicone lens is placed within the capsule bag in Figs. 1.222 to 1.229.

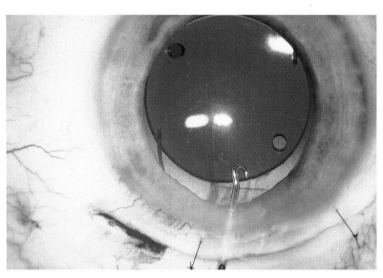

FIG. 1.205

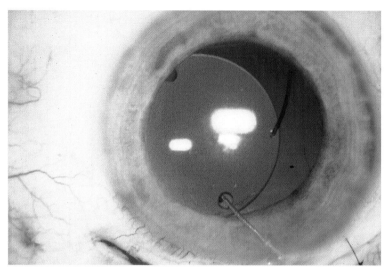

FIG. 1.206

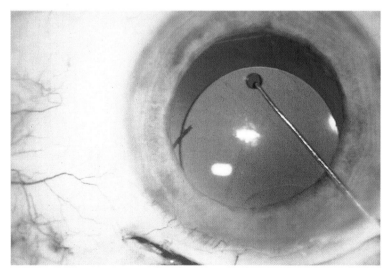

FIG. 1.207

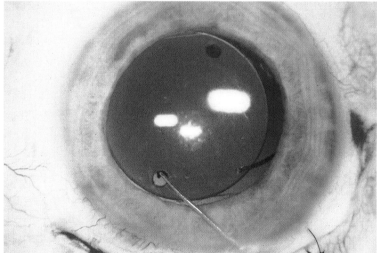

FIG. 1.208

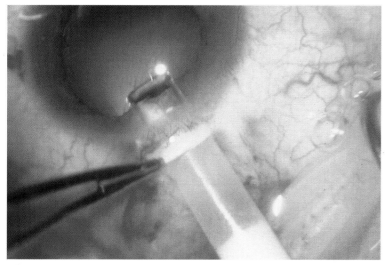

FIG. 1.209

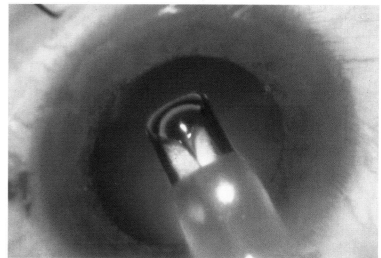

FIG. 1.210

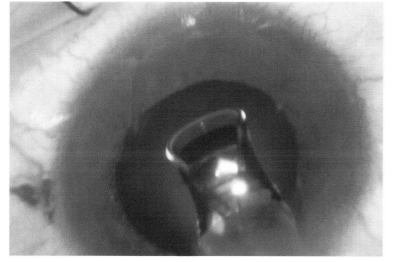

FIG. 1.211

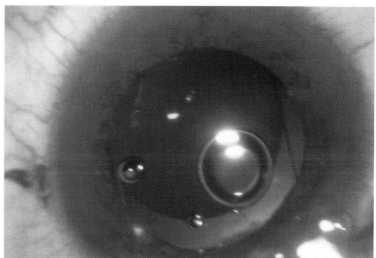

FIG. 1.212

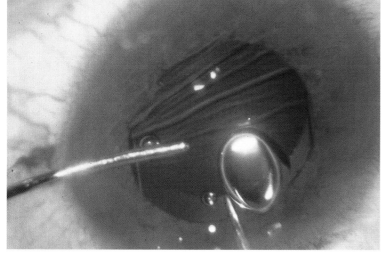

FIG. 1.213

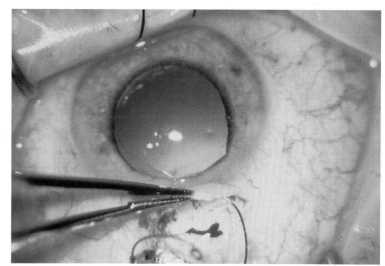

FIG. 1.214

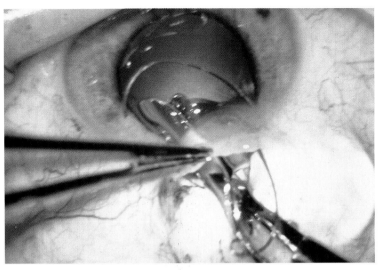

FIG. 1.215

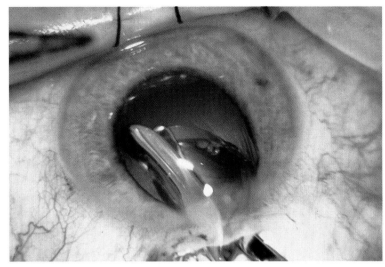

FIG. 1.216

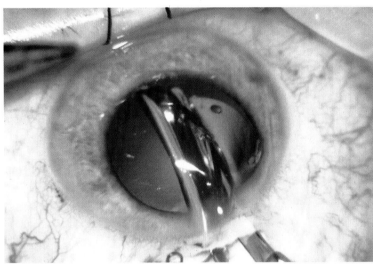

FIG. 1.217

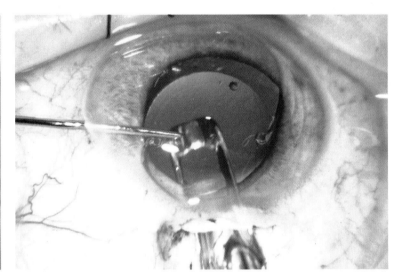

FIG. 1.218

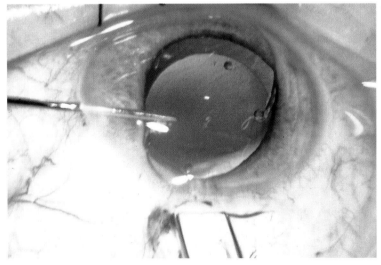

FIG. 1.219

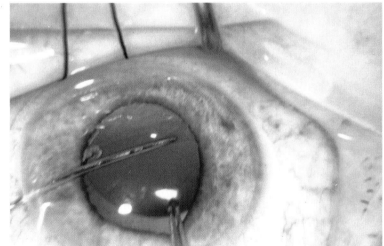

FIG. 1.220

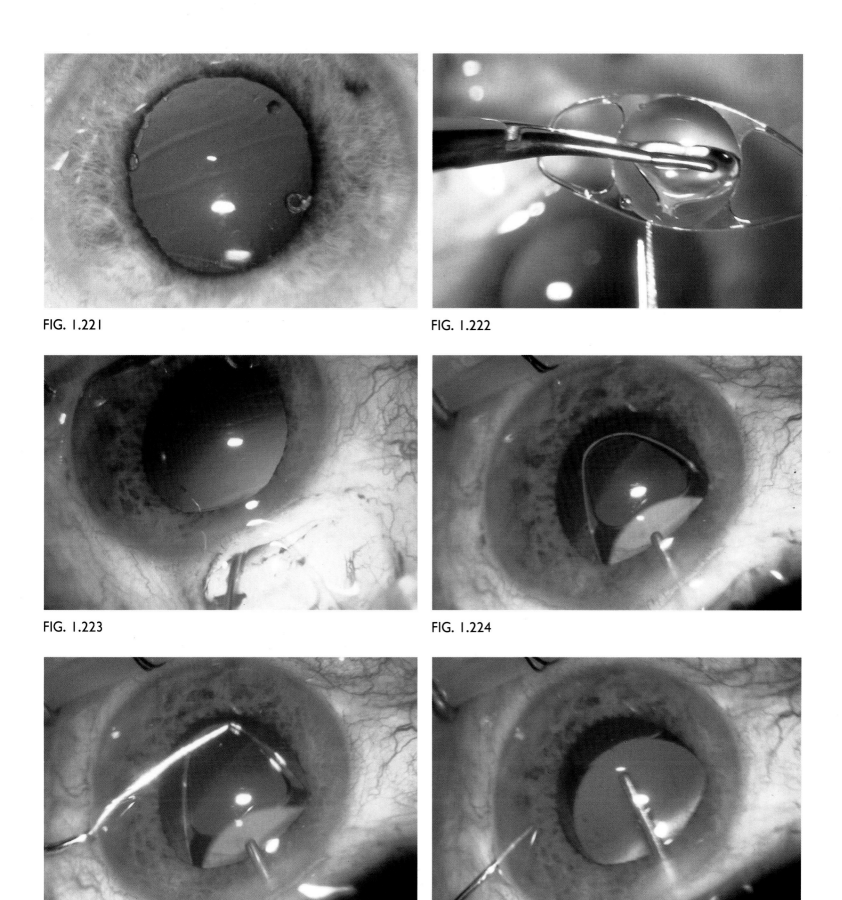

FIG. 1.221

FIG. 1.222

FIG. 1.223

FIG. 1.224

FIG. 1.225

FIG. 1.226

CILIARY SULCUS VERSUS CAPSULAR BAG FIXATION OF POSTERIOR CHAMBER LENSES

Currently more than 90% of cataract extractions performed in the United States are done by the extracapsular method, nearly always with a posterior chamber lens. The advantages of this technique were clearly recognized by surgeons employing sulcus fixation of the intraocular lens. The short-term results were highly satisfactory. At the inception of this method, several theoretical disadvantages were postulated. Within a short time, some of these became realities. As a result, surgeons began to turn to capsular bag fixation in order to avoid some of these problems. It is emphasized that this represents an ultrarefinement of a highly successful procedure.

Some of the alleged and real disadvantages of sulcus fixation are outlined below.

DECENTRATION

Although sulcus-fixated posterior chamber lenses ultimately assume a stable intraocular position, a significant number are found to be decentered. This results from one of several mechanisms, such as asymmetric sealing of anterior capsular flaps to the posterior capsule, the forces of proliferating lens epithelium, one loop in the bag and one out of the bag, and the poor memory of polypropylene loops. A variety of decentrations is observed, including sunset syndrome (Fig. 1.230), sunrise syndrome (Fig. 1.231), horizontal decentration (Fig. 1.232), and windshield wiper syndrome. The latter is the result of an inadequately sized lens in an eye with larger-than-average sulcus-to-sulcus dimensions. Optical disturbances by decentrated lenses are sometimes caused by the presence of the drill holes of the optic in the pupillary space (Figs. 1.233 and 1.234). Some of these problems are minimized with all-PMMA lenses with single-piece technology since the loops have greater plastic memory than polypropylene loops and tend to resist deformation and decentration forces. Most of these problems are eliminated with posterior chamber lenses placed in the capsular bag.

PUPIL CAPTURE

This was more of a problem with the earlier uniplanar J-loop lenses than with current lenses with more flexible loops and anterior angulation. Examples are shown in Figs. 1.279 and 1.280. Pupillary capture is still encountered with inflammation and in some cases where an iridoplasty has been performed. Capsular bag fixation lessens the chance of pupillary capture.

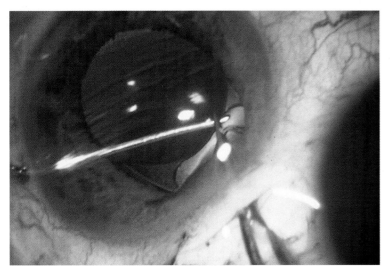

FIG. 1.227

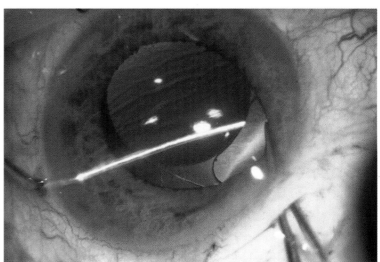

FIG. 1.228

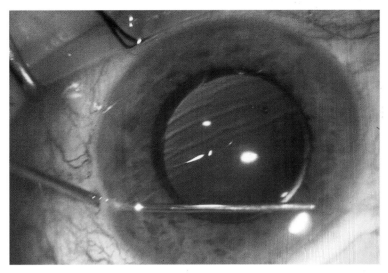

FIG. 1.229

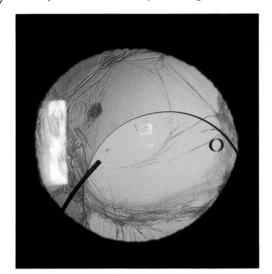

FIG. 1.230

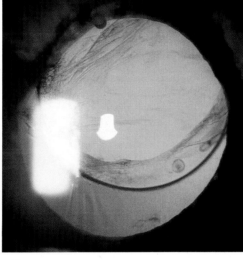

FIG. 1.231

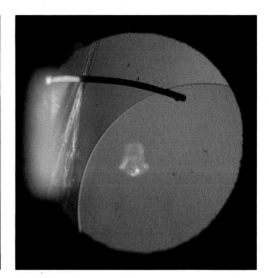

FIG. 1.232

Ciliary Sulcus Versus Capsular Bag Fixation: Decentration

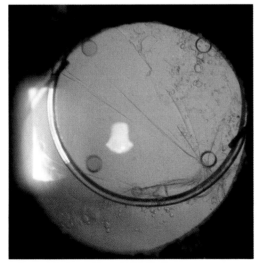

FIG. 1.233

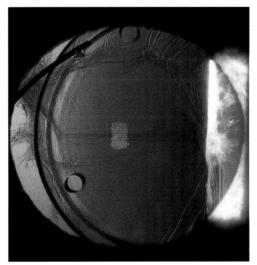

FIG. 1.234

POSTERIOR SYNECHIAE AND SYNECHIAE AT THE MARGINS OF THE OPTIC

These result from chronic inflammation and are related to contact of the lens equator with the pigment epithelium of the iris or the iris margin with the optic (Fig. 1.235).

POSTERIOR IRIS CHAFING SYNDROMES

These occur in two forms. In the first, iris transillumination defects and microhyphemas occur. These are associated with intermittent blurring of vision resembling amaurosis fugax. These are known as "white-out" attacks, and are due to white cells liberated by contact of sulcus-fixated, angulated loops with the back of the iris (Fig. 1.236). This is very rare with capsular bag fixation. A second form is caused by pigment dispersion resulting in glaucoma. An example is shown in Fig. 1.237 where the optic is seen through the iris

against its posterior surface. The extensive loss of pigment is shown by transillumination in Fig. 1.238. A histologic example of pigment deposition in the anterior chamber angle is seen in Fig. 1.239. Once again, this problem is less frequent with capsular bag fixation.

EROSION AND PERFORATION OF THE CILIARY BODY

The anatomic region known as the ciliary sulcus is inexact and poorly defined for the surgeon. The ciliary processes vary widely in their morphology. They may completely obstruct access of the loop of the lens implant to the sulcus. The ciliary sulcus is an area of high metabolic activity. Erosion and perforation of the ciliary body by the loop disrupts the blood–aqueous barrier (Fig. 1.240). The major arterial circle of the iris is in close proximity. The loop may perfo-

▽ Ciliary Sulcus Versus Capsular Bag Fixation: Posterior and Optical Margin Synechiae

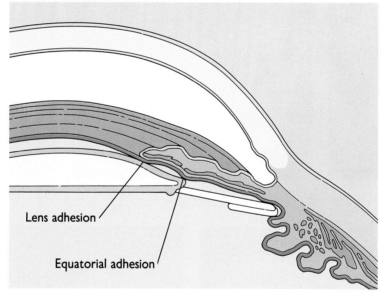

Lens adhesion

Equatorial adhesion

FIG. 1.235

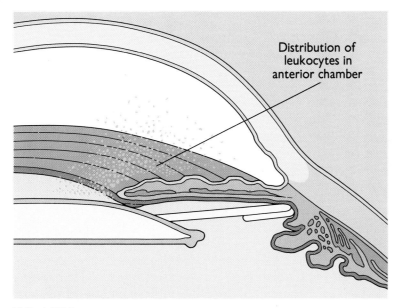

FIG. 1.236

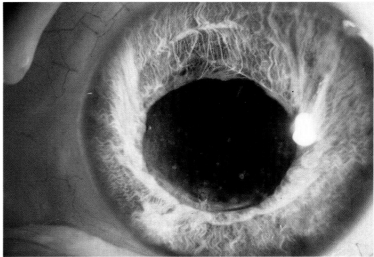

FIG. 1.237

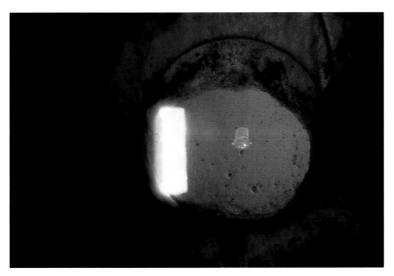

FIG. 1.238

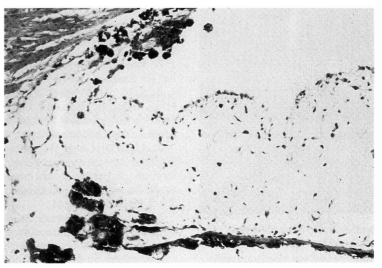

FIG. 1.239

Ciliary Sulcus Versus Capsular Bag Fixation: Ciliary Body Erosion and Perforation

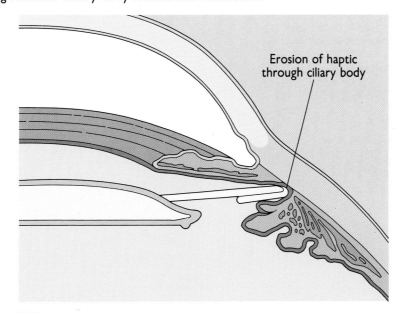

FIG. 1.240

rate the pars plicata (Fig. 1.241) or the muscularis (Fig. 1.242), or merely erode the surface of the ciliary sulcus. Figure 1.243 shows a loop imbedded in the ciliary body surrounded by a foreign body giant cell reaction. Figure 1.244 shows a thrombosis of the major arterial circle of the iris as a result of loop perforation of the ciliary body. A variety of complications is possible under these situations.

Blood–Aqueous Barrier Breakdown

The integrity of this barrier depends on intact surfaces. Erosion of this surface will result in an inflow of inflammatory mediators. These include complement proteins that are activated by contact with the biomaterials of an intraocular lens. In the short term, sulcus-fixated lenses show significantly greater breakdown than capsular bag-fixated lenses.

Perforation of the Ciliary Body

Due to the proximity of the aberrant loop to the greater arterial circle of the iris, the major vessels of the plexus may become occluded (Fig. 1.244), they may hemorrhage, and hemorrhage may occur during explantation of the lens.

Uveitis-Glaucoma-Hyphema (UGH) Syndrome

This has been described only with sulcus-fixated lenses. The region of the ciliary sulcus is spared these problems when the lens is safely sequestered inside the capsule bag as shown with a Simcoe lens in Fig. 1.245 and a Sinskey lens in Fig. 1.246. This is compared with a sulcus-fixated Sinskey lens in Fig. 1.247.

HEMORRHAGE IN PATIENTS WITH HEMATOLOGIC DISORDERS

This includes patients with blood dyscrasias, patients on anticoagulants, coagulopathies, and hematologic malignancies. This danger may not be present at the time of the original surgery but may occur later in patients who develop these systemic disorders postoperatively. Capsular bag-fixated lenses are unlikely to result in these complications.

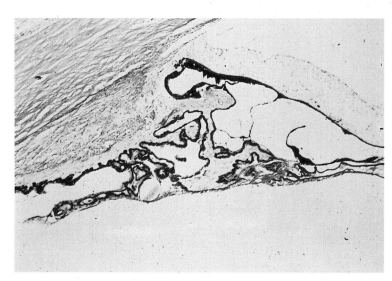

FIG. 1.241

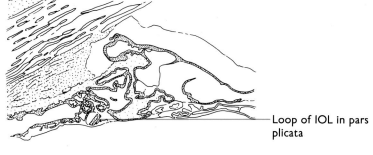

Loop of IOL in pars plicata

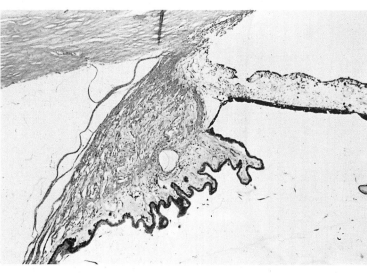

FIG. 1.242

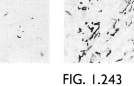

FIG. 1.243

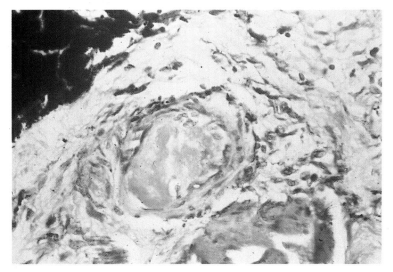

FIG. 1.244

Ciliary Sulcus Versus Capsular Bag Fixation: Uveitis-Glaucoma-Hyphema Syndrome

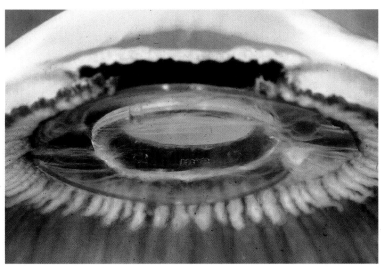

FIG. 1.245

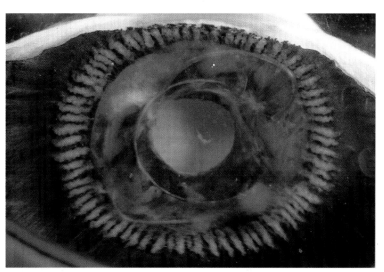

FIG. 1.246

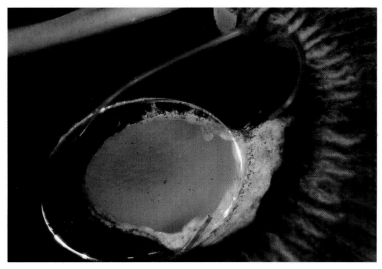

FIG. 1.247

LOOP PERFORATION THROUGH A PERIPHERAL IRIDECTOMY

This problem is encountered with sulcus-fixated lenses as shown in Fig. 1.248. Figure 1.249 shows a perforation of the iris by the distal end of a sulcus-fixated lens. The end of the blue loop is seen in the slit beam on the iris at the left.

The position of a capsular bag-fixated lens is deeper than that of the crystalline lens or a sulcus-fixated lens. Note the relationship between the anterior surface of the crystalline lens and the slit beam on the iris in Fig. 1.250. In the opposite eye of the same patient (Fig. 1.251), note the large space between the slit beam on the iris and the anterior surface of the capsular bag-fixated lens. Figure 1.252 shows an eye with a sulcus-fixated lens. Note the closeness of the anterior surface of the lens to the iris. A capsular bag-fixated lens was implanted in the opposite eye of this patient (Fig. 1.253). Note the distance between the iris and the anterior surface of the lens.

While the disadvantages of sulcus-fixated lenses enumerated above appear to justify the increasing popularity of capsular bag fixation, it is emphasized that they occur infrequently. Additionally, there are advantages in sulcus fixation. They are as follows:

1. Surgery is easier
2. It is safer in eyes with disorders associated with zonular weakness (e.g., pseudoexfoliation syndrome)
3. It can be used with surgical complications, such as rupture of the posterior capsule and zonular dialysis
4. It is safer in eyes with positive vitreous pressure
5. A secondary posterior chamber lens can only be placed in the ciliary sulcus
6. Explantation is easier

LASER RIDGE

When Hoffer introduced the laser ridge concept, it was thought that this would act as a barrier to the migration of lens epithelium into the pupillary space, thereby inhibiting posterior capsular opacification. There is some verification of this premise in an animal model (Fig. 1.254). In this example, the capsule is covered by an opaque membrane peripheral to the laser ridge and the capsule in the pupillary region is clear. However, after considerable experience with laser ridge lenses, I have not been aware of a lowering of the incidence of posterior capsule opacification com-

Ciliary Sulcus Versus Capsular Bag Fixation: Peripheral Iridectomy Loop Perforation

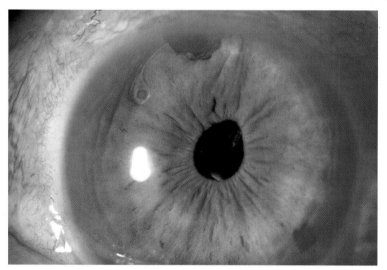

FIG. 1.248

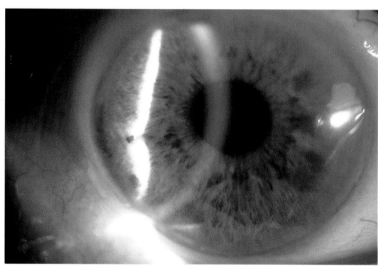

FIG. 1.249

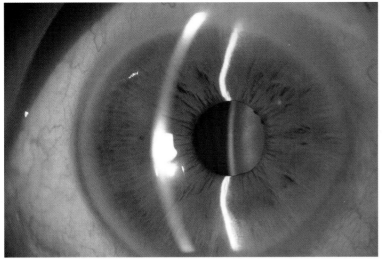

FIG. 1.250

FIG. 1.251

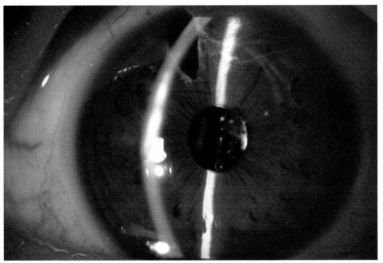

FIG. 1.252

FIG. 1.253

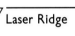 Laser Ridge

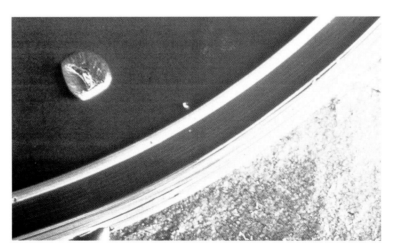

FIG. 1.254

pared to lenses without a laser ridge. The laser ridge does provide a space between the posterior surface of the optic of the lens implant and the posterior capsule. It is felt that this facilitates the use of the YAG laser and that there is less likelihood of leaving marks on the optic. It is known that the energy created by the laser is transmitted anteriorly (Fig. 1.255) and that the amount of energy burst anteriorly depends on the amount of millijoules used (Fig. 1.256). When a lens with a laser ridge is implanted, it is easy to visualize the surfaces of the optic. Marks left on the optic after a YAG laser capsulectomy are seen in Fig. 1.257. These are confined to the area of the laser bursts. The latter eye is shown by retroillumination in Fig. 1.258. The marks are shown dramatically in the slit lamp view in Fig. 1.259.

Four surfaces are visible with a Jaffe lens with a laser ridge (Fig. 1.260). From left to right they are the anterior surface of the optic, posterior surface of the optic, posterior capsule, and anterior surface of the vitreous. The laser ridge

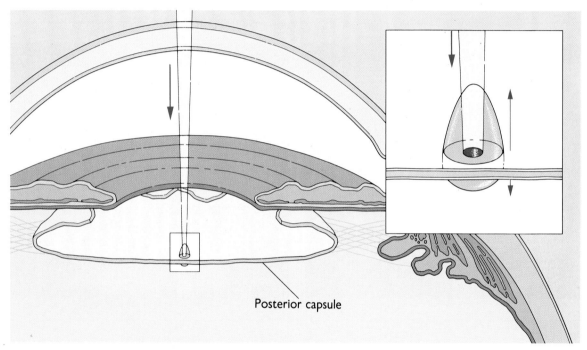

FIG. 1.255

Posterior capsule

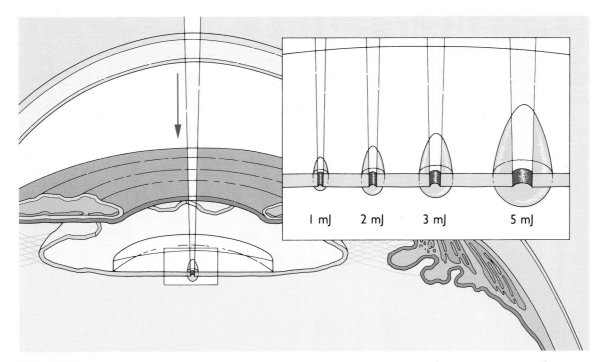

FIG. 1.256

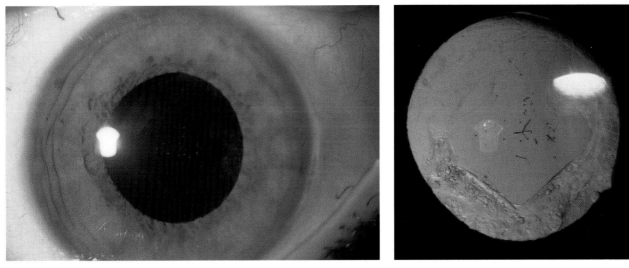

FIG. 1.257

FIG. 1.258

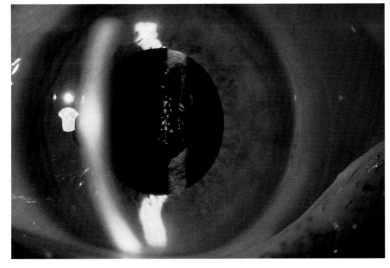

FIG. 1.259

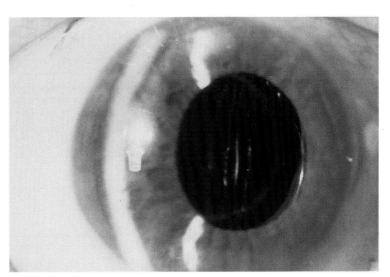

FIG. 1.260

space is clearly visible. This is demonstrated again with a Simcoe lens with a laser ridge (Fig. 1.261). Figures 1.262 and 1.263 show additional examples of Jaffe lenses with laser ridges. Figure 1.264 demonstrates that the space is visible at the slit lamp even with a small pupil. An interesting example of the space created by the laser ridge is shown in Fig. 1.265, where a vertically oval hole is seen in the posterior capsule. A slit lamp view through this portion of the pupil demonstrates a space between the optic and the anterior surface of the vitreous (Fig. 1.266). With the slit lamp

beam directed slightly to the right, the edge of the torn capsule is seen (Fig. 1.267). With the beam moved further to the right, the posterior capsule becomes visible behind the optic (Fig. 1.268). Figure 1.269 demonstrates the difficulty in identifying the surfaces of the optic in an eye with a lens without a laser ridge. In the opposite eye of the same patient, the surfaces are clearly visible since a laser ridge lens is present (Fig. 1.270). While an interrupted laser ridge can also create a space behind the optic, it may allow a greater migration of lens epithelium into the pupillary

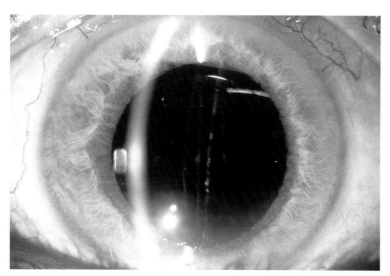

FIG. 1.261

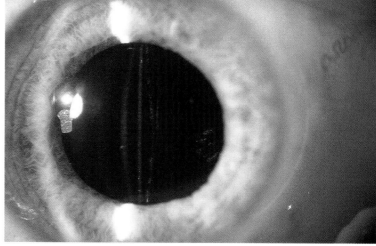

FIG. 1.262

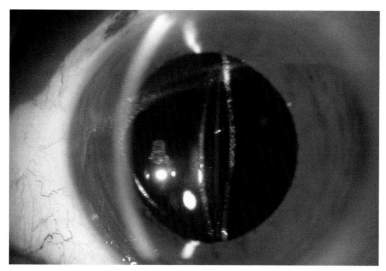

FIG. 1.263

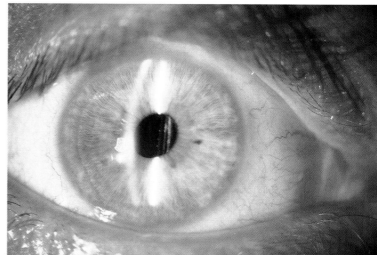

FIG. 1.264

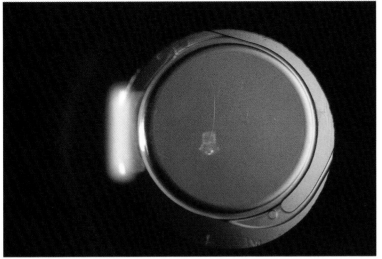

FIG. 1.265

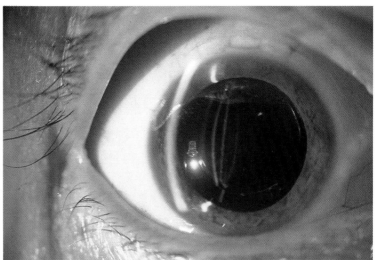

FIG. 1.266

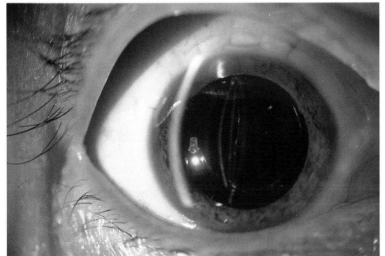

FIG. 1.267

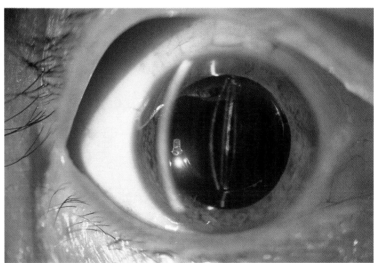

FIG. 1.268

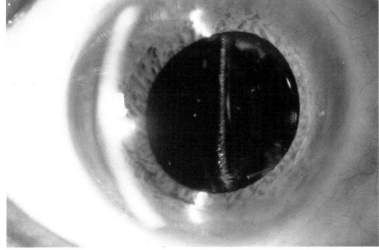

FIG. 1.269

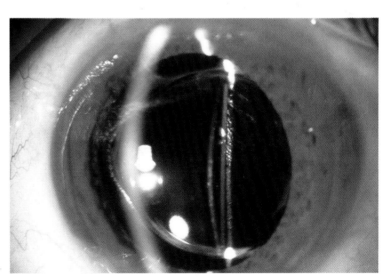

FIG. 1.270

space through the interruptions in the ridge compared to a lens with a complete laser ridge or one without a laser ridge (Fig. 1.271).

The creation of the laser ridge space has opened the possibility of material such as exudate and blood gaining access to this space. Figures 1.272 and 1.273 illustrate the eye of a patient who developed *Staphylococcus epidermidis* endophthalmitis 2 weeks postoperatively. During aspiration of the hypopyon for smear and culture, the exudate inadvertently passed behind the lens into the laser space. I have termed this hypopyon of the laser space. One week later, some absorption of the exudate has occurred and it can clearly be seen that the optic is anterior to the exudate (Fig. 1.274). Further absorption of the exudate is seen 4 weeks (Fig. 1.275) and 5 weeks postoperatively (Fig. 1.276). A hyphema of the laser space is seen one day postoperatively

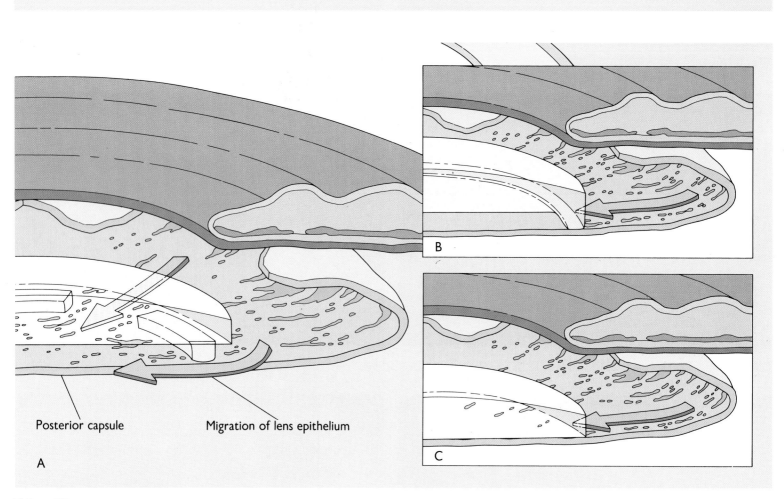

Posterior capsule   Migration of lens epithelium

A

B

C

FIG. 1.271

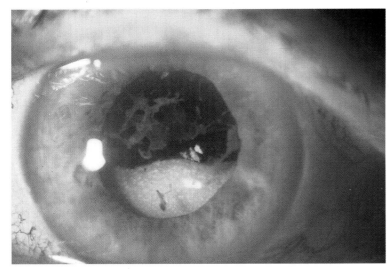

FIG. 1.272

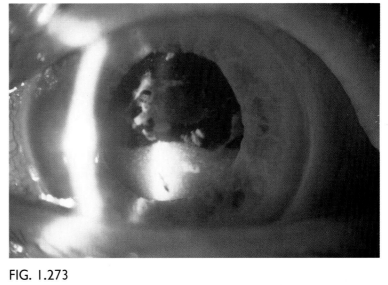

FIG. 1.273

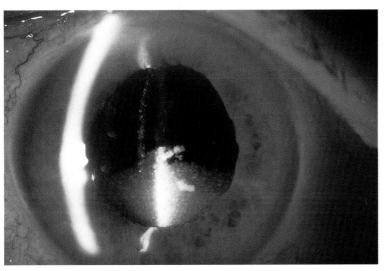

FIG. 1.274

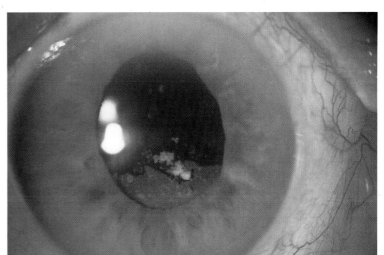

FIG. 1.275

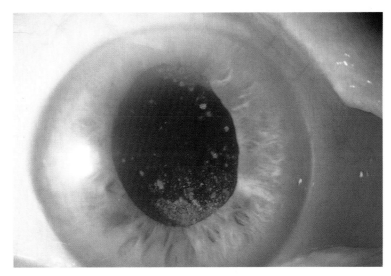

FIG. 1.276

in Figs. 1.277 and 1.278. The terms hypopyon and hyphema are used loosely since the exudate and blood are not in the anterior chamber. They are used because of their resemblance to a true hypopyon and a true hyphema.

MALPOSITIONS OF INTRAOCULAR LENSES: POSTERIOR CHAMBER LENSES

PUPILLARY CAPTURE

Pupillary capture exists when part (Fig. 1.279) or all (Fig. 1.280) of the optic of the posterior chamber lens finds its way anterior to the iris. If discovered within a few weeks of the surgery, it can often be corrected by dilating the pupil and constricting it if the optic falls back into the posterior chamber. In some cases it may be necessary to introduce a needle into the anterior chamber through the limbus and tap the optic back into place. If the capture is discovered many weeks or months postoperatively, posterior synechiae usually exist and the optic cannot easily be moved poste-

riorly. In such a case it is best to leave the lens in this position (Fig. 1.281). Pupillary capture is found less frequently since the popularity of angulated haptics and capsular bag fixation.

SUNSET SYNDROME

This is a form of decentration of a posterior chamber lens where the optic is displaced toward 6 o'clock. It may be disturbing to the patient since a portion of the pupil is pseudophakic and another portion aphakic (Fig. 1.282). There are four methods of correcting a sunset syndrome, depending on the seriousness of the displacement. The first two methods are particularly effective if there is little or no vitreous in the anterior chamber. Figure 1.283 demonstrates such a case. The entire optic fell behind the inferior iris. It was corrected by creating an intentional pupillary capture (Fig. 1.284). This is done by drawing the lens up toward 12 o'clock with a Jaffe or Sinskey hook and tilting the optic anterior to the iris at each horizontal meridian. Once in this

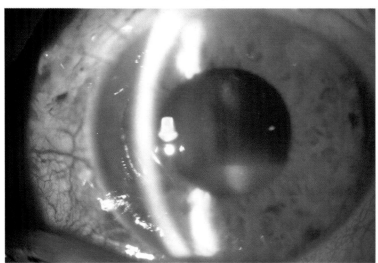

FIG. 1.277

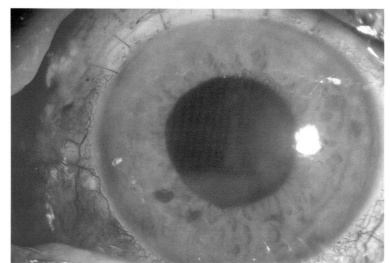

FIG. 1.278

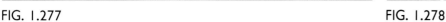

Malpositions of Intraocular Lenses: Pupillary Capture

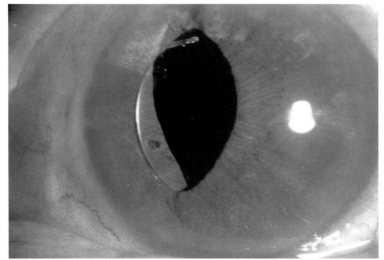

FIG. 1.279

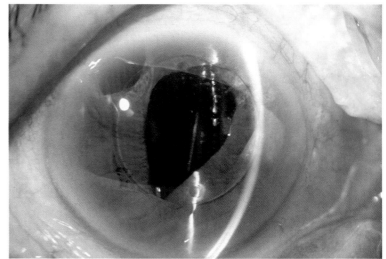

FIG. 1.280

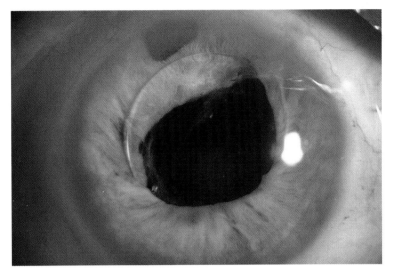

FIG. 1.281

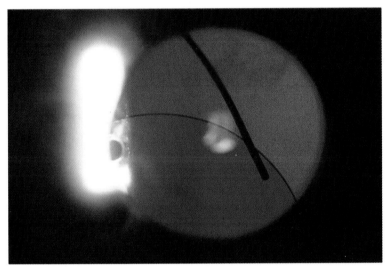

FIG. 1.282

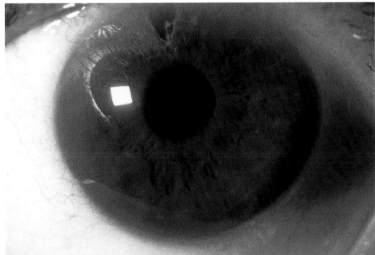

FIG. 1.283

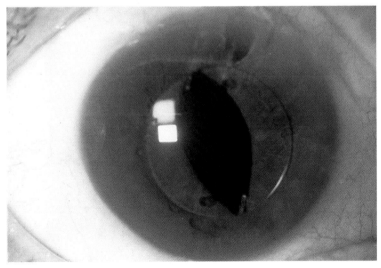

FIG. 1.284

position, the optic rarely falls back behind the iris. An alternate method is to draw the lens up into correct position and secure the superior haptic with a McCannel suture. Figure 1.285 shows an eye with a sunset syndrome. The site of the primary posterior capsulotomy is seen and there is no vitreous in the anterior chamber. The same eye is shown in Fig. 1.286 photographed at the slit lamp. The lens was drawn up into position with a hook and a McCannel suture secured the superior haptic to the edge of a peripheral iridectomy. The blue polypropylene suture is visible in Fig. 1.287. If the anterior chamber is filled with vitreous, as in Fig. 1.288, it is probably best to explant it, perform an automated partial anterior vitrectomy, and implant an anterior chamber lens (Fig. 1.289). A postmortem view of an eye with a partial pupillary capture is shown in Fig. 1.290. Sunset syndrome usually occurs when an inferior zonular dialysis occurs but is unrecognized at the time of surgery. It is prevented by using a McCannel suture at the time of surgery when a zonular dialysis or posterior capsule rupture is seen. The most serious form of sunset syndrome is seen when the entire lens falls back into the vitreous. It may be brought back up into position through the pars plana. However, if a haptic becomes imbedded in the vitreous base, it is best not to remove the lens. Some surgeons have implanted an anterior chamber lens in such cases.

SUNRISE SYNDROME

This is another form of decentration that usually occurs when the lower haptic is in the capsule bag and the upper haptic is outside the bag (Figs. 1.291 to 1.294). This is less serious than the sunset syndrome since there is little danger of the lens falling back into the vitreous. If the optical problems caused by a sunrise syndrome are intolerable, the surgeon may attempt to pull the lower haptic out of the bag and place it in the ciliary sulcus.

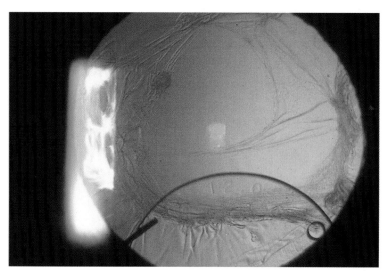

FIG. 1.285

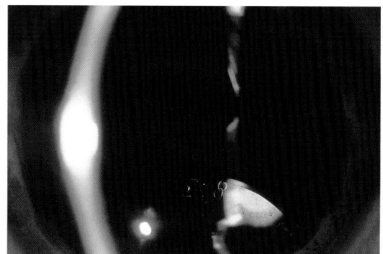

FIG. 1.286

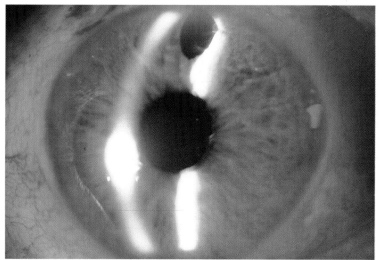

FIG. 1.287

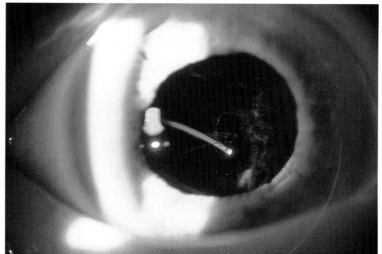

FIG. 1.288

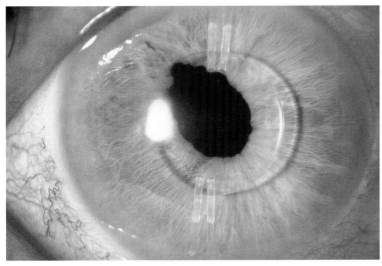

FIG. 1.289

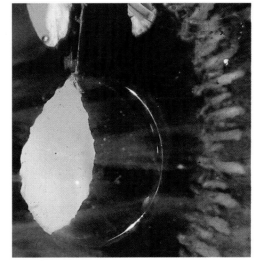

FIG. 1.290

Malpositions of Intraocular Lenses: Sunrise Syndrome

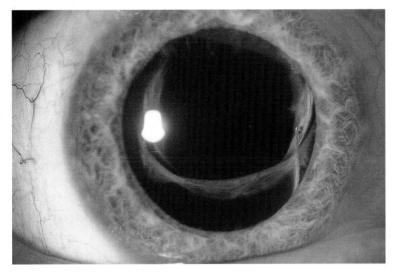

FIG. 1.291

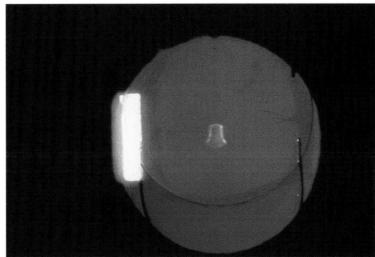

FIG. 1.292

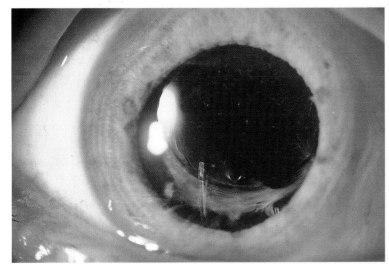

FIG. 1.293

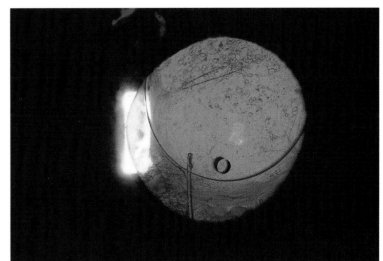

FIG. 1.294

HORIZONTAL DECENTRATION

This condition is again caused by one haptic in the capsular bag and the other haptic outside the bag. However, it may also be caused by intraocular inflammation. An example of a horizontal decentration that was left as found is shown in Figs. 1.295 and 1.296. When serious optical disturbances occur due to fibrosed posterior capsules, the lens may have to be explanted and replaced by an anterior chamber lens.

A membranectomy and vitrectomy are usually necessary. One such case is shown in Figs. 1.297 and 1.298. An anterior chamber lens was implanted following removal of the decentered posterior chamber lens (Fig. 1.299). Another case is seen in Figs. 1.300 and 1.301. It was treated in the same manner (Fig. 1.302). Lenses with polypropylene loops are more likely to decenter than those with PMMA loops. For example, the eyes in Figs. 1.303 to

Malpositions of Intraocular Lenses: Horizontal Decentration

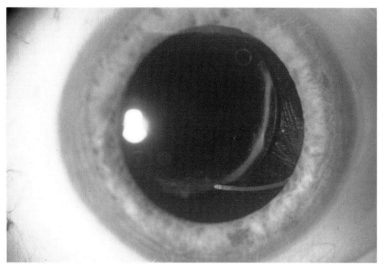

FIG. 1.295

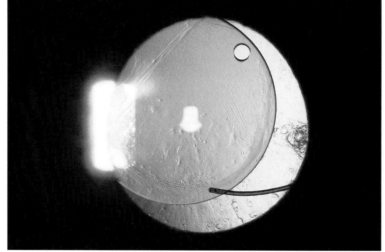

FIG. 1.296

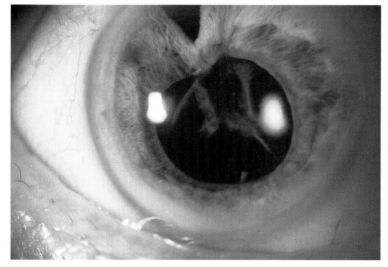

FIG. 1.297

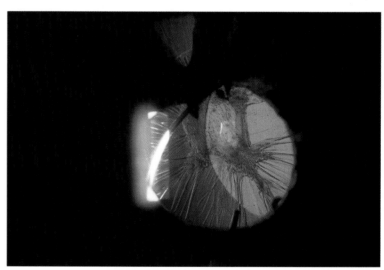

FIG. 1.298

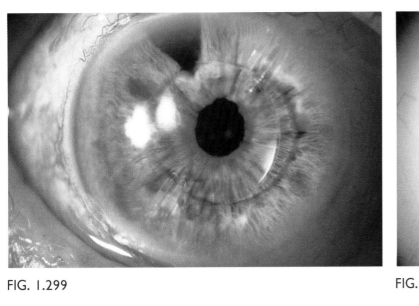

FIG. 1.299

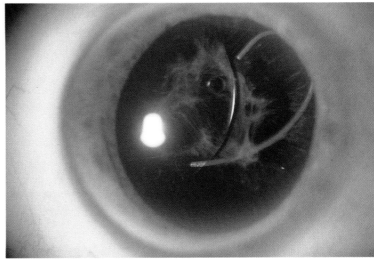

FIG. 1.300

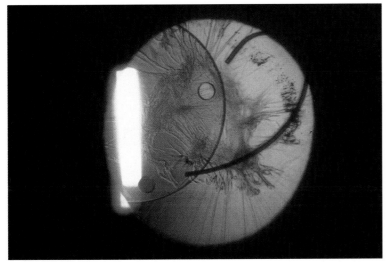

FIG. 1.301

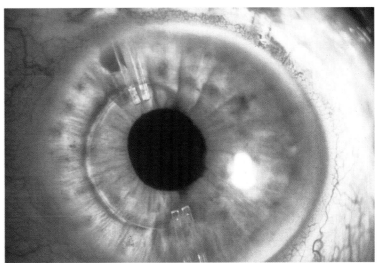

FIG. 1.302

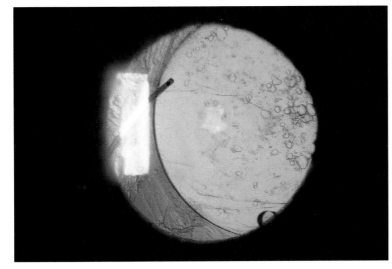

FIG. 1.303

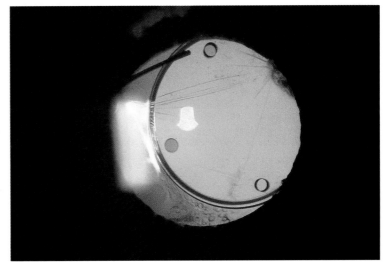

FIG. 1.304

1.305 show decentration of lenses with polypropylene loops due to asymmetric placement in the capsular bag or due to one loop being outside the bag. On the contrary, the eye with a one-piece all-PMMA loop in Fig. 1.306 has a well-centered lens, in spite of asymmetric anterior capsule flaps. Other examples are seen in Figs. 1.307 to 1.310. A postmortem specimen of a well-centered Sinskey lens with capsular bag fixation is shown in Fig. 1.311 and a Simcoe lens in Fig. 1.312. Fig. 1.313 shows a subluxation of a lens following the use of the YAG laser. Fig. 1.314 shows a luxation of a lens behind a rupture of the posterior capsule due to trauma.

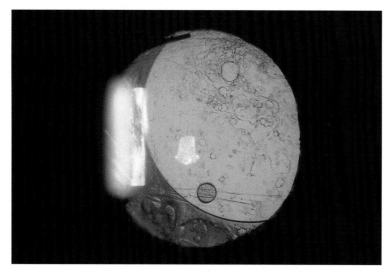

FIG. 1.305

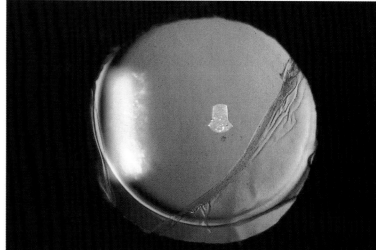

FIG. 1.306

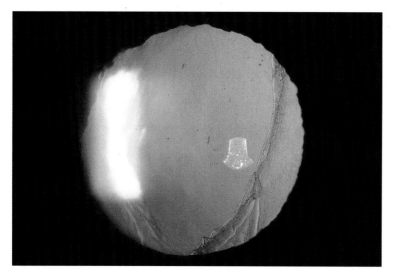

FIG. 1.307

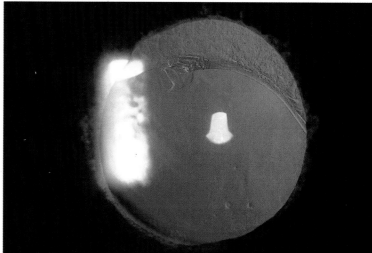

FIG. 1.308

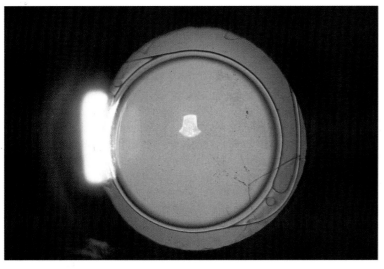

FIG. 1.309

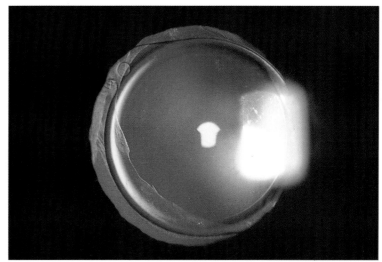

FIG. 1.310

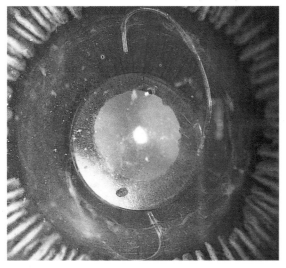

FIG. 1.311

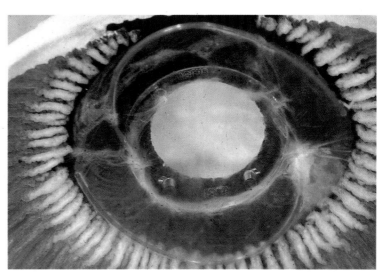

FIG. 1.312

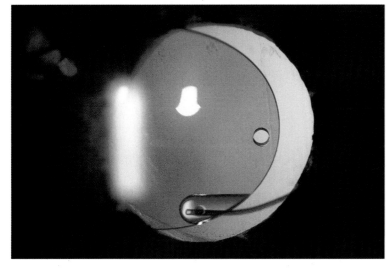

FIG. 1.313

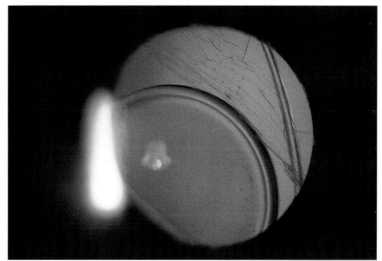

FIG. 1.314

ANTERIOR CHAMBER LENSES AND SECONDARY LENS IMPLANTATION

Anterior chamber lenses are ideally suited for three situations:

1. In conjunction with an intracapsular cataract extraction
2. In case of rupture or zonular dialysis of the posterior capsule
3. Secondary lens implantation

There are three types of anterior chamber lenses:

1. Rigid [Choyce Mark VIII (Fig. 1.315), Mark IX, and Kelman tripod (Fig. 1.316)]
2. Semiflexible [Hessburg (Fig. 1.317)]
3. Flexible [Kelman Multiflex (Fig. 1.318)]

The advantages of the rigid lens are a long history of tolerance within the eye when well manufactured, less tendency toward formation of goniosynechiae, less tendency to vault, and ease of explantation. The disadvantages are greater occular tenderness, possibly higher incidence of pupillary block, and less margin for error with faulty sizing.

Most surgeons currently prefer semiflexible and flexible anterior chamber lenses. They cause much less ocular tenderness than rigid lenses and they are more forgiving for sizing errors, but the semiflexible lenses may vault if they are too large. A serious problem that results with some of these lenses is the development of goniosynechiae, which may result in chronic inflammation and which makes explantation difficult. An example of this is shown in Fig. 1.319. The superior loop of a Leiske lens is surrounded by a fibrous tissue capsule and the loop is imbedded in the iris near the arterial circle. Figure 1.320 shows an explanted Leiske lens from an eye with a UGH (uveitis-glaucoma-hyphema) syndrome. Note that in order to remove the lens without causing an iridodialysis or serious damage to the angle, both distal loops were cut with scissors and the optic was then removed. Each remaining loop was then slid out of its fibrous tissue tunnel. Note the residual inflammatory debris on the optic and the haptics. The postoperative result is shown in Fig. 1.321. The patient now uses a contact lens.

It has been said that anterior chamber lenses are easy to insert but difficult to insert correctly so that the haptics rest at the scleral spur. Figure 1.322 shows an erosion of the ciliary body and angle recession. Endothelium lines the ero-

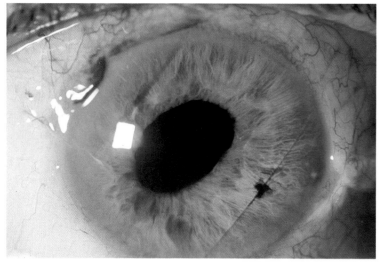

FIG. 1.315

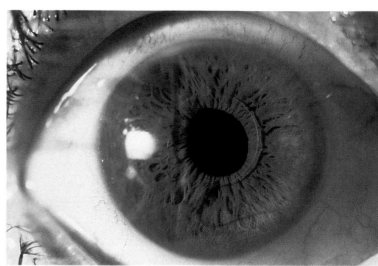

FIG. 1.316

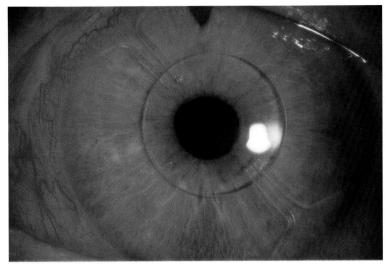

FIG. 1.317

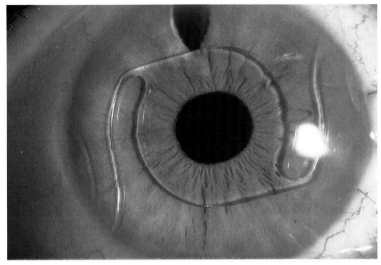

FIG. 1.318

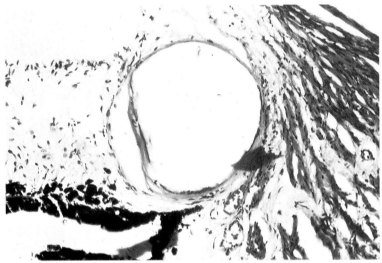

FIG. 1.319

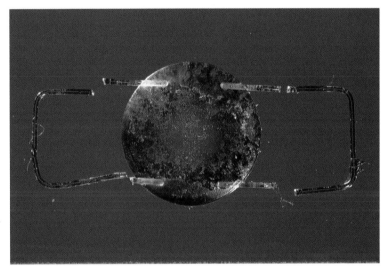

FIG. 1.320

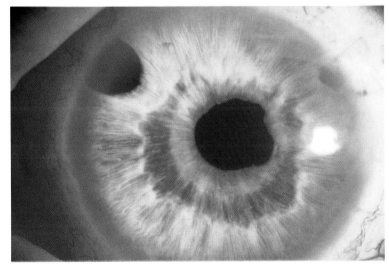

FIG. 1.321

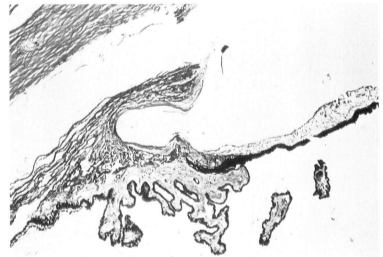

FIG. 1.322

sion and the anterior surface of the iris. A clinical example is shown in Figs. 1.323 and 1.324. A Leiske lens was implanted so that the lower loop caused a separation of the iris root. The pupil is updrawn. The superior loop is well located at the scleral spur. The gonioscopic view in Fig. 1.324 indicates that the lens was probably too large for the eye. Figure 1.325 shows erosion of the loop of an anterior chamber lens into the ciliary body. Figure 1.326 also shows a loop in the ciliary body. Figure 1.327 demonstrates an angle recession with endothelialization and descemetization. Figure 1.328 shows the same eye with extension of endothelium and Descemet's membrane over the iris. Figure 1.329 shows another example of fibrosis of the angle with endothelialization and descemetization. Figure 1.330 demonstrates iris tuck. Figure 1.331 shows iris tuck with the haptic penetrating through the peripheral iridectomy.

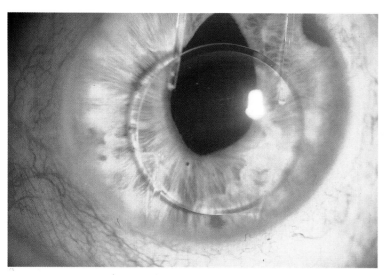

FIG. 1.323

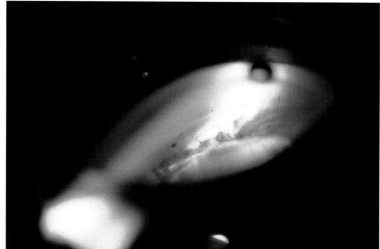

FIG. 1.324

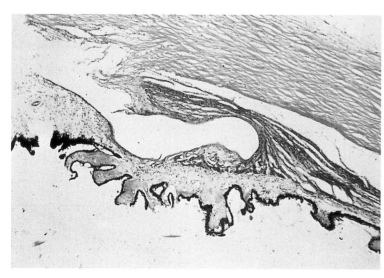

FIG. 1.325

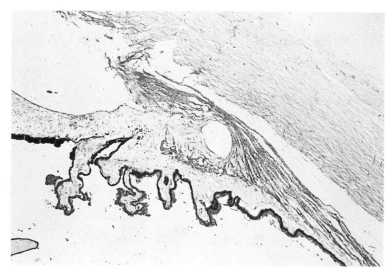

FIG. 1.326

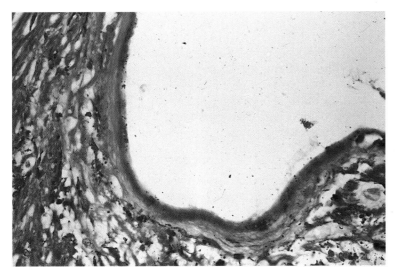

FIG. 1.327

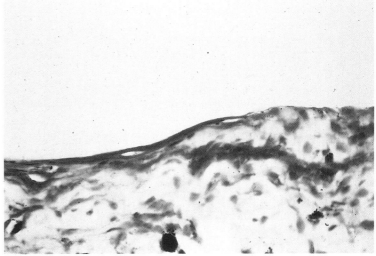

FIG. 1.328

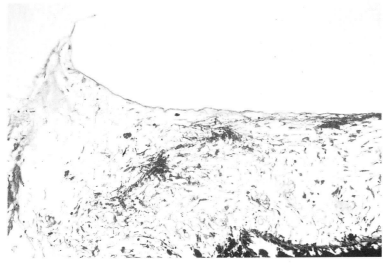

FIG. 1.329

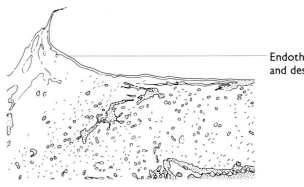

Endothelialization and descemetization

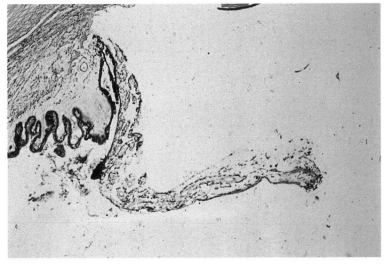

FIG. 1.330

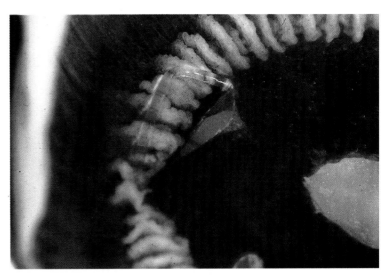

FIG. 1.331

Figure 1.332 demonstrates the loop of a lens in the conjunctiva. Figure 1.333 shows a Kelman Omnifit lens with one haptic entering the peripheral iridectomy. The lower haptic was tilted forward and rested against the back of the inferior cornea. The tilt was caused by an adhesion of the penetrating loop to the ciliary body. The adhesion did not separate easily and the loop was cut, leaving a small portion attached to the ciliary body (Fig. 1.334). The lens was removed and a Kelman Multiflex lens was inserted horizontally (Fig. 1.335). Figure 1.336 shows another anterior chamber lens with the haptic entering the peripheral iridectomy, resulting in a decentered lens.

It is seen from the above that haptics of anterior chamber lenses find their way into aberrant locations. The following photographs demonstrate highly satisfactory secondary lens implantations, a true blessing for the patient who cannot tolerate a contact lens. In most instances, these lenses are placed horizontally in order to avoid the original cataract incision and peripheral iridectomies. Peripheral anterior synechiae are more likely superiorly at the site of the original incision. The surgeon should examine the angle carefully to avoid peripheral anterior synechiae in other locations. The corneal endothelium should be evaluated in questionable cases. Small amounts of vitreous in the anterior chamber may be ignored since such vitreous has usually lost its fibroblastic potential. If most of the anterior chamber is filled with vitreous, a vitrectomy is usually performed before the lens is inserted. However, this should not be too extensive.

Figure 1.337 shows a secondary Kelman tripod lens. Figure 1.338 shows a secondary Kelman Multiflex lens. Figure 1.339 shows a secondary Hessburg lens. Figure 1.340 shows a secondary Hessburg lens in an eye that had an intracapsular cataract extraction with a wide sector iridectomy. Figure 1.341 shows an obliquely placed secondary Hessburg lens. It was placed in this position in order to avoid the peripheral iridectomy and peripheral anterior synechiae between 1 and 3 o'clock.

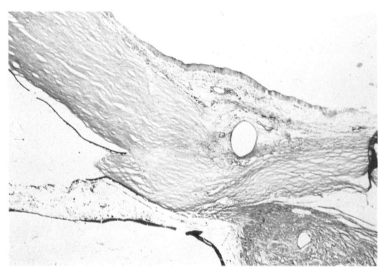

FIG. 1.332

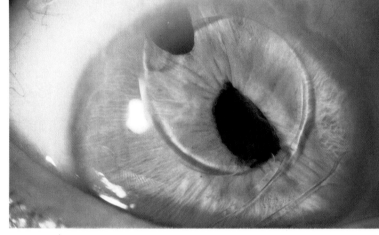

FIG. 1.333

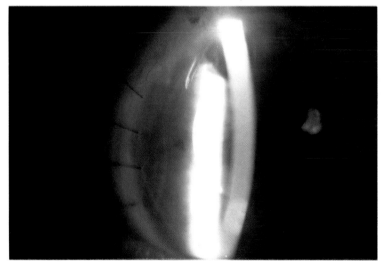

FIG. 1.334

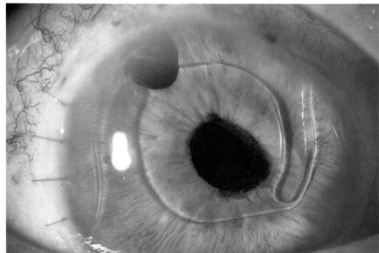

FIG. 1.335

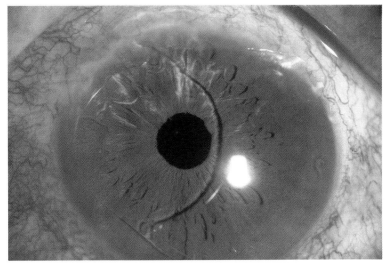

FIG. 1.336

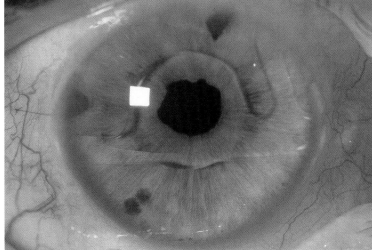

FIG. 1.337

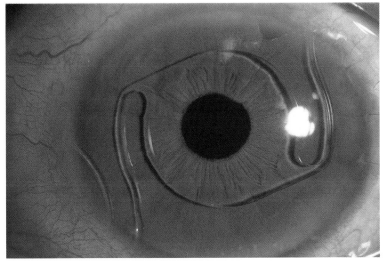

FIG. 1.338

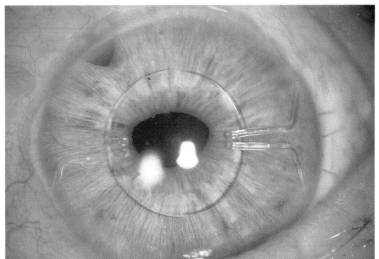

FIG. 1.339

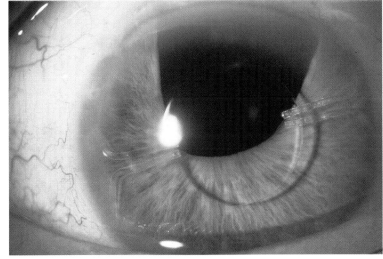

FIG. 1.340

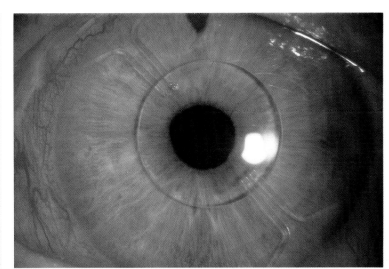

FIG. 1.341

TECHNIQUE OF SECONDARY LENS IMPLANTATION

In most instances it is best to perform a secondary lens implantation with an anterior chamber lens from the temporal side. This avoids the peripheral iridectomy and any peripheral anterior synechiae in the region of the original cataract incision. In Fig. 1.342 an eye is shown 4 years after a phacoemulsification. A large peripheral iridectomy is seen and a posterior capsulotomy was performed through which some vitreous has entered the anterior chamber. A white-to-white measurement is made with calipers (Fig. 1.343). It measures less than 11.5 mm. A grooved incision is made at the limbus on the temporal side of the eye and an ab externo incision is made with a diamond knife (Fig. 1.344). Acetylcholine (Miochol) is injected into the anterior chamber (Fig. 1.345). There occurs an immediate constriction of the pupil (Fig. 1.346). A viscoelastic material is injected into the anterior chamber through the same opening (Fig. 1.347). The incision is enlarged to the left along the previously prepared groove (Fig. 1.348). A Kelman Multiflex anterior chamber lens (Cooper-Cilco) is held with Blaydes forceps (Fig. 1.349). It is passed through the incision and into the anterior chamber until the leading edge reaches the opposite angle at the scleral spur (Figs. 1.350 to 1.352). The sclera is retracted with toothed forceps and the "knee" of the trailing haptic is passed behind the scleral edge of the incision (Fig. 1.353). The lens is in good position (Fig. 1.354). The viscoelastic material is aspirated (Fig. 1.355).

The final position of the lens is shown and the sutured incision is seen (Fig. 1.356).

OPACIFICATION OF THE POSTERIOR CAPSULE

Opacification of the posterior capsule is inevitable in a significant number of eyes following any form of extracapsular cataract extraction. It is erroneous to speak of opacification of the posterior capsule since the opacity consists of a membrane that covers the capsule, the capsule itself remaining clear. However, opacification of the posterior capsule is a description that is still commonly used.

An anterior capsulectomy creates a situation in which the remaining rim of the anterior capsule becomes adherent to the underlying posterior capsule. Lens epithelium lining the residual anterior capsule and the equatorial zone of the capsule becomes sequestered inside this sealed area (Fig. 1.357). Replicating epithelium may escape this trap and grow along the intact posterior capsule (Fig. 1.358A) and over the anterior surface of the remaining anterior capsule (Fig. 1.358B). Finally, a dense membrane consisting of clusters of lens epithelium, known as Elschnig's pearls, covers the posterior capsule (Fig. 1.358C). This represents lens epithelium's capacity to form new lens fibers. The opacification may consist of metaplastic fibrous tissue, pearls, or both.

Technique of Secondary Lens Implantation

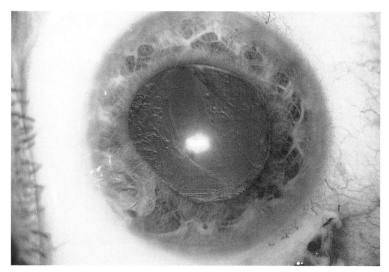

FIG. 1.342

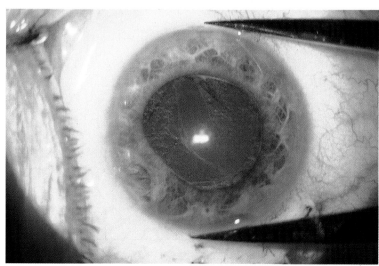

FIG. 1.343

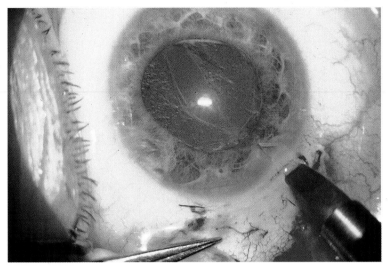

FIG. 1.344

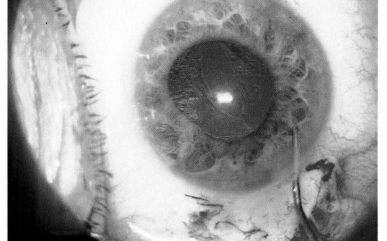

FIG. 1.345

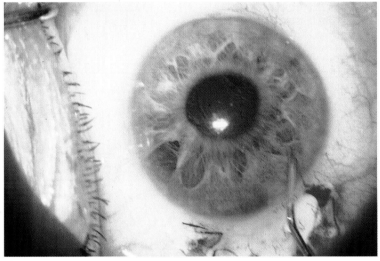

FIG. 1.346

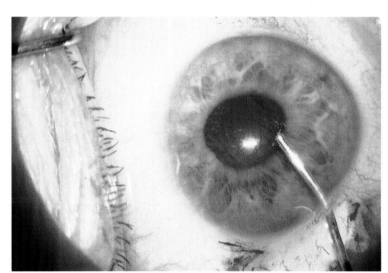

FIG. 1.347

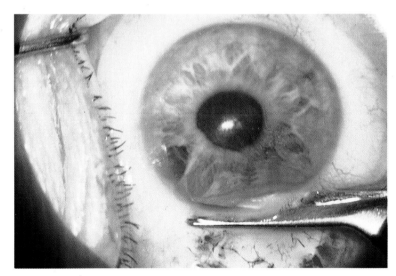

FIG. 1.348

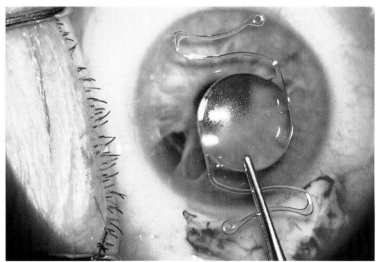

FIG. 1.349

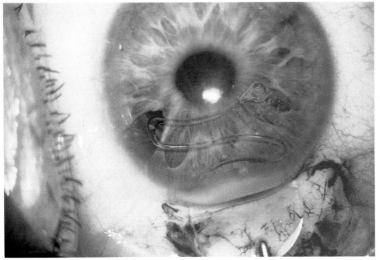

FIG. 1.350

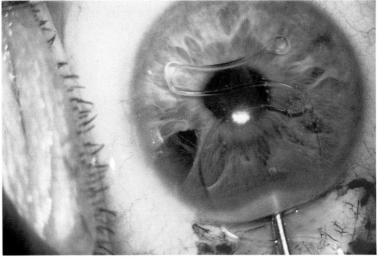

FIG. 1.351

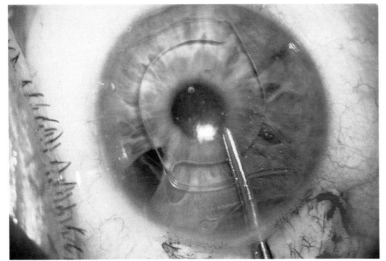

FIG. 1.352

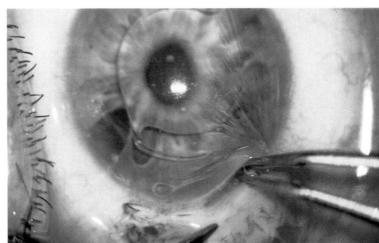

FIG. 1.353

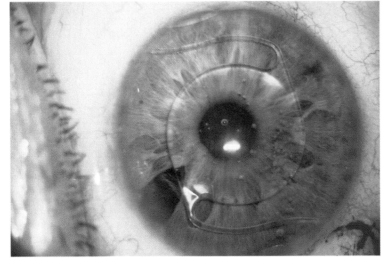

FIG. 1.354

FIG. 1.355

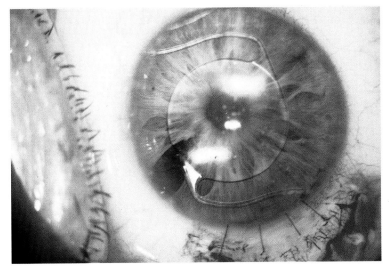

FIG. 1.356

Opacification of the Posterior Capsule

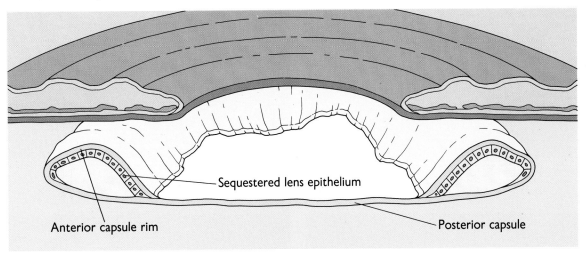

Sequestered lens epithelium

Anterior capsule rim

Posterior capsule

FIG. 1.357

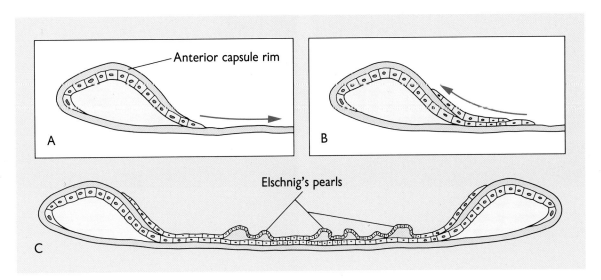

Anterior capsule rim

A

B

Elschnig's pearls

C

FIG. 1.358

The seam that occurs when the border of the incised anterior capsule becomes adherent to the posterior capsule is shown clinically in Figs. 1.359 and 1.360. The dense opacity that can result is seen in Fig. 1.361. An eye with Elschnig's pearls is shown in Fig. 1.362. The thickness of the membrane is shown in Fig. 1.363. The eye illustrated in Figs. 1.364 to 1.366 underwent a phacoemulsification and developed the membrane shown within 9 months. The patient was 31 years of age. The advancing membrane frequently stops abruptly at the margins of a posterior capsulotomy. The eye illustrated in Figs. 1.367 and 1.368 underwent a phacoemulsification with a primary posterior capsulotomy. Note that the only portion of clarity is the oval opening in the posterior capsule near the upper part of the

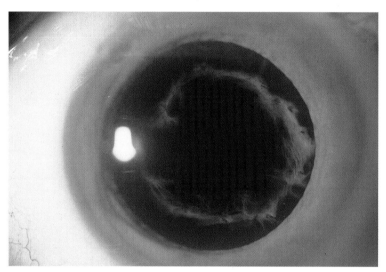

FIG. 1.359

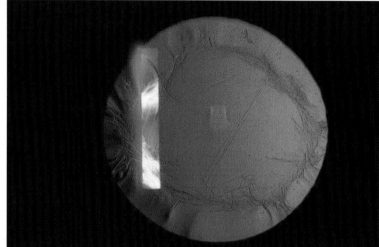

FIG. 1.360

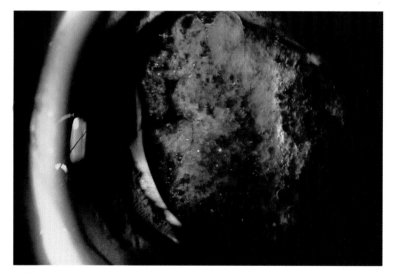

FIG. 1.361

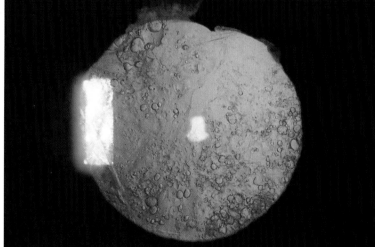

FIG. 1.362

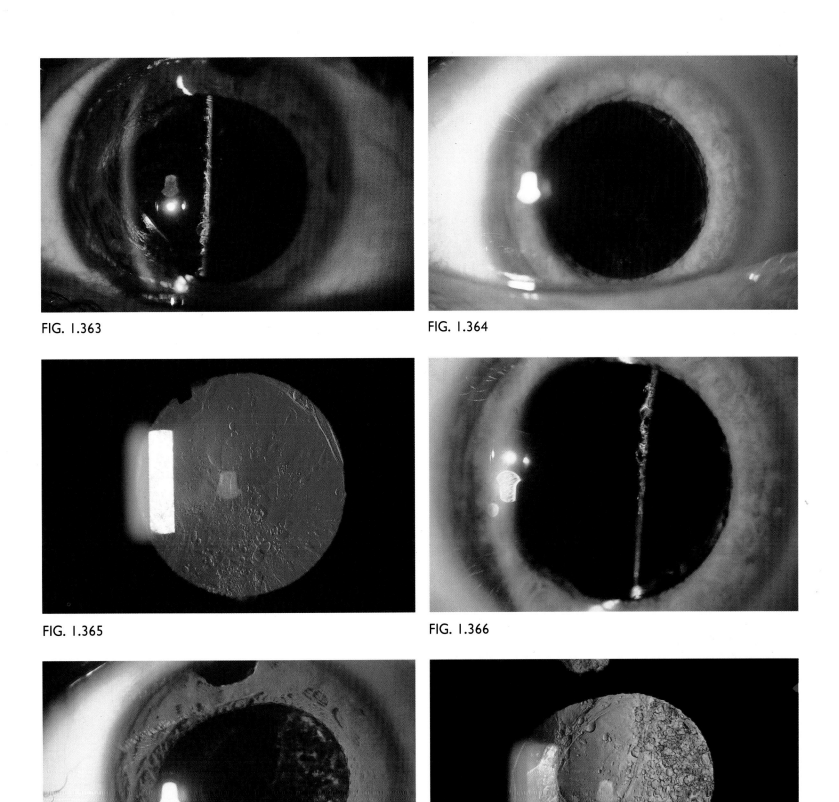

FIG. 1.363

FIG. 1.364

FIG. 1.365

FIG. 1.366

FIG. 1.367

FIG. 1.368

pupillary space where the primary posterior capsulotomy was performed. With the use of the YAG laser, an opening can be made in the membrane and posterior capsule, usually resulting in a dramatic improvement of vision (Fig. 1.369).

The proliferation of lens epithelium may result in a thick structure that sometimes has the appearance of a string of sausages. This is clearly shown in Fig. 1.370. Since this is an eye with aniridia, the entire structure is visible. Note that a posterior capsulotomy was performed. This structure is known as a Soemmering's ring. It represents an attempt of replicating lens epithelium to form a new lens. The Soemmering's ring is shown histologically in Figs. 1.371 to 1.373. Note that the inner border of the ring is limited by the seam of the anterior and posterior capsules. The ring appears to contain a nucleus. Also, note that there is an epithelial lining (Fig. 1.373) but, unlike the normal crystalline lens, the epithelium is not limited to the anterior and equatorial zones. It lines the entire structure.

Loose residual cortex usually absorbs. However, it can result in opaque dense bundles of lens material. It may also obstruct outflow channels of the eye, resulting in glaucoma (Fig. 1.374).

When the posterior capsule opacifies after an extracapsular cataract extraction, sufficient to interfere with clear vision, an opening is made in the capsule. This is usually performed with the Neodymium-YAG laser. Because of the expense of the equipment, some surgeons make the opening with a knife needle or a cystotome. An example of an opacified posterior capsule after a phacoemulsification with implantation of a Jaffe posterior chamber lens is shown in Fig. 1.375. The result after use of the Neodymium-YAG laser is shown in Fig. 1.376 and the slit lamp view in Fig. 1.377.

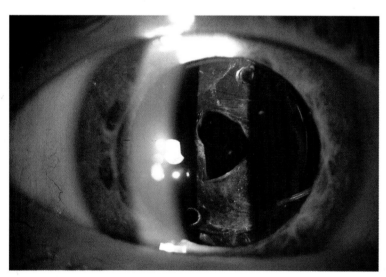

FIG. 1.369

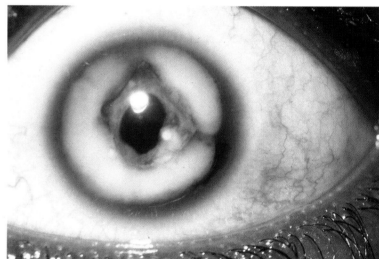

FIG. 1.370

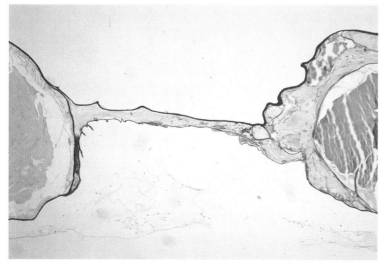

FIG. 1.371

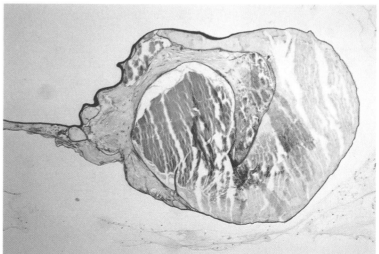

FIG. 1.372

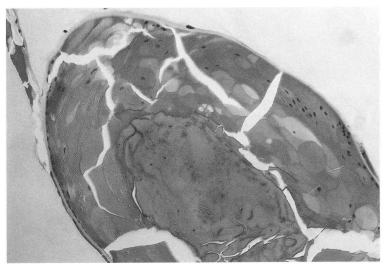

FIG. 1.373

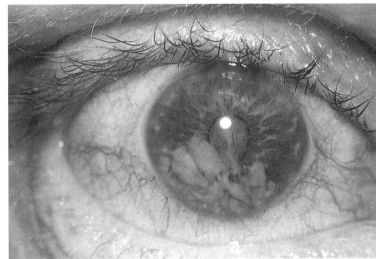

FIG. 1.374

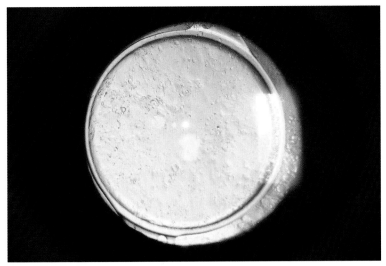

FIG. 1.375

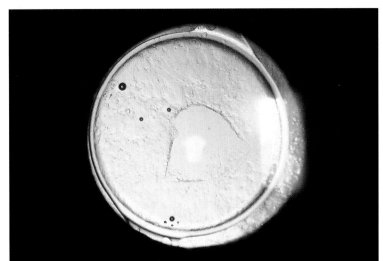

FIG. 1.376

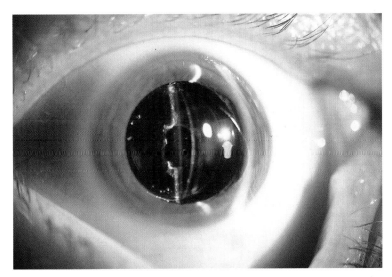

FIG. 1.377

POSTOPERATIVE ENDOPHTHALMITIS

Postoperative endophthalmitis is one of the most serious complications of cataract surgery. It has a varied etiology. It may be classified as follows:

1. Aseptic endophthalmitis
   a. Lens-induced
   b. IOL-induced
2. Septic endophthalmitis
   a. Aerobic
   b. Anaerobic
   c. Fungal

ASEPTIC ENDOPHTHALMITIS

Lens-Induced

The prototype for this is phacoanaphylactic endophthalmitis. It is currently thought to be allergic in nature. In certain patients with a peculiar immunologic makeup, exposure to one's own lens protein, when an extracapsular cataract extraction is performed, results in a severe antigen–antibody response. The onset is usually delayed, weeks to months postoperatively. Initially, there is a good response to steroids but this eventually becomes ineffective. Figure 1.378 shows an eye that developed a postoperative uveitis 10 weeks after cataract surgery with a capsular bag-fixated posterior chamber lens. The eye was free of inflammation after topical steroid therapy. Figure 1.379 shows the same eye 11 months later after numerous recurrences of inflammation. Keratic precipitates (KP) are clearly visible. A diagnosis of phacoanaphylactic endophthalmitis was finally established. The lens and intact posterior capsule were removed with cessation of inflammation. The onset of this disorder is often quite benign. The vitreous may show mild involvement as seen in Fig. 1.380. Figure 1.381 shows still another eye with the same diagnosis 16 months after cataract surgery with posterior chamber lens implantation. A fibrinous exudate covers the implant and the vitreous is involved. In some cases after recurrences, the eye becomes more seriously involved and hypopyon is usually found (Fig. 1.382). Procrastination in the management of phacoanaphylactic endophthalmitis usually leads to loss of vision and even enucleation. The only effective treatment is removal of all lens remnants. In cases with an intact posterior capsule, the entire capsule must be removed. Lens remnants in the vitreous should be removed by vitrectomy. If a posterior chamber lens is present, it must be removed with the posterior capsule. Viscoelastic material and alpha-chymotrypsin are useful adjuncts to the surgery. If the diagnosis is correct, recovery is dramatic.

An important lesson is learned in the case shown in Fig. 1.383. An extracapsular cataract extraction with implantation of a posterior chamber lens was performed. The white material represents an inflammatory infiltrate. Six months postoperatively and 1 week before explanation of the lens implant, mutton fat KP are seen (Fig. 1.384). Eighteen months later, the eye is shown in Fig. 1.385. An organized

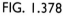
Postoperative Lens-Induced Aseptic Endophthalmitis

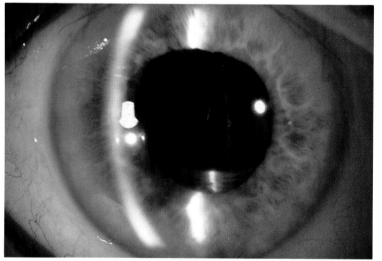

FIG. 1.378

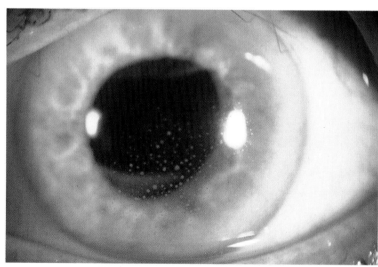

FIG. 1.379

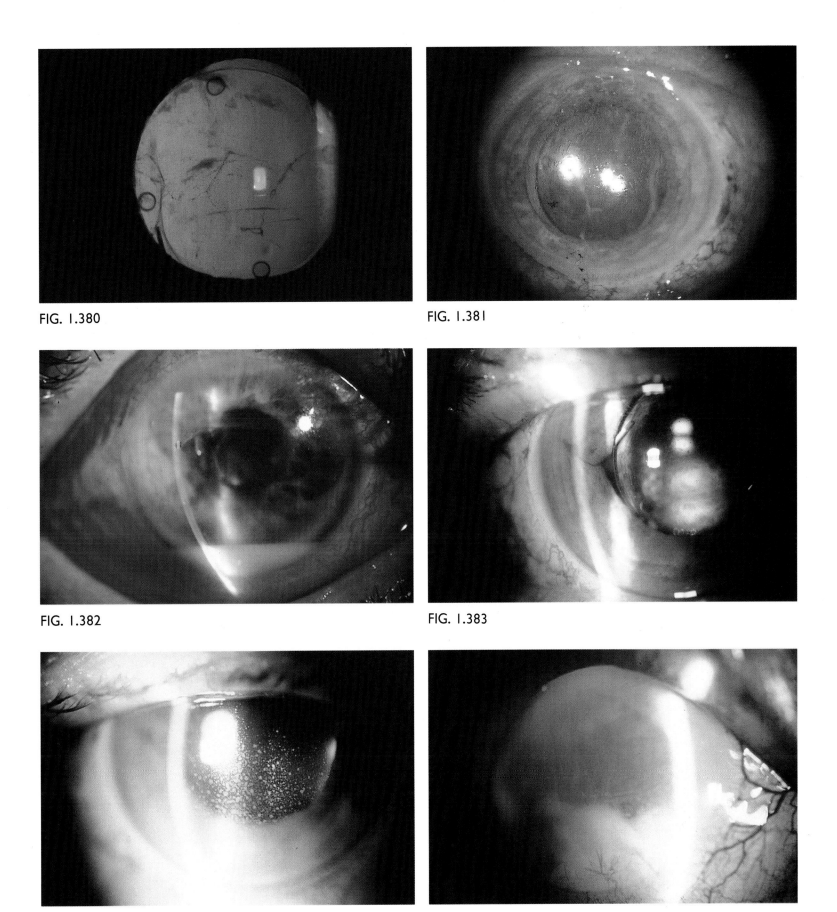

FIG. 1.380

FIG. 1.381

FIG. 1.382

FIG. 1.383

FIG. 1.384

FIG. 1.385

hypopyon is seen and the cornea is cloudy. One week later the eye was enucleated. The globe is shown in Fig. 1.386. Note the organized inflammatory infiltrate occupying the position formerly held by the crystalline lens. Note the organized pericyclitic membrane and the organized hypopyon. The posterior segment of the globe is relatively free of inflammation, in contrast to what one would see in sympathetic ophthalmitis. This case underscores the fact that procrastination is an incorrect course. Following explantation of the implant, if there is no improvement in the clinical picture, one must rid the eye of all residual lens material. Figure 1.387 shows another case of phacoanaphylactic endophthalmitis in which a large piece of lens nucleus was left in the eye. A total iris bombé resulted.

The histologic picture of phacoanaphylactic endophthalmitis is quite specific. Figure 1.388 shows a section from a globe mistakenly enucleated because of an erroneous diagnosis of sympathetic ophthalmitis. The iris is seen at the left. An overwhelming inflammatory response is seen surrounding lens material. In the zone immediately surrounding residual lens material, the cells consist of polymorphonuclear leukocytes (Fig. 1.389). More peripherally, the cells are of a chronic inflammatory nature: lymphocytes, epithelioid cells, and plasma cells (Fig. 1.390). The amorphous pink bodies in Fig. 1.391 are Russell bodies, which represent the end stage of plasma cell degeneration.

IOL-Induced

Most cases of this nature, such as residual polishing agents left on the implant and other instances of "hot lots," have been eliminated by greatly improved quality control. However, the problem of complement activation by components of the intraocular lens remains. Complement proteins consist of a large group of proteins found in serun in an inactive state. These proteins cross the blood–aqueous barrier during intraocular surgery. It has been shown that nylon and polypropylene, both haptic polymers, are capable of causing complement activation. It appears that inflammatory mediators that agglutinate on the surface of the PMMA optic are also capable of complement activation.

The following case illustrates this problem. A 68-year-old female had an uneventful extracapsular cataract extraction on 9/25/80. Corrected vision was 20/20. Four months later the eye became painful and red and a diagnosis of iritis was made. During the next 3 months there were several recurrences, each one responding less effectively to steroids. The vitreous became involved and vision was reduced to 20/60 on 4/16/81. Hypopyon was noted on 12/16/81. This cleared rapidly with steroid therapy but there were two recurrences of hypopyon. On 3/12/82, 18 months postoperatively, vision was reduced to counting fingers at two feet. The implant was removed without loss of vitreous. Some of the lens material adherent to the implant was removed

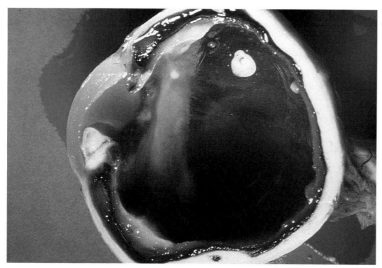

FIG. 1.386

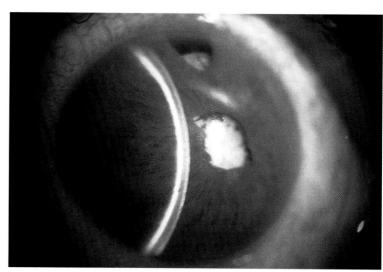

FIG. 1.387

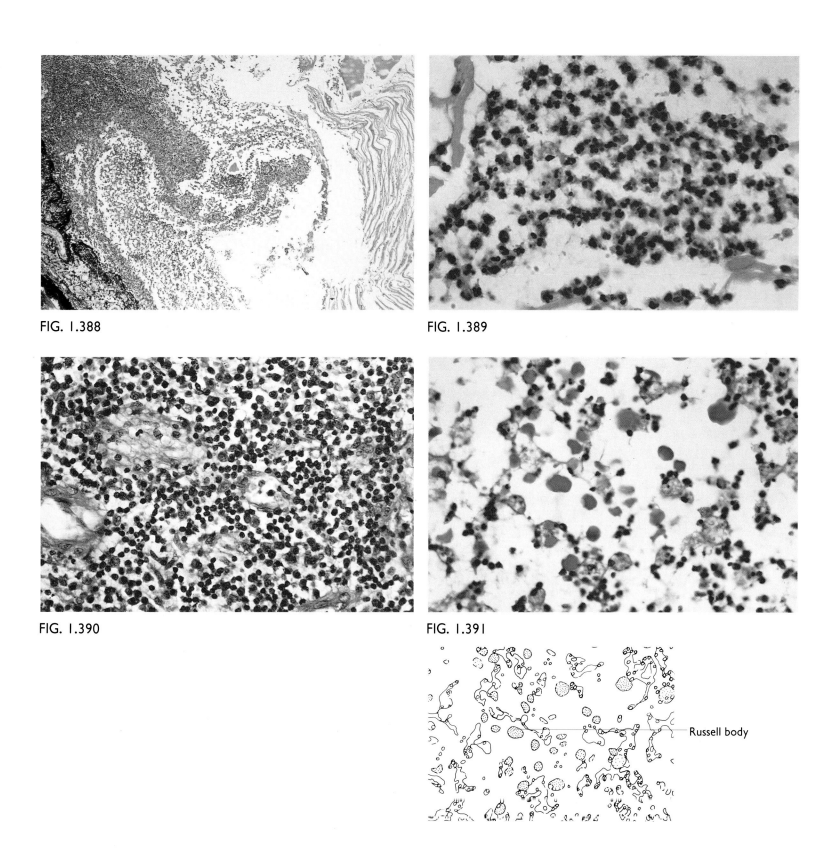

FIG. 1.388

FIG. 1.389

FIG. 1.390

FIG. 1.391

Russell body

along with the implant. However, considerable lens material, along with the posterior capsule, was left inside the eye. The surface of the optic was covered with inflammatory exudate and the polypropylene loops were bent out of shape and showed focal areas of deterioration (Fig. 1.392). The superior part of the iris sphincter was damaged during explantation, resulting in an eccentric pupil (Fig. 1.393). The eye quickly recovered during the first postoperative days and there has not been a single recurrence of inflammation through January 1987, more than 6 years after the original cataract surgery. Vision with contact lens correction was 20/25. An important decision was required when the cataract in the second eye progressed. Because the author was convinced that the problem in the first eye was related to the lens implant and not to residual lens material, a phacoemulsification with implantation of an all-PMMA lens was performed on 12/1/83. There has been no intraocular inflammation in the second eye to the present. The eye is shown in Fig. 1.394. The implant is seen by retroillumination in Fig. 1.395. Vision is 20/20.

SEPTIC ENDOPHTHALMITIS

The signs and symptoms of microbial endophthalmitis vary, probably according to the virulence of the organism. The surgeon should have a high level of suspicion in any case of sudden onset of inflammation. An important symptom is toxic visual loss, i.e., a severe decrease in vision out of all proportion to other signs. An important sign is involvement of the vitreous. Pain, chemosis, and ptosis of the upper eyelid are present in many cases but one cannot depend on their presence in making the diagnosis. The most important lesson is to diagnose early and treat early.

An early acute inflammation (within 48 hours of surgery) is usually due to a highly virulent organism, e.g., *Staphylococcus aureus, Streptococcus* species, Enterobacteriaceae *(Enterobacter, Klebsiella, Proteus, Serratia)*. *Staphylococcus epidermidis* may also cause an early acute infection but the inflammation is less severe, although a more serious inflammation may occur (Fig. 1.396). The onset of signs and symptoms of infection may be modified by prophylactic antibiotic and steroid therapy. A delayed subacute or chronic inflammation is usually due to an organism of relatively low virulence, e.g., *S. epidermidis, Propionibacterium acnes, Nocardia, Mycobacterium,* yeasts, and filamentous fungi. In cases with mild onset, a few hours of a topical steroid (every 30 minutes) and a cycloplegic may be justified. The eye should be reevaluated after four to six hours. If there is any question, there should be no further delay in obtaining material for smear and culture from the aqueous

and the vitreous. Anaerobic and fungal cultures must be included. At the same time, intraocular therapy should be administered. The preferred intravitreal antibiotics initially are cefazolin 2.5 mg or vancomycin 1.0 mg and gentamicin 0.1 mg. This covers the most likely causes of bacterial infection. Intravitreal dexamethasone 0.4 mg may also be administered. While awaiting the results of culture and sensitivity, topical, periocular, and systemic therapy should begin. In severe cases with marked vitreous involvement, a pars plana vitrectomy is justified. B-scan ultrasonography is useful in cases where visibility is poor due to corneal stromal edema and fibrinous exudate in the anterior chamber. If there is an intraocular lens present, it usually does not require removal unless it interferes with visibility for vitrectomy or if a fungal etiology is established.

A new dilemma confronts the surgeon in presumed microbial endophthalmitis and its differential diagnosis. A sharp increase in the number of cases of *Propionibacterium acnes* endophthalmitis is being reported. The onset is typically delayed due to sequestration of the organism within the lens capsule, the residual cortex, or host inflammatory cells. This is an anaerobic organism. I have a suspicion that some cases of presumed phacoanaphylactic endophthalmitis that improve dramatically with removal of the posterior chamber lens and posterior capsule may be infected with *Propionibacterium acnes.* The following case illustrates this.

A 66-year-old male underwent a left phacoemulsification with implantation of an all-PMMA posterior chamber lens on 7/31/84. There have been no postoperative complications and vision has been 20/20. On 8/8/85 the same procedure was performed on the right eye. The postoperative course was uneventful until 10/21/85 when there was a sudden onset of pain and photophobia. The symptoms abated with the use of topical steroid therapy. On 12/3/85 a diagnosis of iritis was made but vision was 20/20. Topical steroid therapy was again given and the response was excellent. On 12/31/85 there were no cells visible in the anterior chamber. On 1/10/86, 5 months postoperatively, the patient presented with a red, painful eye and hypopyon (Fig. 1.397). Anterior chamber and vitreous samples were taken and intraocular antibiotics were given: cefazolin 2.5 mg and gentamicin 0.1 mg. Cultures were negative. The condition improved over the next few months but topical steroids were required to control the inflammation. The patient's vision decreased to 20/200 on 5/19/86. A presumptive diagnosis of phacoanaphylactic endophthalmitis was made. Discrete white lesions were noted on the posterior capsule and these were enlarging. The posterior chamber lens and the posterior capsule were removed without loss of vitreous on 6/12/86, ten months after the original

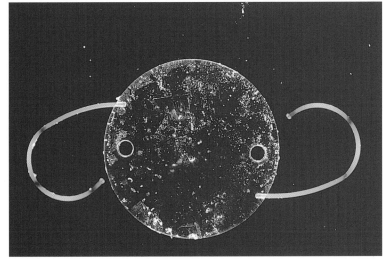

FIG. 1.392

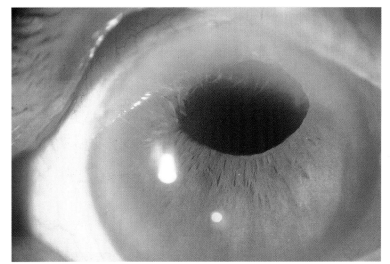

FIG. 1.393

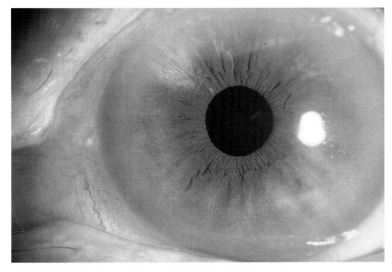

FIG. 1.394

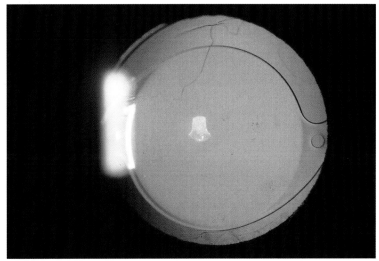

FIG. 1.395

Postoperative Septic Endophthalmitis

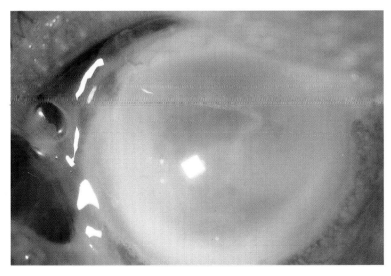

FIG. 1.396

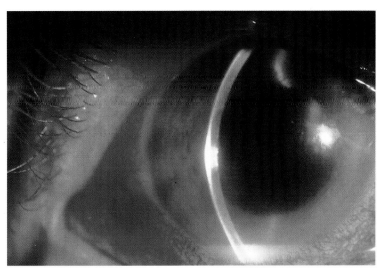

FIG. 1.397

surgery. A Kelman Multiflex anterior chamber lens was implanted at the same time (Fig. 1.398). Intraocular antibiotics were not used but periocular cefazolin 100 mg and gentamicin 20 mg were given at the conclusion of the surgery. The capsule specimen was submitted for histologic examination and cultures, including an anaerobic culture. *Propionibacterium acnes* grew in the anaerobic medium. The capsule specimen and inflammatory cells are shown in Fig. 1.399. There have been no recurrences of iritis although cystoid macular edema has persisted. Vision has varied during subsequent examinations between 20/25 and 20/40. Figure 1.400 shows the capsule specimen removed in a similar case. Inflammatory cells are shown sequestered inside the capsule. *Propionibacterium acnes* was cultured anaerobically.

As stated above, one wonders how many cases of presumed phacoanaphylactic endophthalmitis that improve after removal of the lens capsule are really cases of *P. acnes* endophthalmitis. The possibility also exists that the organism may be an adjunct in a phacoanaphylactic reaction. Ophthalmologists should be alerted to this since the organism is found in nearly 50% of normal eyes.

EPITHELIAL INVASION OF THE ANTERIOR CHAMBER

The invasion of the anterior chamber by epithelium after cataract surgery has been recognized since the 19th century, but its diagnosis and management still confront ophthalmic surgeons with a severe challenge. Fortunately, with improvements in surgical techniques, it occurs less frequently.

A classification of epithelial growths within the anterior chamber was provided 50 years ago by Perera:

1. Pearl tumors of the iris
2. Posttraumatic cysts of the iris
3. Epithelialization of the anterior chamber

PEARL TUMORS

Iris epithelial pearl tumors are almost exclusively discovered after accidental trauma, and usually result from the implantation of a hair follicle or piece of skin into the anterior chamber coincident with a perforating injury. These growths usually remain small and are confined to the iris. They appear as solid pearly tumors or opaque white cysts on the surface of the iris and are not connected with the wound of entry into the anterior chamber (Fig. 1.401). They usually grow slowly, rarely exceed 2 to 3 mm in diameter, and are fairly firm in consistency, encapsulated, and consist of layers of stratified or cuboidal epithelium, sometimes closely resembling that of the cornea or conjunctiva.

EPITHELIAL CYSTS

These are caused by invasion of the anterior chamber by a double continuous layer of epithelium that forms a closed cyst. Although they are usually in contact with the wound of entry or the cataract incision, this continuity may be broken by the interposition of scar tissue. The pathogenesis of these cysts appears to be related primarily to faulty wound closure. There is often a history of delayed formation of the anterior chamber associated with defective wound closure. Iris, lens debris, vitreous, and particulate matter may become lodged in the wound.

Epithelial cysts appear as translucent or grayish cysts connected with the area of penetration into the anterior chamber (Figs. 1.402 and 1.403). The cysts may remain dormant for many years and cause no disturbance. Shown in Fig.

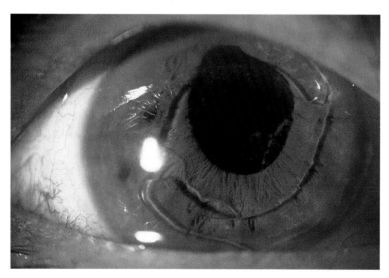

FIG. 1.398

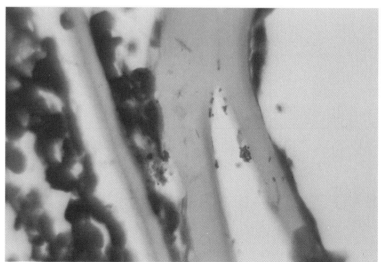

FIG. 1.399

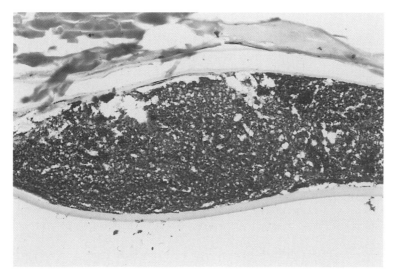

FIG. 1.400

Epithelial Invasion of the Anterior Chamber: Pearl Tumors

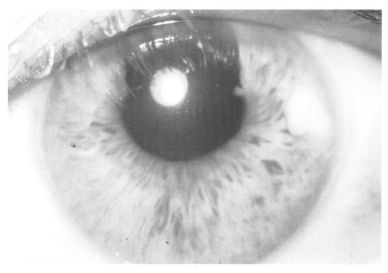

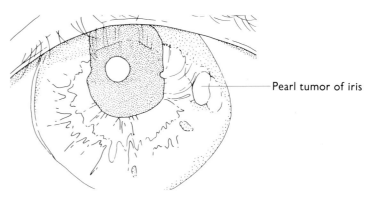

Pearl tumor of iris

FIG: 1.401

Epithelial Invasion of the Anterior Chamber: Epithelial Cysts

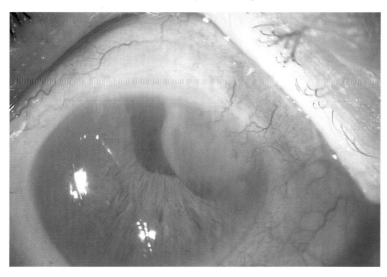

FIG. 1.402

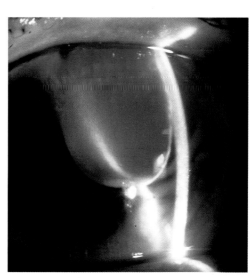

FIG. 1.403

1.404 is an epithelial cyst that caused no loss of vision 5 years later (Fig. 1.405). The only significant change was ectropion uvea. The pupil is dilated with a mydriatic in Fig. 1.404. The pupil was not dilated in Fig. 1.405. On the other hand, these cysts may become huge, occupying almost the entire anterior chamber. Figure 1.406 shows a multiloculated epithelial cyst filling the entire anterior chamber. Band keratopathy is present. Secondary glaucoma and iridocyclitis usually are present when growth of the cyst is active. A thin-walled epithelial cyst is shown histologically in Fig. 1.407. The epithelial cyst is usually more multilay- ered where it is in contact with uveal tissue than where it is in contact with the cornea. This is shown in Fig. 1.408. Note that continuity of the cyst with the wound is broken. A multiloculated cyst is shown in Fig. 1.409 (trichrome stain). The posterior wall of the cyst is often partially pigmented, especially where the cyst is in contact with the iris. The cyst may enter the posterior chamber through an iridotomy or even by eroding through the iris. Figure 1.410 shows such an erosion. With the pupil dilated, it has the appearance of a pigmented lesion and may be mistaken for a melanoma (Fig. 1.411). This eye was enucleated and Fig.

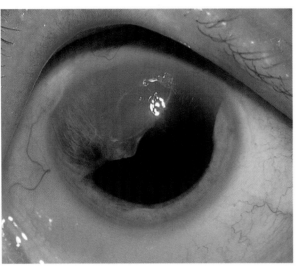

FIG. 1.404

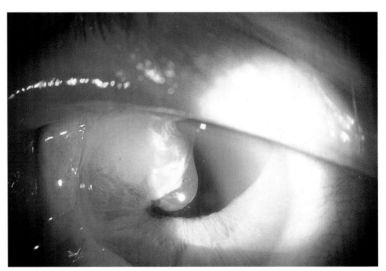

FIG. 1.405

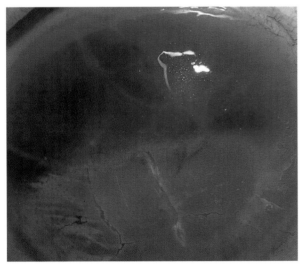

FIG. 1.406

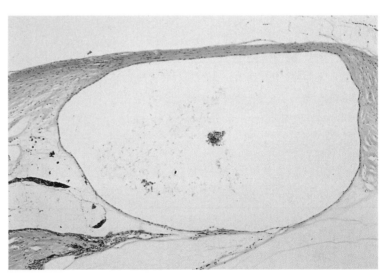

FIG. 1.407

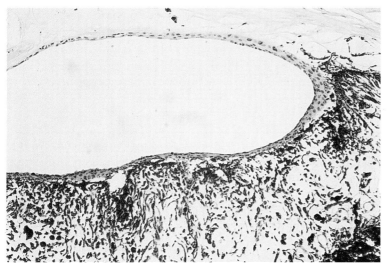

FIG. 1.408

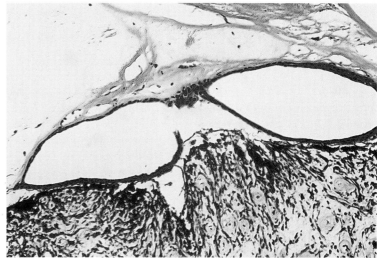

FIG. 1.409

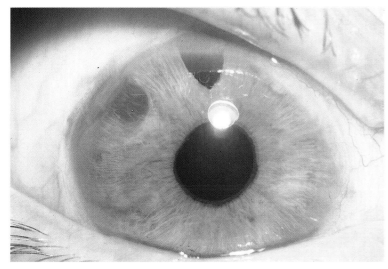

FIG. 1.410

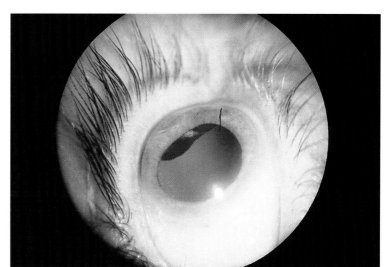

FIG. 1.411

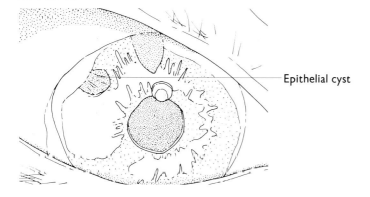

Epithelial cyst

1.412 shows the lesion. The erosion through the iris is plainly visible. An enlarged view of the cyst is seen in Fig. 1.413.

Many methods have been reported for the treatment of epithelial cysts but most recent reports involve cryosurgery. Ferry and Naghdi employed a cryosurgical technique to treat an epithelial cyst that filled one-third of the anterior chamber. The posterior wall was adherent to iris stroma. The cyst was perforated with a fine needle. The needle was removed and a cryostylet was placed within the sac. A temperature of 0° to −10° F was applied for 15 seconds. The sac of the cyst and the adherent iris were then exteriorized and excised. A safer modification of this method consists of aspiration of cyst contents (Fig. 1.414). The anterior vitre-ous is excised using a small-diameter vitrectomy probe to provide a larger fluid-filled space for introduction of a large air bubble (Fig. 1.415). The air bubble compresses the cyst remnants against the inner wall of the eye and provides thermal insulation for a translimbal cryothermy (inset).

EPITHELIAL DOWNGROWTH

This is a far more serious complication than an epithelial cyst. As with epithelial cysts, the cause is faulty wound closure. The main prerequisite is a cut proliferating edge of epithelium in contact with a fistula into the anterior chamber. The wound must remain open for some time, and there must be some contact between the wound and adjacent

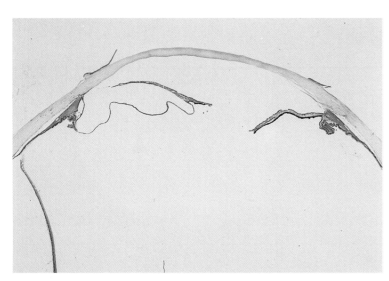

FIG. 1.412

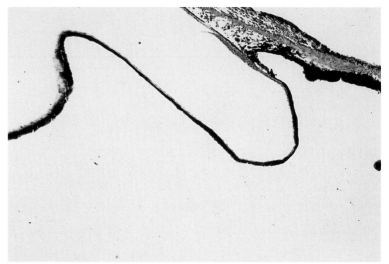

FIG. 1.413

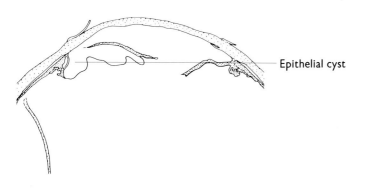

Epithelial cyst

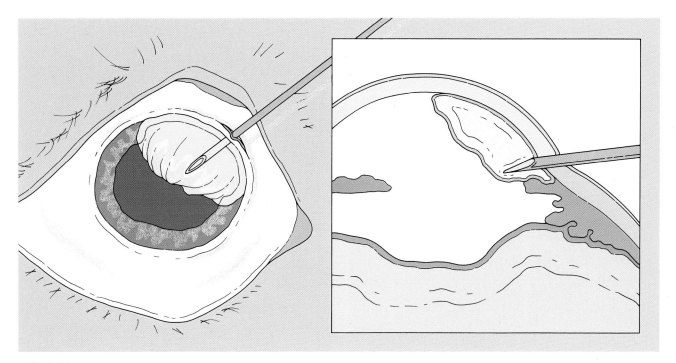

FIG. 1.414

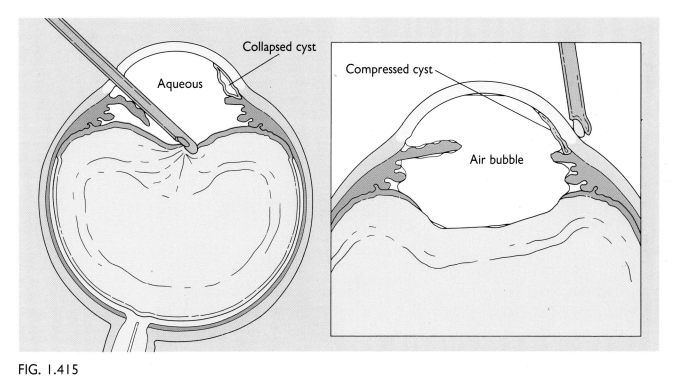

FIG. 1.415

uveal tissue. Figure 1.416 shows a histologic section of defective wound closure during cataract surgery. The section was taken just astride a fistula. Note the downgrowth of epithelium in a more magnified view (Fig. 1.417).

The epithelium grows over the back of the cornea as a sheet. The advancing edge is marked by a gray line (Figs. 1.418 and 1.419). Note the filtering bleb at 11:30 o'clock in Fig. 1.420. A faint gray line is present. Figure 1.421 shows an eye with a positive Seidel's sign and highlighting of the gray line by the fluorescein dye. The reason for the gray line is a heaping up of epithelium at the advancing margin of the epithelial sheet (Fig. 1.422). Epithelium lines

Epithelial Invasion of the Anterior Chamber: Epithelial Downgrowth

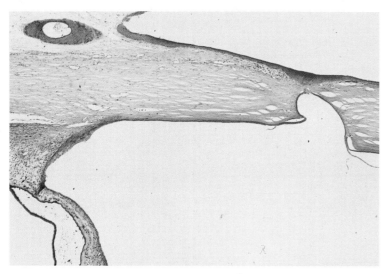

FIG. 1.416

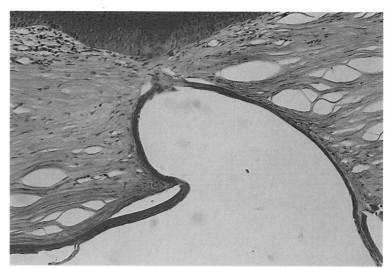

FIG. 1.417

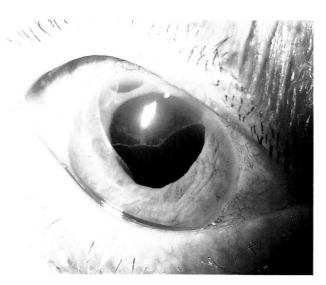

FIG. 1.418

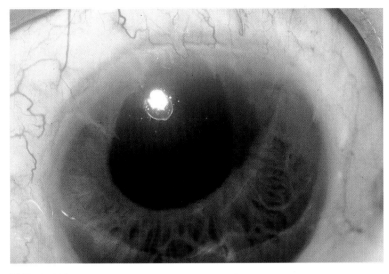

FIG. 1.419

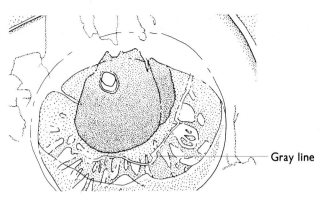

Gray line

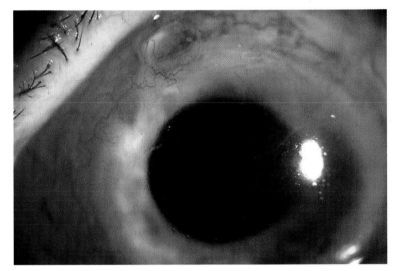

FIG. 1.420

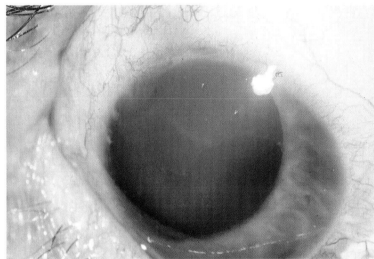

FIG. 1.421

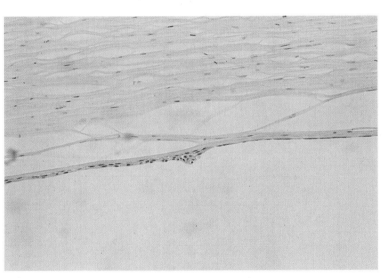

FIG. 1.422

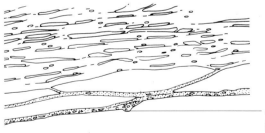

Advancing edge of
gray line

the back of the cornea to the left of the gray line and endothelium is seen to the right of the gray line. The epithelium lines the angle of the anterior chamber and the anterior surface of the iris (Fig. 1.423). It also covers the face of the vitreous after an intracapsular cataract extraction (Fig. 1.424). The epithelial membrane over the vitreous is usually one or two layers thick (Fig. 1.425), as it is over the back of the cornea. However, the membrane is many layers thick where it covers the more vascularized uveal tissue. This is clearly shown with a trichrome stain in Fig. 1.426. The illustration shows the red epithelial cells covering the back of the cornea, the anterior chamber angle, and the vitreous.

FIBROUS INGROWTH

Fibrous outgrowth is often confused with epithelial downgrowth, occurs at least as frequently, and is usually diagnosed by the pathologist. It is characterized by an ingrowth of connective tissue elements into the anterior chamber and aided and abetted by poor wound healing and incarceration of tissue such as vitreous, iris, or lens remnants into the surgical incision. It has also been referred to as stromal overgrowth, fibroblastic ingrowth, fibrocytic ingrowth, and fibrous metaplasia.

The source of the fibroblasts responsible for fibrous ingrowth is controversial. The most likely sources are the following:

1. Subepithelial connective tissue
2. Corneal or limbal stroma
3. Metaplastic endothelium

Normally, bridging of the inner wound by endothelium seems to confine fibroplasia to the stromal defect, even when its inner edge gapes. A defect in the endothelium predisposes to a fibroblastic retrocorneal membrane that may be difficult to differentiate from epithelial downgrowth. The extent of fibroplasia is variable. As in epithelial invasion, the structures of the anterior segment, such as the iris, angle, and vitreous face, may become involved.

Many consider the fibrous ingrowth to arise from the stromal keratocytes, which convert to fibroblasts. If such is the case, the stroma itself would be the source of the fibroplasia of the anterior segment of the eye. It is extremely difficult to determine the source by histologic examination. Most specimens make it appear as if the fibrous tissue in the anterior chamber is continuous with the corneal stroma on both sides of the wound. However, one can also implicate the subepithelial connective tissue in these same histologic specimens.

The third possibility involves fibrous metaplasia. In some cases, regeneration of incised or injured corneal endothelium is not normal but is characterized by an excessive amount of Descemet's membrane production. This is accomplished by conversion of endothelial cells into a fibroblast-like cell that produces fibrous tissue in addition to basement membrane.

Fibrous ingrowth may assume many of the characteristics of epithelial downgrowth. The connective tissue invasion may clothe the back of the cornea. Figure 1.427 shows an exuberant fibrous ingrowth from a cataract incision that extends over the back of the cornea. It may cover the chamber angle. Figure 1.428 shows a fibrous ingrowth from a cataract incision filling the anterior chamber and extending into the chamber angle in an eye that suffered an iris pro-

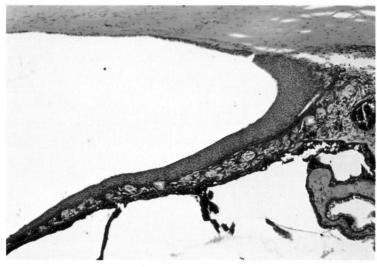

FIG. 1.423

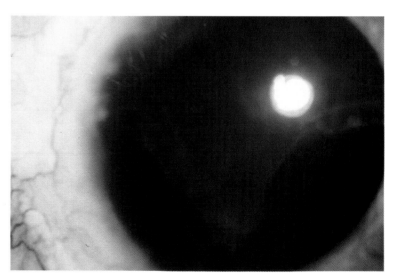

FIG. 1.424

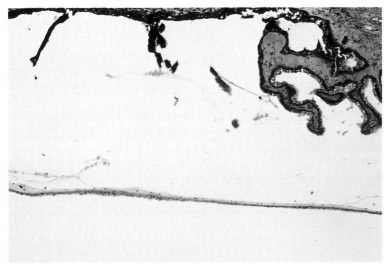

FIG. 1.425

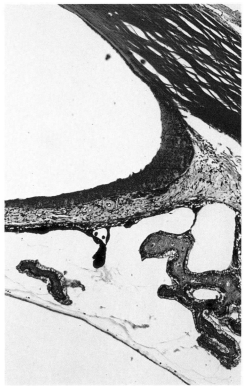

FIG. 1.426

Fibrous Ingrowth

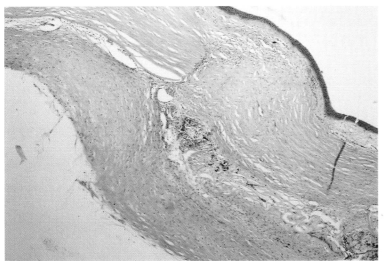

FIG. 1.427

FIG. 1.428

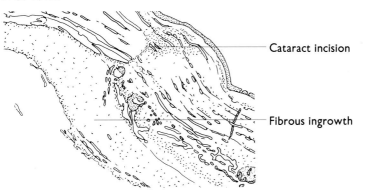

Cataract incision

Fibrous ingrowth

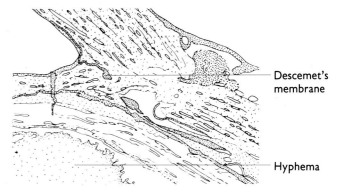

Descemet's membrane

Hyphema

lapse after cataract surgery. The prolapse was treated by cryothermy. An extensive hyphema is also seen. It may cover the surface of the iris. Figure 1.429 shows a fibrous ingrowth extending from a cataract incision onto the anterior surface of the iris. Figure 1.430 shows fibrous tissue growing over the anterior and posterior surfaces of the iris after cataract extraction. Artifactitious separation of the pigment epithelium of the iris has occurred. It may cover the anterior surface of the vitreous and may even extend so far as to adhere to the retina.

The pathogenesis of fibrous ingrowth includes the following:

1. Malapproximation of the wound edges characterized by posterior gaping or overriding of the wound may cause persistent irritation and slow recovery. In some patients, this alone is sufficient stimulus for an exuberant, reparative overgrowth. The greater the extent of the wound gape facing the anterior chamber, the greater the likelihood of fibrous ingrowth in the favorable milieu provided with the eye.

2. Incarceration of vitreous, iris (Fig. 1.428), or lens matter in the wound increases the possibility of fibrous ingrowth. Figure 1.431 shows an exuberant fibrous ingrowth extending down from the corneal wound. Many of these cases involve a history of operative loss of vitreous. The inevitable protuberance of vitreous strands between the lips of the wound or, at the least, lining the posterior portion of the wound provides a framework for downward growth of fibrous tissue elements. This fibroplastic response results in many of the unfavorable sequelae after loss of formed vitreous during cataract surgery.

3. Intraocular inflammation, if prolonged and of low intensity, may cause an excessive reparative response. Excessive repair can seriously disable the eye because the limitations of space in the eye do not permit an overabundance of any tissue without interfering with ocular physiology.

4. Excessive bleeding into the anterior chamber may occasionally cause a fibroplastic response in the anterior chamber. It remains questionable whether this bleeding encourages a fibrous ingrowth.

Although the pathogenesis and clinical features of fibrous and epithelial downgrowth have some similarities, the former tends to be self-limiting in many cases, and the appearance of the membrane is different. In epithelial downgrowth the membrane on the back of the cornea shows a well-defined border, but the advancing edge of the fibrous membrane appears frayed, with irregular tonguelike strands running ahead (Fig. 1.432). Detachment of Descemet's membrane, glaucoma, bullous keratopathy, retinal detachment, and phthisis bulbi are associated with fibrous ingrowth. Figure 1.433 shows a massive fibrous ingrowth in an eye with phthisis bulbi. Fibrous tissue is seen surrounding the iris. There is no known treatment for fibrous ingrowth, although its sequelae (glaucoma, bullous keratopathy, and retinal detachment) may be treatable.

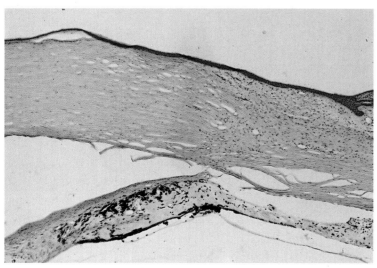

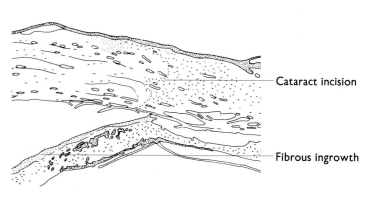

Cataract incision

Fibrous ingrowth

FIG. 1.429

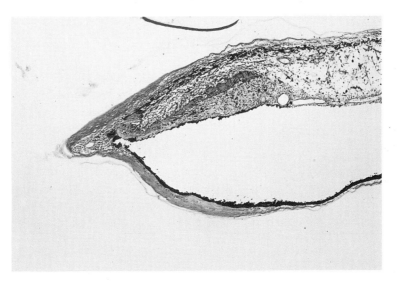

FIG. 1.430

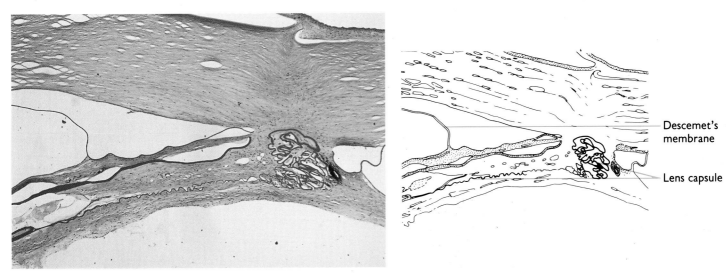

FIG. 1.431

Descemet's membrane

Lens capsule

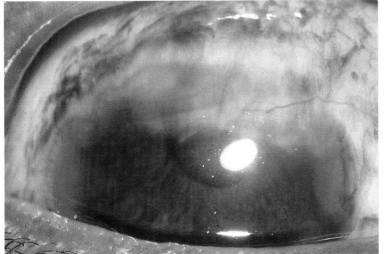

FIG. 1.432

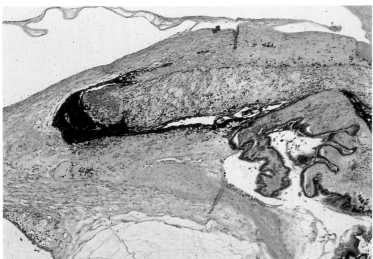

FIG. 1.433

CORNEAL ENDOTHELIAL PROLIFERATION

When Descemet's membrane and corneal endothelium are incised or injured, repair occurs rapidly, but not as rapidly as for epithelium. Due to its elasticity, Descemet's membrane retracts and curls into a spiral directed forward, exposing an area of posterior stroma. There is a migration of neighboring endothelial cells increasing in size up to twice their diameter. Descemet's membrane is eventually secreted by the endothelium in uncomplicated cases. This is a slow process. A new Descemet's membrane does not appear for several weeks and does not reach its peak for several months. The membrane may never reach its original thickness.

In addition to this process of repair, it is known that corneal endothelium has a tendency to cover free surfaces and to surround and enclose anything in contact with it. This includes foreign bodies, calcified lens remnants, and rolled up portions of Descemet's membrane. It may grow along vitreous strands and zonular fibers, in which case it forms tubular structures known as Descemet's tubes. As the endothelium grows along these structures, it secretes a new Descemet's membrane. For some as yet unexplained reason, the endothelium peripheral to Schwalbe's line also proliferates, but fortunately does not elaborate a glass membrane.

Glass membranes on the anterior surface of the iris do not result in tubular structures, but instead form sheet-like membranes. This more closely resembles the anterior chamber invasions associated with epithelial downgrowth and fibrous ingrowth. This usually occurs only after the peripheral cornea has come in contact with iris or scar tissue overlying the iris. Anterior adhesions of iris to the peripheral cornea form a "false angle" over which endothelial cells grow readily. These are usually eyes with very extensive pathological changes such as advanced glaucoma and long-standing chronic iridocyclitis.

DESCEMET'S TUBES

These are usually seen in children after the obsolete needling procedures. They are also seen after injuries, shelving corneal incisions, and improper cyclodialysis. The incision or wound must be central to Schwalbe's line. The tube may enclose vitreous, zonular fibers, fibrin strands, and particulate matter. They usually develop some years after the original surgery or injury. Endothelium grows down for some time and stops, leaving a tube reaching only partway down. The tube consists of the enclosed material, the newly secreted Descemet's membrane, and endothelium.

Figure 1.434 shows the eye of an elderly man who had cataract surgery at age 14 years. Note a typical Descemet's tube that is pigmented and casts a shadow on the iris. Note a flaring out of vitreous below the tube. Figure 1.435 shows the opposite eye of the same patient. A Descemet's tube is seen extending partway down an enclosed vitreous strand. Figure 1.436 shows another Descemet's tube in the eye of a patient who had surgery for a congenital cataract at age 4 years. The tube encloses a vitreous strand and reaches only partway down the strand. Figure 1.437 shows a Descemet's tube in the eye of an elderly man who had multiple needlings for congenital cataracts about 60 years previously. A dense tube-like structure extends about two-thirds of the way to the pupil and is attached to the cornea at the old scar. Vitreous can be seen extending from the posterior end of the tube into the pupil. The original photograph is on the left and a retouched photograph is on the right. Figure 1.438 shows a histologic section of a vitreous tube. It consists of the enclosed material, Descemet's membrane, and endothelium. Figure 1.439 shows the anterior segment of an eye that suffered a perforating injury. A stump of iris is adherent to the area of perforation. Endothelial proliferation and newly formed Descemet's membrane are shown on zonular fibers. Figure 1.440 shows a high-power view of tubes, showing a core of zonular fibers, newly formed Descemet's membrane, and proliferated endothelium on its surface.

Corneal Endothelial Proliferation: Descemet's Tubes

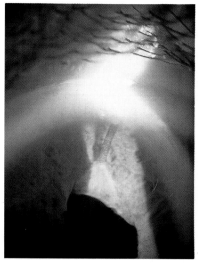 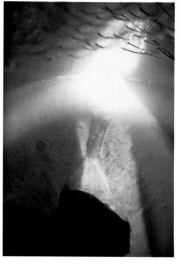 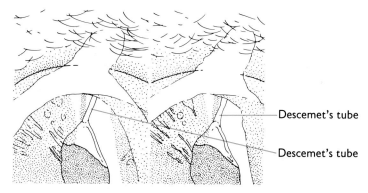

Descemet's tube

Descemet's tube

FIG. 1.434

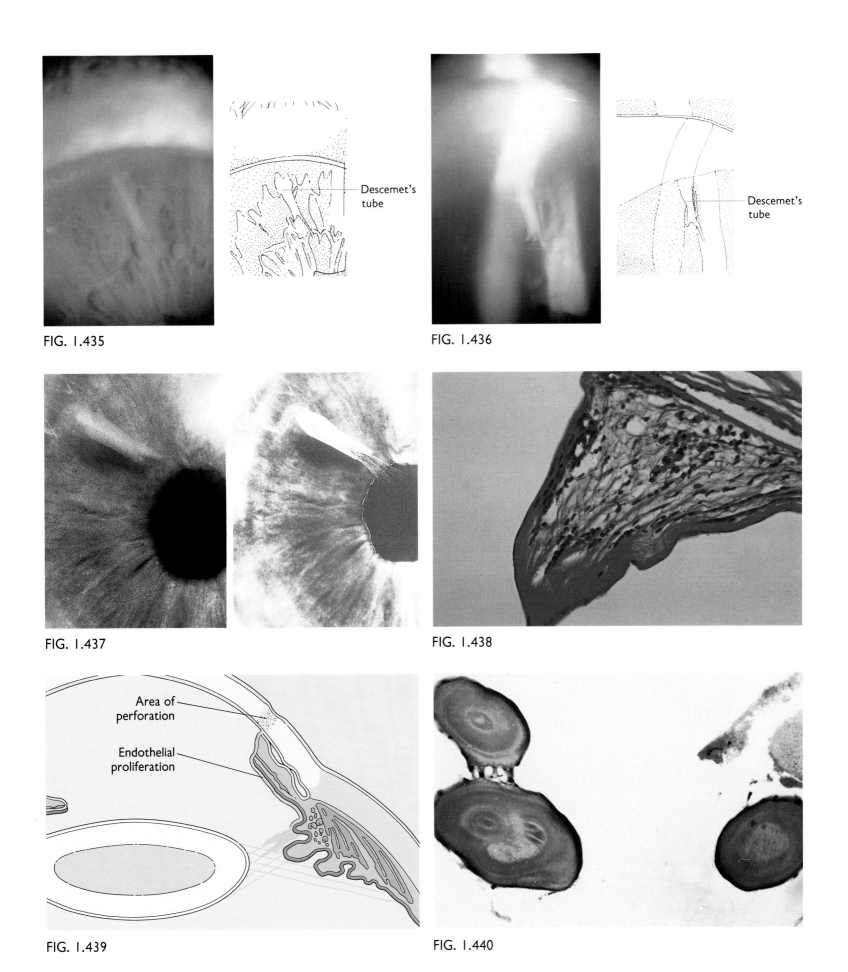

FIG. 1.435

FIG. 1.436

Descemet's tube

Descemet's tube

FIG. 1.437

FIG. 1.438

FIG. 1.439

Area of perforation

Endothelial proliferation

FIG. 1.440

ANTERIOR CHAMBER DEPTH ABNORMALITIES

The most important clinical situations associated with abnormalities of anterior chamber depth are hypotension, choroidal detachment, and aphakic pupillary block.

HYPOTENSION

Although ocular hypotension causes less concern than hypertension because it is less severe and generally carries a more favorable prognosis, its recognition and treatment may prevent an unhappy ending to an otherwise successful cataract extraction.

Causes of ocular hypotension are numerous, but, in general, prolonged changes in the intraocular pressure may be produced by changes in the resistance to the outflow of aqueous and changes in the rate of formation of aqueous.

Most cases of a shallow anterior chamber in the early postoperative period are due to a leaky wound. However, if aqueous secretion equals aqueous drainage, the anterior chamber may be of normal depth. However, there is usually a net aqueous loss and the chamber may be shallow or absent. A wound is swabbed with fluorescein solution. Using the cobalt filter at the slit lamp, aqueous drainage is demonstrated as seen in Fig. 1.441. After a few minutes, aqueous may be detected in the anterior chamber (Fig. 1.442). Persistent postoperative hypotension may be due to hyposecretion of aqueous caused by a detachment of the ciliary body and choroid. In some cases the ciliary body is detached up to but not including the scleral spur. In others the scleral spur may also be detached and a cyclodialysis cleft is present. A distinction between the two may be made by performing the test illustrated in Fig. 1.443. If a cleft is present, injection of a dilute solution of fluorescein into the anterior chamber will flow into the supraciliary space. A supraciliary incision made well away from the cleft will show leakage of the dye. When a cleft is not present (inset), dye will not be recovered from the supraciliary space but an undyed fluid may be present.

The patient with ocular hypotension may have no unusual symptoms, and the eye may retain its function indefinitely. However, in most cases, signs of irritation and ciliary congestion associated with an irritative iridocyclitis may become evident. The eye may become intermittently painful. In extreme cases phthisis bulbi may result. The patient's vision may become blurred. This was usually attributed to macular edema but it is now known that some patients develop loss of central vision as a result of marked irregular folding of the choroid and pigment epithelium.

The following case is a classic example of postoperative hypotension attributed to aqueous hyposecretion. Figure 1.444 shows the eye of a 71-year-old patient who underwent an uneventful intracapsular cataract extraction with sector iridectomy in 1969. During annual examinations, visual acuity was correctible to 20/20 and intraocular pressures were normal. In 1977, visual acuity decreased to 20/70 and applanation pressure was 2 mm. Note the loose strand of pigment over the iris at 1 o'clock. A detachment of the ciliary body was detected by gonioscopy (Fig. 1.445).

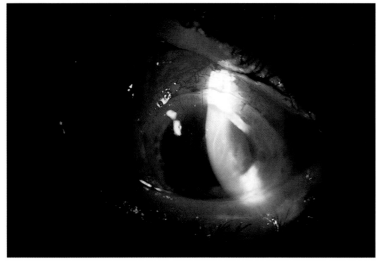

FIG. 1.441

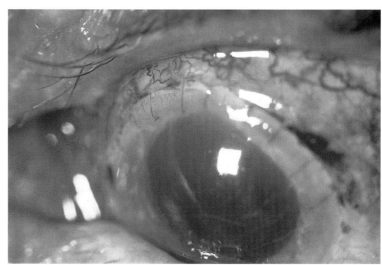

FIG. 1.442

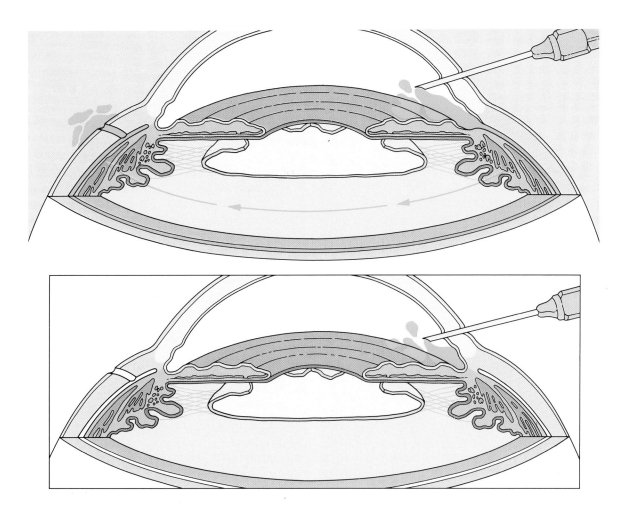

FIG. 1.443

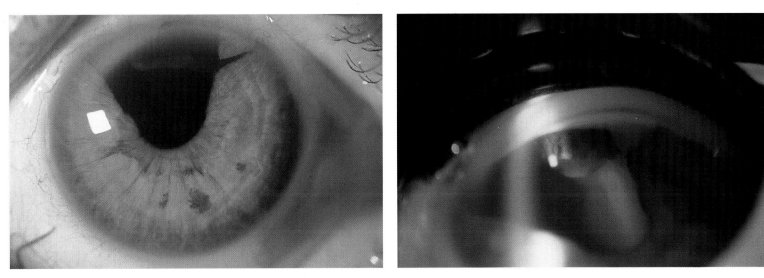

FIG. 1.444

FIG. 1.445

In addition, two well-defined cyclodialysis clefts were found. These are demonstrated in Fig. 1.446. Fundus examination of the patient revealed the characteristic choroidal folds consisting of alternating yellow and dark streaks (Fig. 1.447). The elevated portions of crests of the folds appear yellow, in contrast to the darker appearance of the troughs, or depressions of these layers. These folds are dramatically seen in this patient with fluorescein angiography. Hyperfluorescent lines corresponding to the yellow lines observed in the fundus are plainly visible. They are the result of the relative thinning of the pigment epithelium on the crest, the greater thickness of the pool of choroidal dye beneath the crest, and the shorter course of the incident blue and reflected yellow-green light through the pigment epithelium on the crest. The troughs of the folds appear relatively hypofluorescent (Fig. 1.448). Choroidal folds are shown in another case of hyposecretion hypotension in Fig. 1.449. The characteristic angiography pattern is shown in Fig. 1.450. These folds are also seen in other ocular conditions, the most common being extreme hypermetropia. Such an eye is shown in Figure 1.451. The axial length was 19.1 mm. Papilledema may be present in some cases. This is seen in Fig. 1.452.

The treatment of ocular hypotension depends on the cause. If an external fistula is present, it might be closed by applying a pressure dressing over the operated eye. It may be advisable in a resistant case to occlude the opposite eye to eliminate the blink reflex. If this fails, the wound leak should be identified in the operating room and the wound should be sutured.

The treatment of hyposecretion is usually more complex. Unless danger signs such as choroidal folds at the macula and decreased vision appear, it is best to simply observe the eye and not treat it. If one is compelled to intervene, the following approach is useful. A search for a cyclodialysis cleft is made by the use of a gonioscopic lens. This is best done with the pupil constricted. A painstaking examination is necessary, since the opening may be no more than a pinhead in width. If none is found, the anterior chamber is filled with balanced salt solution to increase the intraocular pressure and deepen the chamber. This facilitates gonioscopy with a Koeppe lens and the surgical microscope. The cleft is more easily located in this manner. If it is still not located, a weak solution of fluorescein (2% fluorescein diluted three or four times with normal saline solution) is injected into the anterior chamber. A scratch incision is made through the sclera over the ciliary body perpendicular to the limbus in the inferior temporal quadrant. If the fluid that escapes is tinged with fluorescein, a cleft must be present (see Fig. 1.443). If it is not, all the fluid should be milked out by exerting pressure on the globe well away from the incision while the lips of the incision are spread with fine forceps. Air or balanced salt solution may then be placed in the anterior chamber through a limbal wound. This may terminate the hypotension if the ciliary body becomes reattached. If a cleft is present but cannot be

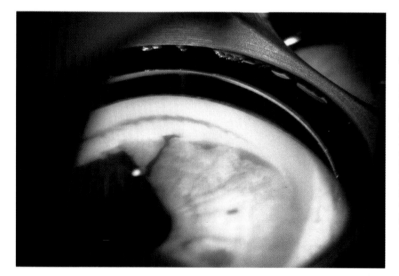

FIG. 1.446

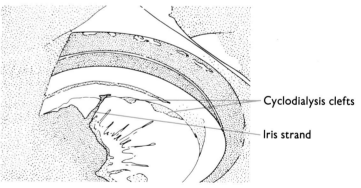

Cyclodialysis clefts

Iris strand

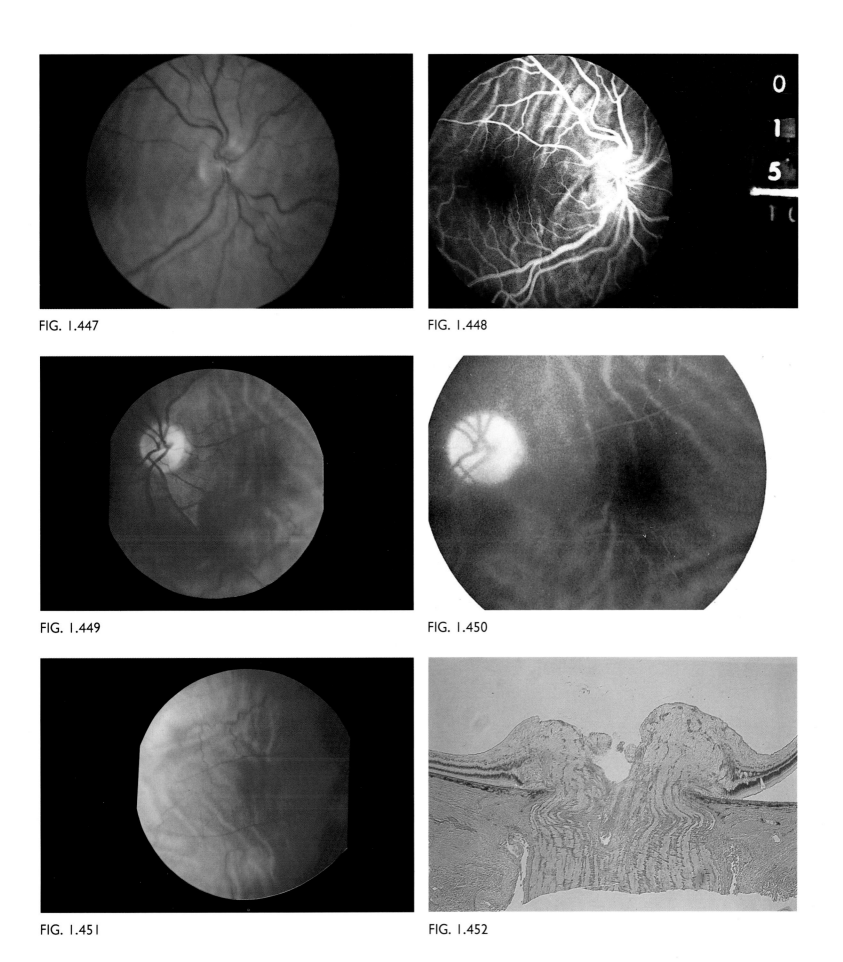

FIG. 1.447

FIG. 1.448

FIG. 1.449

FIG. 1.450

FIG. 1.451

FIG. 1.452

located, the anterior chamber is again filled with balanced salt solution and another search is made. If the cleft is found, it may be closed with a McCannel suture as shown in Figure 1.453. A 10-0 polypropylene suture swaged on to a sharp needle is used. The needle is passed through the cornea overlying the cleft and engages the periphery of the iris and is brought through the sclera at the posterior limbal border. A stab wound is made at the limbus overlying the suture. The trailing end of the suture is brought out of the anterior chamber using an iris hook. The suture is then tied. The best treatment may be the use of the argon laser. A Goldmann goniolens is used to direct the burns to the area of the iris and ciliary spur surrounding the cleft and into the depth of the cleft.

CHOROIDAL DETACHMENT

A study of the anatomy of sclerochoroidal relationships reveals that the perichoroidal space is a very narrow cleft that lies between the inner surface of the sclera and the outer surface of the uvea. It is really a potential space that becomes a true space when filled with blood or fluid. It extends from the ciliary spur anteriorly to the optic nerve posteriorly, although the space probably ceases altogether some distance in front of the nerve, especially on the temporal side in the region of the fovea. The choroid and ciliary body are bound to the sclera by suprachoroidal and supraciliary lamellae that ramify throughout the perichoroidal space in an almost random distribution, which provides a system of intercommunicating spaces.

The topography of a ciliochoroidal detachment is determined by the nature of the attachment of the uvea to the sclera. The attachments are much more secure posteriorly than anteriorly. In Figs. 1.454 and 1.455, the choroid and ciliary body are detached anteriorly to the scleral spur. The choroid is attached more posteriorly. The more secure posterior relationship is attributed to the vortex veins, short posterior ciliary arteries, and nerves passing between sclera and choroid, which augment the suprachoroidal lamellae in holding the posterior choroid to the sclera. Even in the case of a suprachoroidal hemorrhage (Fig. 1.456), the blood fills the suprachoroidal space more anteriorly. The firm attachment of the choroid to the sclera at the ampullae of the four vortex veins causes the typical quadrilobed appearance of a large choroidal detachment. Two of these lobes are plainly visible in Fig. 1.457. The attachment of the sclera to the

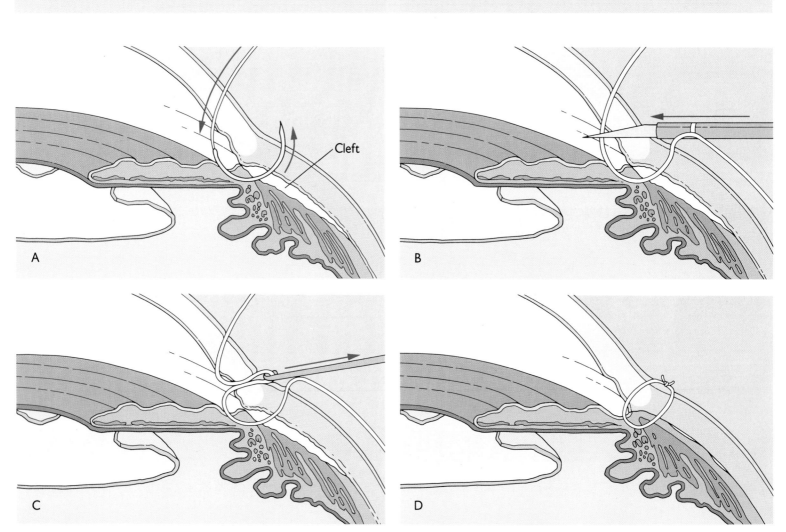

FIG. 1.453

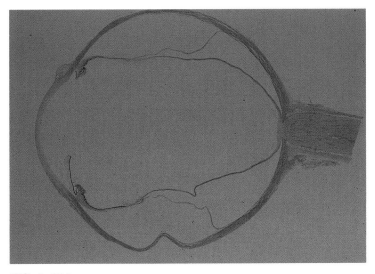

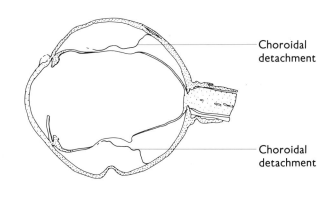

Choroidal detachment

Choroidal detachment

FIG. 1.454

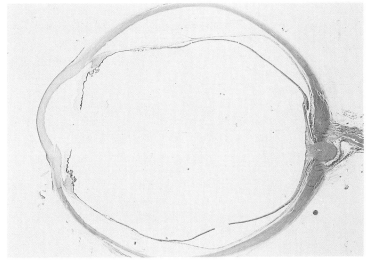

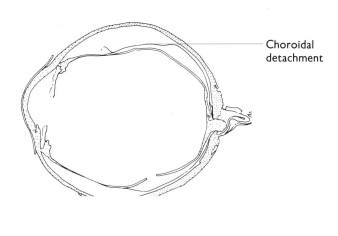

Choroidal detachment

FIG. 1.455

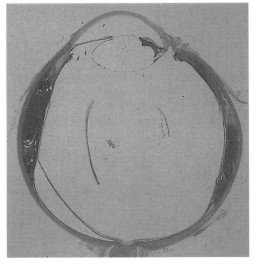

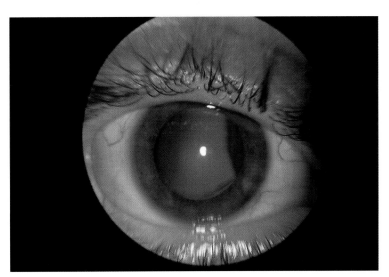

FIG. 1.456

FIG. 1.457

choroid is also secure at the optic nerve. Anteriorly, the attachment is negligible, since here the long, thin suprachoroidal lamellae run in a very oblique manner. Thus transudate from the choroidal vessels becomes distributed mainly throughout the supraciliary space and posteriorly between the choroid and sclera to the entrance of the vortex veins.

Three main forces influence the transudation of fluid from the choroidal vessels:

1. Intraocular pressure, which acts against transudation. During surgical decompression of the globe, this pressure falls to that of the atmosphere.

2. Intravascular pressure, which favors transudation. Since transudation occurs primarily at the capillary level, the pressure in the choroidal capillaries is to be considered. Blood pressure at the arterial end is about 32 mm Hg, whereas at the venous end it is 12 mm Hg.

3. Intravascular oncotic pressure, or colloid osmotic pressure, which is an osmotic force exerted by the protein colloids of the plasma and tends to draw fluids from the tissues into the vascular tree. The oncotic force is especially active at the venous end where the plasma is more concentrated in colloids because water and electrolytes are forced out at the arterial end. The fluid transudate tends to reenter the vascular bed at the venous end without the aid of lymphatics. The normal oncotic pressure measures 25 to 30 mm Hg.

Surgical decompression causes a drop in intraocular pressure. Surgical trauma causes capillary damage with leakage of colloids. This lowers the intravascular oncotic pressure. These factors play principal roles in the pathogenesis of a choroidal detachment.

The cause of the flat or shallow anterior chamber in an eye without a wound leak but with a choroidal detachment is not always clear. Theoretically, for the anterior chamber to become shallow, the iris has to move forward, and it must be pushed from behind by some force exerted against it. When a large bullous choroidal detachment is present, it is not difficult to imagine that the mass compresses the vitreous which in turn pushes the iris forward. However, what about eyes in which a thin suprachoroidal cleft is present? The shallowing may be due to a rotation of the ciliary processes to the degree that they lie in the plane of the cornea. The ciliary structures are under tension and, when the intraocular pressure is reduced, they tend to cause the ciliary body to curl inward.

There are fundus alterations occasionally observed with long-standing choroidal detachments. Lobular detachments are separated by deep valleys, probably caused by anchorages of vortex veins. If a choroidal detachment persists for a long time, two types of pigmentary disturbances may be observed on fundus examination. One consists of widespread atrophy of the retinal pigment epithelium, with clumping of pigment confined to the area of the choroidal detachment. This is seen in Fig. 1.458. A second consists of streaks of pigment that may appear even after the lesion has subsided for some time. They are said to be pathognomonic of this condition. They may result from ridgelike hyperplasia of the pigment epithelium that had accumulated in the creases formed in the choroid during detachment. However, this is speculative. An example of the pigment streak is shown in Fig. 1.459.

Immediate choroidal detachments were once considered very common after cataract surgery. However, this is unlikely. It is possible that early observers confused choroidal detachment with a fundus picture described by Kirsch and Singer in 1973 (Kirsch RE, Singer JA: Ocular fundus immediately after cataract extraction. *Arch Ophthalmol* 1973; 90:460–464). With binocular indirect ophthalmoscopy and fluorescein angiography they observed striking fundus changes immediately after delivery of the cataract. These consisted of full-thickness infoldings of the sclera, choroid, and retina. They were not choroidal detachments. They closely resembled the appearance of buckles in scleral buckling procedures. There was no evidence of suprachoroidal fluid extravasation, the infoldings did not increase in size, and they disappeared as a result of various anterior segment maneuvers. The phenomenon was attributed to ocular hypotension. These folds have also been observed with open-sky partial anterior vitrectomy but not with closed-system vitrectomy. A fundus photograph taken on the operating table is shown in Fig. 1.460. The fluorescein angiogram also taken on the operating table is shown in Fig. 1.461. The white areas in the angiogram correspond to the yellow areas in the fundus photograph. They represent the crests of the folds. The dark areas represent the troughs.

The presence of a choroidal detachment is of no serious consequence as long as the shallowing of the anterior chamber does not favor peripheral anterior synechiae. If the angle is obliterated by the shallowing, surgical correction is necessary. A small meridional incision is made through the sclera in the region of the choroidal detachment. This can be made anywhere between the pars plana and the equator of the globe. An escape of yellow-tinged fluid occurs. With the tip of a muscle hook or the end of an iris spatula the sclera is stroked toward the incision to milk out additional fluid. If this is continued, other bullous areas will finally empty through the same opening. The anterior chamber is filled with air introduced through a limbal stab wound. This treatment is usually successful in reversing the choroidal detachment.

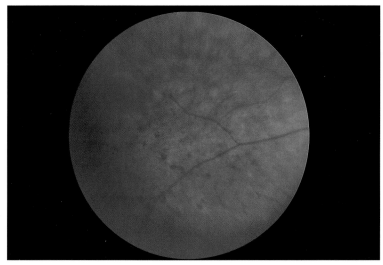

FIG. 1.458

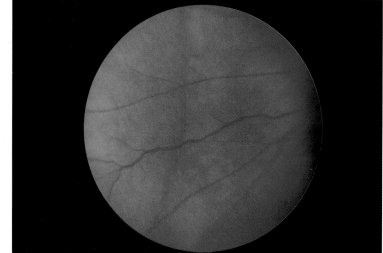

FIG. 1.459

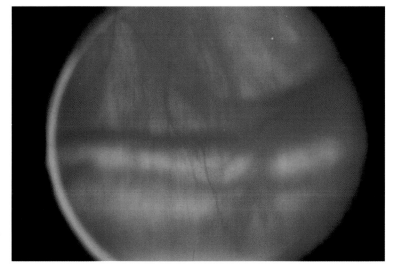

FIG. 1.460

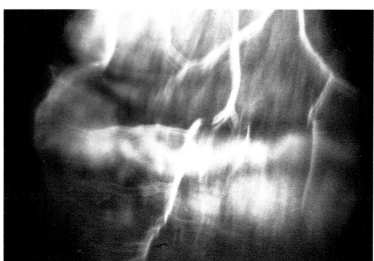

FIG. 1.461

PUPILLARY BLOCK

Pupillary block is a more frequent complication following intracapsular than extracapsular cataract extraction. This is because the intact posterior capsule prevents forward movement of the vitreous. However, most causes of pupillary block are common to both methods.

Pathophysiology

Causes of pupillary block after cataract extraction include the following:

1. Leaky wound
2. Postoperative iridocyclitis
3. Posterior vitreous detachment associated with pooling of retrovitreal aqueous
4. Dense, impermeable anterior hyaloid membrane
5. Pupillary block by air
6. Inadequate iris openings
7. Swollen lens material behind the iris
8. Choroidal detachment and hemorrhage
9. Scleral collapse
10. Free vitreous block
11. Anterior chamber hemorrhage

A leaky wound is probably the commonest cause of early pupillary block. It permits the anterior hyaloid membrane or the posterior capsule to adhere to the iris and to any surgical openings made in the iris. This can cause a misdirection of aqueous into the vitreous or into the retrovitreal space, as shown in Fig. 1.462. Pooling of aqueous in these two areas creates a force that pushes the vitreous forward, thus shallowing the anterior chamber (inset).

The sizes of both the anterior and posterior chambers undergo wide variations in pupillary block. This is illustrated after an intracapsular cataract extraction. In Fig. 1.463A the anterior chamber is of normal depth due to mushrooming of vitreous into the anterior chamber. The anterior chamber may be slightly smaller when there is less vitreous in it (Fig. 1.463B). It may be practically flat, as shown in Fig. 1.463C.

Even in the presence of a wound leak, the anterior chamber may show a variable depth. In Fig. 1.464A, the anterior chamber is shallow. A wound leak is present (upper arrow) and there is continued aqueous secretion (lower arrows). The shallowness of the anterior chamber is due to a net aqueous loss. In Fig. 1.464B, there is a wound leak and hyposecretion of aqueous. The anterior chamber is even more shallow. However, in the presence of a wound leak and continued aqueous secretion, but with free communication of aqueous between the anterior and posterior chambers (no pupillary block), the anterior chamber may be of normal depth because there is no net aqueous loss (Fig. 1.464C).

The posterior chamber may also undergo wide variations

Anterior Chamber Depth Abnormalities: Pupillary Block Pathophysiology

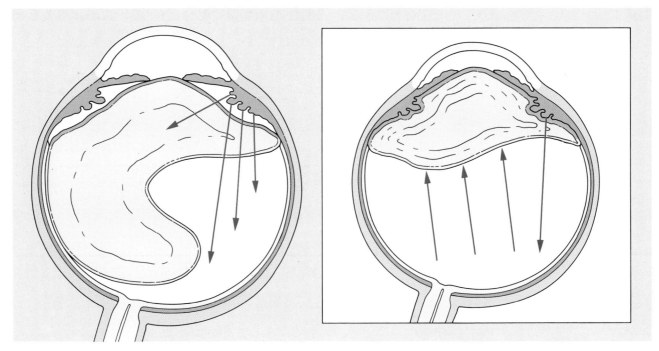

FIG. 1.462

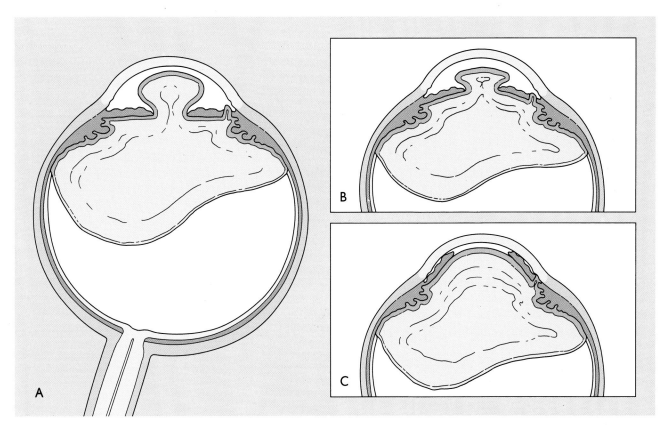

FIG. 1.463

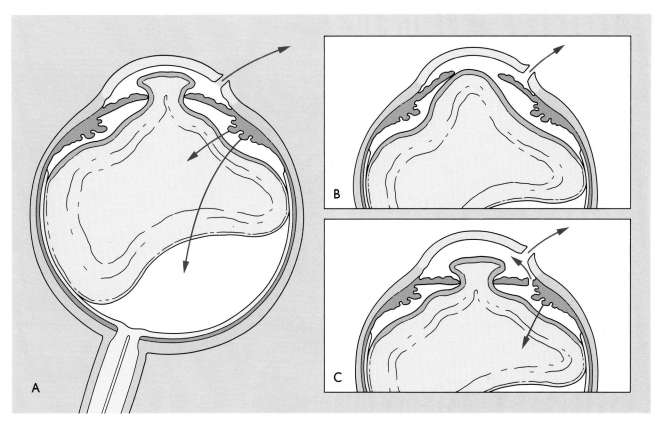

FIG. 1.464

in size. The anterior chamber may be deep in the center but shallow peripherally where the iris is more convex. This creates an iris bombé. The pooling of aqueous in the posterior chamber creates this effect. This is seen in Fig. 1.465. In Fig. 1.466, the posterior chamber is wide on the left where aqueous has pooled, but shallow on the right where aqueous has been misdirected posteriorly. The inset shows a total absence of the posterior chamber. The entire posterior surface of the iris is lined by the anterior hyaloid membrane. There is a uniform shallowing of the anterior chamber. This situation is often seen as a result of intraocular inflammation.

The vital role played by the pooling of vitreous in the retrovitreal space in aphakic pupillary block is emphasized by considering the same mechanism in malignant glaucoma and acute narrow angle glaucoma in phakic eyes. In malignant glaucoma the anterior chamber remains very shallow or absent and the intraocular pressure is high after a peripheral iridectomy, a cyclodialysis, or a filtering procedure. The lens–iris diaphragm moves anteriorly. The vitreous likewise moves forward and may lie anterior to the lens equator and even the ciliary processes. Removal of the lens

is usually insufficient to remedy the situation, since the vitreous then occupies the space formerly held by the lens, and the pupil remains blocked. Aqueous continues to pool behind the vitreous. Treatment of pupillary block is described below.

Treatment
Medical. Treatment consists of dilating the pupil as widely as possible. As shown in Fig. 1.467, this permits aqueous to enter the anterior chamber, thereby breaking the block. Pupillary dilation may be facilitated by the systemic administration of a hyperosmotic agent. Dehydration of the vitreous may displace the anterior hyaloid membrane posteriorly from its closely apposed position against the back of the iris, thus allowing mydriasis to occur.

Surgical. Iridectomy is probably the most frequently performed surgical procedure for aphakic pupillary block. It works best when fluid is trapped in the posterior chamber, as shown in Fig. 1.468. The iridectomy may be performed surgically or with the laser.

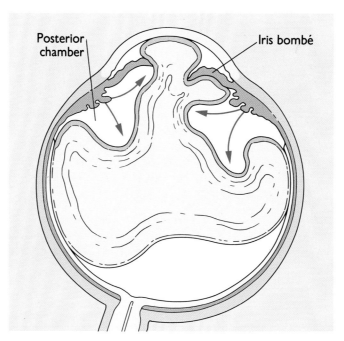

FIG. 1.465

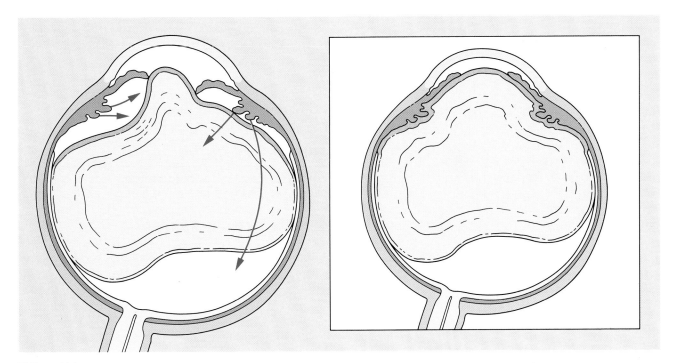

FIG. 1.466

▽ Anterior Chamber Depth Abnormalities:
Pupillary Block Medical Treatment

▽ Anterior Chamber Depth Abnormalities:
Pupillary Block Surgical Treatment

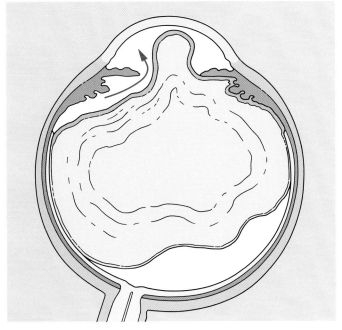

FIG. 1.467

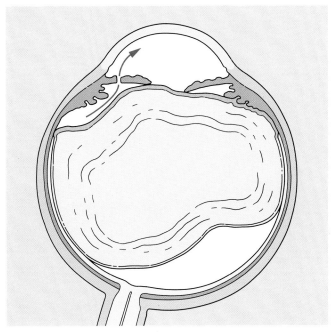

FIG. 1.468

In cases in which the anterior hyaloid membrane appears unduly thickened or is covered by a membrane after iridocyclitis or hyphema, a simple incision of the anterior vitreous face may release a gush of pooled aqueous and terminate the block. This is shown in Fig. 1.469.

A through-and-through incision of the vitreous is required in most cases, since fluid is usually trapped behind the vitreous. This is effective in malignant glaucoma. The vitreous is penetrated with a 22-gauge, 1.5-in needle attached to a syringe, from the anterior hyaloid membrane to the retrovitreal space through a limbal approach. This is shown in Fig. 1.470. When the retrovitreal space is reached, aspiration of fluid into the syringe is possible. The needle is moved from side to side as it is withdrawn to create a wide communication between the anterior chamber and the retrovitreal space. The result is shown in the inset.

A logical surgical approach to aphakic or pseudophakic pupillary block is to perform a peripheral iridectomy. If fluid enters the anterior chamber from the posterior chamber, the anterior chamber will deepen. This may be curative. If no fluid is present in the posterior chamber, a 22-gauge needle should be passed through the iridectomy, through the vitreous, and into the retrovitreal space to create the communication between the anterior chamber and the retrovitreal space described above.

With contemporary cataract surgery techniques, a pars plana vitrectomy may be the most reliable surgical solution to pupillary block. This is especially useful with an intact posterior capsule and a posterior chamber lens implant.

LENS EXTRACTION IN SPECIAL SITUATIONS
LENS DISPLACEMENT

Lens displacement or ectopia lentis may be classified as follows: heritable, spontaneous, and traumatic.

Heritable Ectopia Lentis
This is usually associated with other systemic or ocular anomalies but may appear as an isolated anomaly.

Marfan's syndrome is the most common type and is characterized by a triad of skeletal, cardiovascular, and ocular anomalies. The most characteristic ocular anomaly is ectopia lentis, which is found in 70% to 80% of cases, is nearly always bilateral, is usually partial, is rarely progressive, and the lens is characteristically displaced superiorly and temporally. In Fig. 1.471 the lens is displaced superiorly and temporally and the free part of the lens is tilted posteriorly. Vitreous is present in the anterior chamber. A similar displacement is seen in Fig. 1.472, except that the free part of the lens is tilted only slightly posteriorly and there is no vit-

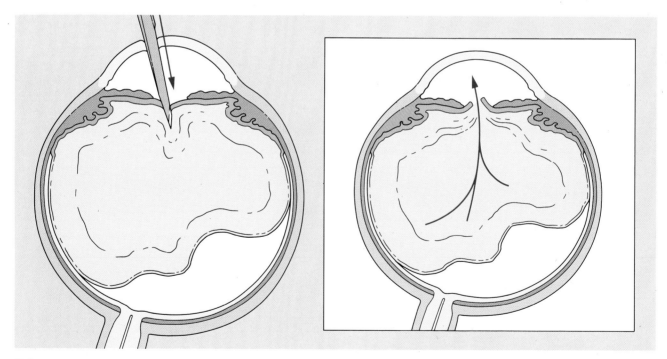

FIG. 1.469

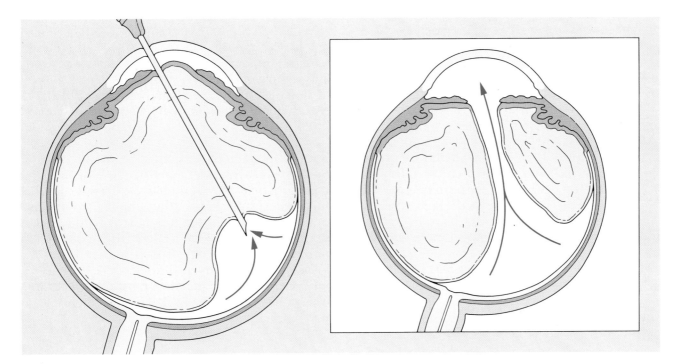

FIG. 1.470

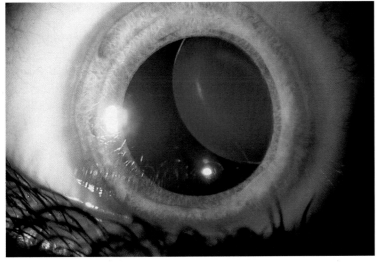

FIG. 1.471

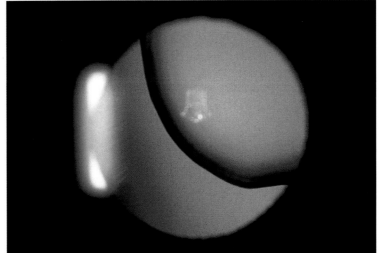

FIG. 1.472

reous in the anterior chamber. Rarely, the lens may be dislocated into the anterior chamber, as seen in Fig. 1.473. Myopia is common and is associated with a lenticular, as well as an axial, component. Retinal detachment is more common in those eyes with high axial length.

Homocystinuria is an inborn error of metabolism of the sulfur-containing amino acids. This enzymopathy may resemble Marfan's syndrome, with at least 50% of patients showing a similar clinical appearance. Mental retardation, not seen in Marfan's syndrome, occurs in 50% of cases and may be progressive. The cardiovascular problems are more common and more serious than those in Marfan's syndrome. Thromboembolic phenomena occur in at least 50% of cases as a result of blood coagulation disorders or increased blood viscosity caused by platelet stickiness. They are more likely to occur after vessel puncture and general anesthesia. Therefore, these patients are at high risk during surgery. Ectopia lentis is a characteristic finding in 90% of cases. Unlike Marfan's syndrome, the lens displacement is usually inferior (Fig. 1.474) and often toward the nasal side.

Weill-Marchesani syndrome, also called spherophakia, is much more rare than Marfan's syndrome. Although it is also a mesodermal dystrophy, there is a marked contrast in the appearance of these patients. The skeletal anomalies consist of brachymorphy, short stature, and spadelike hands and feet. Ectopia lentis in a patient with this syndrome is seen in Fig. 1.475.

Spontaneous Ectopia Lentis
Spontaneous displacements of the lens are slightly more common than the heritable varieties and are related to mechanical stretching of the zonule. In certain middle-aged or older individuals the lens gradually tilts backward as the upper zonules give way and eventually becomes dislocated into the vitreous cavity. This is seen in Fig. 1.476 in a 72-year-old man. A similar dislocation is seen in Fig. 1.477 in a 67-year-old man. Maximal dilation of the pupil is shown. This is seen again in Fig. 1.478 after an intracapsular cataract extraction with a sector iridectomy.

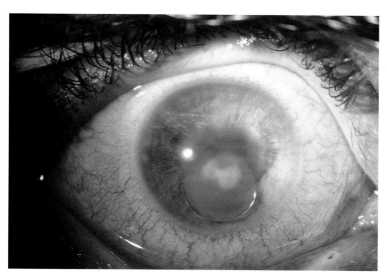

FIG. 1.473

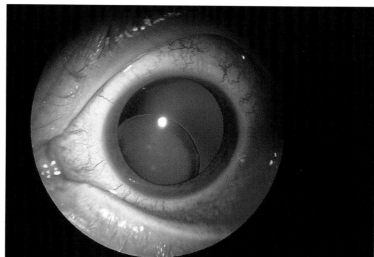

FIG. 1.474

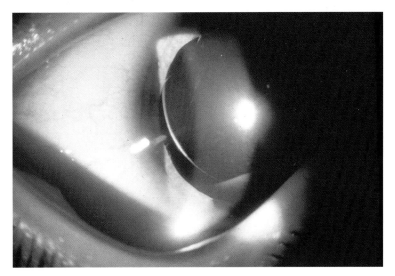

FIG. 1.475

Lens Extraction in Special Situations: Spontaneous Ectopia Lentis

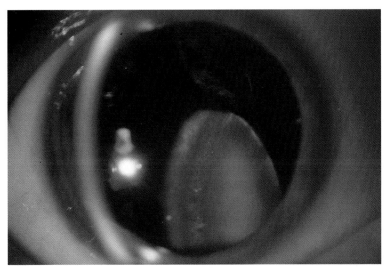

FIG. 1.476

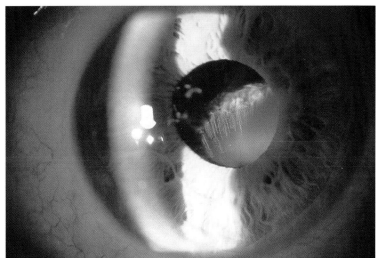

FIG. 1.477

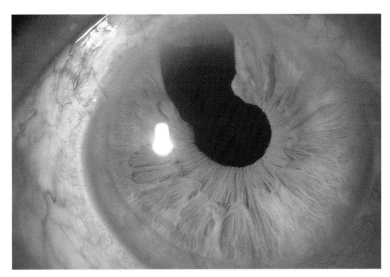

FIG. 1.478

Traumatic Ectopia Lentis

Traumatic lens displacements are frequently associated with other ocular damage, such as recession of the anterior chamber angle, iris laceration, injury to the ciliary body, choroid, and retina, retinal detachment, cataract, intraocular hemorrhage, rupture of the globe, and so on. A subtle traumatic lens displacement is seen in Fig. 1.479. A greater lens displacement is seen in Fig. 1.480.

Surgery for Ectopia Lentis

Lens surgery in ectopia lentis can be difficult and has a high rate of intraoperative and postoperative complications. In general, the following are indications for lens surgery:

1. Dislocation into the anterior chamber with corneal touch
2. Mature or hypermature cataract
3. Lens-induced uveitis
4. Inadequate visual acuity caused by the displaced lens
5. Increasing subluxation of the lens

Subluxated Lens Still in Pupillary Space. If the lens is subluxated in the pupillary space, I tend to leave it in situ even if it becomes cataractous, providing the opposite eye has adequate vision for the patient's needs. If binocular vision is required for occupational reasons, a cataractous lens is removed. If progressive dislocation occurs, the lens should be removed before it luxates completely into the vitreous.

Subluxated Lens in the Anterior Chamber. The lens should be extracted in these cases because of the danger of corneal endothelial damage. Some of these lenses may be displaced through the pupil into the posterior chamber by alternately dilating and constricting the pupil.

Subluxated Lens in the Vitreous. The lens may be fixed to the retina or may be floating freely in the vitreous. If the eye appears to be tolerating the dislocated lens without undue inflammation, as is often the case, no surgery is done. If the lens is fixated to the retina, surgery is contraindicated. However, if a free-floating lens produces lens-induced uveitis or glaucoma, or if it seriously interferes with vision in a one-eyed patient, the dislocated lens should be removed.

Vitreous surgery has offered an improved prognosis in surgery for ectopia lentis. An automated vitrector is useful in preventing the sequelae of vitreous loss in the same way as in operative loss of vitreous in routine cataract surgery. Vitreous surgery may also relieve pupillary block in cases of subluxation of the lens where it may be inadvisable to remove the lens.

The method of lens extraction is determined by the age of the patient and the location of the displaced lens. In patients over the age of 35 years it makes little sense to remove a dislocated lens by any other method than cryoextraction if access to the lens is possible and if the capsule is intact. In children and young adults, lens aspiration is usually effective. In some of these, the lens and vitreous may be simultaneously removed with an automated vitrector. A pars plana approach is often effective in removal of lenses in the vitreous. Caution should be exercised in cases with glaucoma, especially if the dislocation follows trauma. In many of these, the cause of the glaucoma is angle recession, which will not be helped by lens removal. The relatively high risk of retinal detachment postoperatively is seen in Fig. 1.481 in a patient who underwent lens extraction following a traumatic dislocation.

MORGAGNIAN CATARACT

A Morgagnian cataract is a hypermature cataract in which the cortex becomes liquefied to such an extent that its dark brown nucleus sinks to the bottom of the capsule bag. This is seen in Fig. 1.482. A histologic section of a cataract with liquefaction of the cortex is seen in Fig. 1.483. An extreme

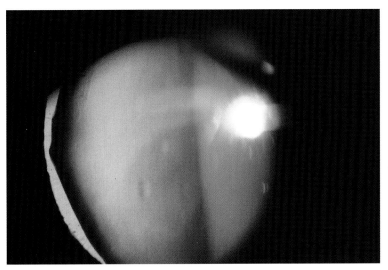

FIG. 1.479

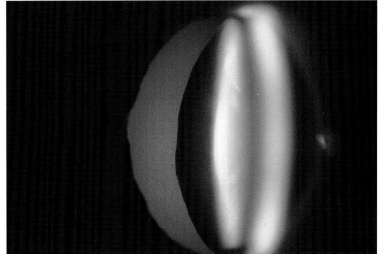

FIG. 1.480

Lens Extraction in Special Situations: Surgery for Subluxated Lens in the Vitreous

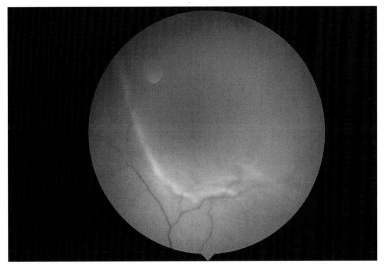

FIG. 1.481

Lens Extraction in Special Situations: Morgagnian Cataract

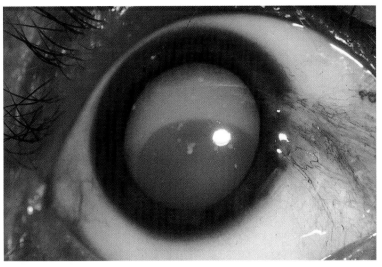

FIG. 1.482

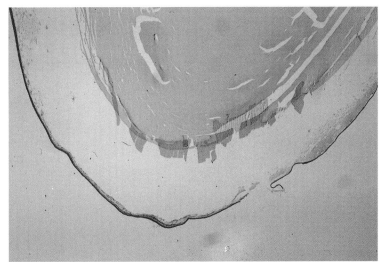

FIG. 1.483

example is seen in Fig. 1.484 in a 49-year-old man. The nucleus has sunk to the bottom of the capsule bag and the remainder of the bag is filled with a relatively clear liquid. Vision was 20/70. Some of the debris present in the liquid is seen easily by transillumination (Fig. 1.485). The collapsed anterior capsule is seen in a slit lamp view in Fig. 1.486. Because of an acute onset of lens-induced uveitis, surgery was performed. These lenses usually have weak zonules. Cryoextraction is difficult to perform because of the liquefied cortex. The anterior capsule is difficult to grasp with intracapsular forceps. Surgery is usually performed by the extracapsular technique. This was performed on the patient just described. The traditional can-opener anterior capsulectomy was difficult to perform because of the laxity of the anterior capsule. A puncture was made in the anterior capsule with a diamond knife. A Vannas scissors anterior capsulectomy was then performed. The cornea was protected with a viscoelastic agent. There were several residual plaques on the posterior capsule that prevented much improvement in vision (Fig. 1.487). Three weeks

later a YAG laser posterior capsulectomy was performed. The result is shown in Fig. 1.488. Vision improved to 20/25. It is possible in a hypermature cataract for liquefaction to involve the entire nucleus as well as the cortex. Such an eye is shown in Fig. 1.489.

PSEUDOEXFOLIATION

The material referred to as pseudoexfoliation deposits itself on the anterior lens capsule. It is seen also at the iris sphincter. Patients with pseudoexfoliation often have an associated glaucoma. This syndrome causes two disturbances that are of importance to the cataract surgeon. The pupils in these eyes do not dilate well and the zonules may be very weak. Zonular dialyses are common during extracapsular cataract extraction. A good example of pseudoexfoliation of the lens capsule is seen in Fig. 1.490. An extreme example of residual material left on the face of the vitreous after an intracapsular cataract extraction is seen in Fig. 1.491.

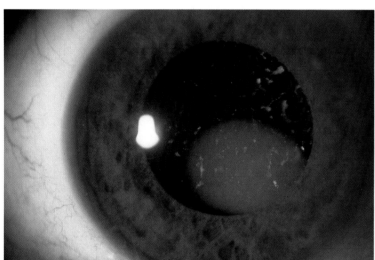

FIG. 1.484

FIG. 1.485

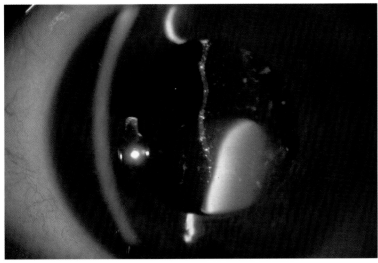

FIG. 1.486

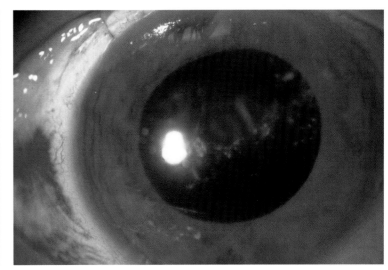

FIG. 1.487

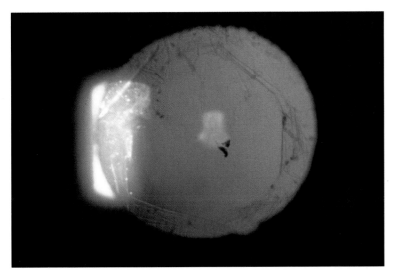

FIG. 1.488

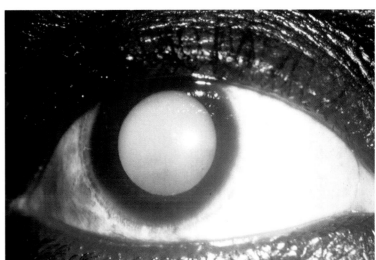

FIG. 1.489

Lens Extraction in Special Situations: Pseudoexfoliation

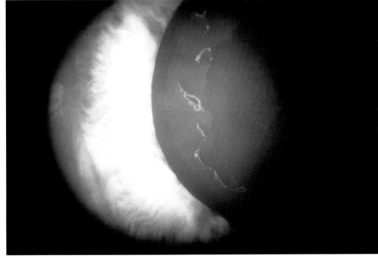

FIG. 1.490

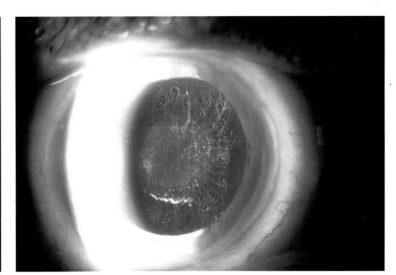

FIG. 1.491

CORNEAL ENDOTHELIAL DYSTROPHY

The association of cataract and corneal endothelial dystrophy (Fig. 1.492) presents the cataract surgeon with a judgment decision. The surgeon must decide whether the cornea can tolerate a cataract extraction without undergoing decompensation. Specular microscopy and corneal pachymetry may assist in the decision. An extracapsular cataract extraction with an intact posterior capsule improves the prognosis if a subsequent penetrating keratoplasty becomes necessary. Most surgeons prefer a triple procedure consisting of a cataract extraction, lens implantation, and penetrating keratoplasty. An example of an eye that underwent a penetrating keratoplasty some time after an extracapsular cataract extraction is shown in Fig. 1.493. Note the iris suture used during the cataract extraction to close a sector iridotomy that was made because of a miotic pupil. Figure 1.494 shows an eye that had a phacoemulsification with a posterior chamber lens implantation 3 years after a penetrating keratoplasty. An example of the more frequently performed triple procedure is shown in Fig. 1.495. The surgical technique of a triple procedure is as follows. A deep trephine groove is made in the recipient cornea (Fig. 1.496). A puncture is made in the groove with a diamond blade (Fig. 1.497). A viscoelastic material is then injected into the anterior chamber (Fig. 1.498). The corneal button is excised with scissors (Figs. 1.499 and 1.500). Anterior

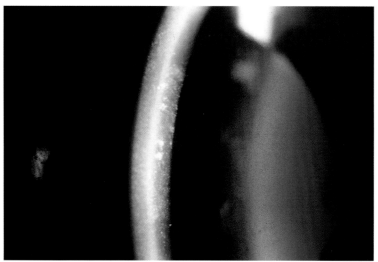

FIG. 1.492

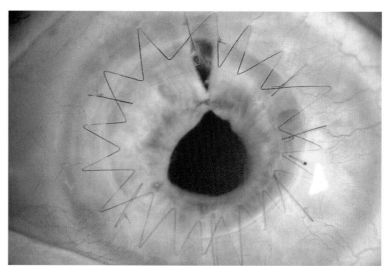

FIG. 1.493

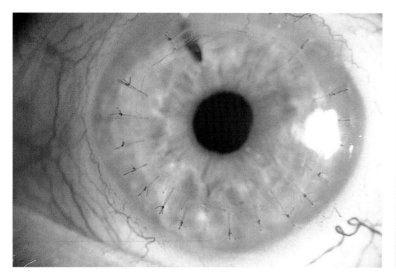

FIG. 1.494

FIG. 1.495

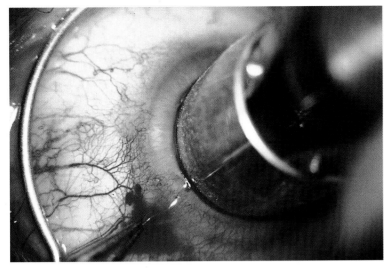

FIG. 1.496

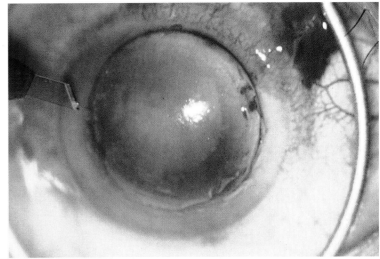

FIG. 1.497

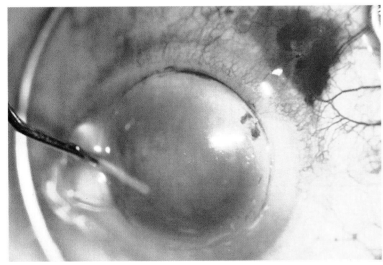

FIG. 1.498

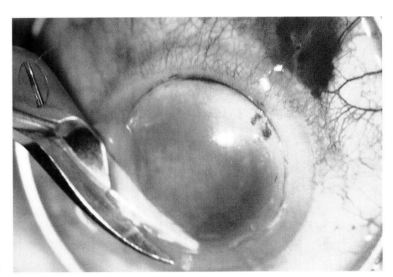

FIG. 1.499

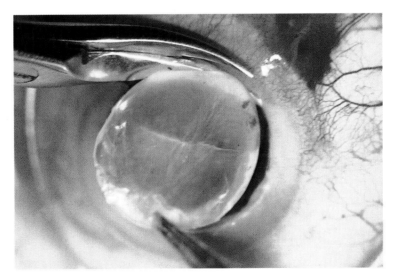

FIG. 1.500

capsulectomy is performed (Figs. 1.501 and 1.502). The surgeon then removes the nucleus of the lens (Figs. 1.503 and 1.504). Irrigation and aspiration of the residual lens cortex is performed in an open system (Figs. 1.505 and 1.506). A Jaffe posterior chamber lens is implanted (Figs. 1.507 to 1.509). The donor button is sutured in place (Fig. 1.510). The postoperative result is shown in Fig. 1.511.

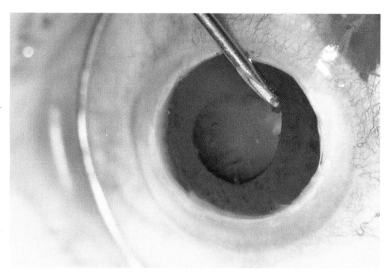

FIG. 1.501

FIG. 1.502

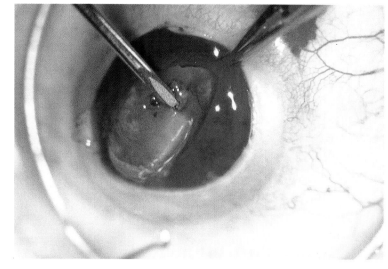

FIG. 1.503

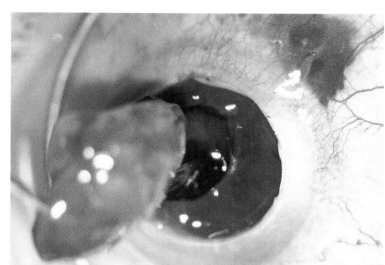

FIG. 1.504

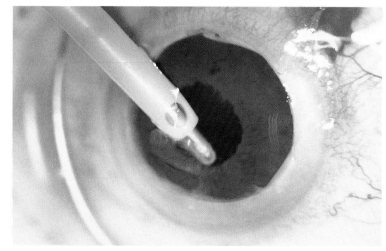

FIG. 1.505

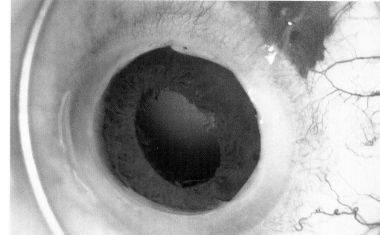

FIG. 1.506

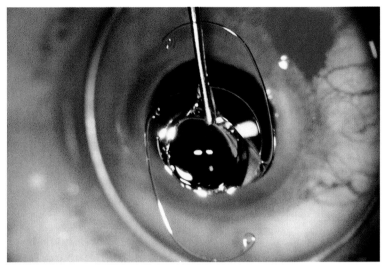

FIG. 1.507

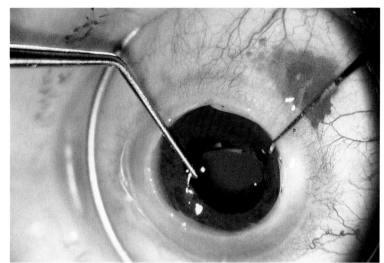

FIG. 1.508

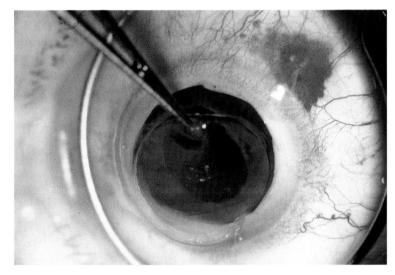

FIG. 1.509

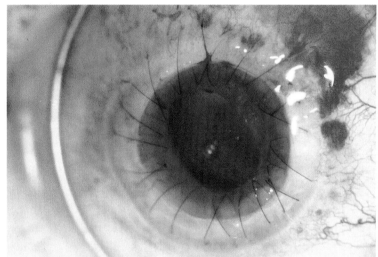

FIG. 1.510

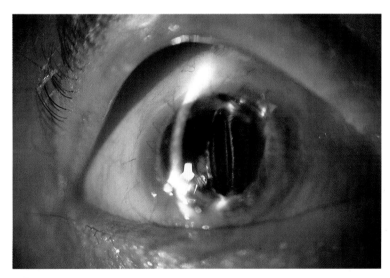

FIG. 1.511

CONGENITAL COLOBOMATA

Occasionally one must perform a cataract extraction in an eye with a congenital coloboma of the iris, retina, and choroid. Until recently it was recommended that an intracapsular cataract extraction be performed because of a defect in the zonules in the region of the iris coloboma. An example is seen in Fig. 1.512, the eye of a 69-year-old female. An intracapsular cataract extraction with a superior iridotomy connecting with the inferior iris coloboma was performed (Fig. 1.513). A fundus view of the coloboma of the retina and choroid is seen postoperatively in Fig. 1.514. Final vision is 20/70. Figure 1.515 shows the eye of a 48-year-old male with a congenital coloboma of the iris, retina, and choroid. A phacoemulsification with implantation of a Clayman posterior chamber lens was performed. The lens was placed in the capsule bag. The postoperative appearance is seen in Fig. 1.516. Final vision is 20/20. Figure 1.517 shows the postoperative appearance of the eye of a

48-year-old female with a congenital coloboma of the iris, retina, and choroid. A phacoemulsification with the in-the-bag implantation of a Jaffe posterior chamber lens was performed. The slit lamp view in Fig. 1.518 shows the two surfaces of the lens and the laser ridge space between the optic and the posterior capsule. The inferior portion of the implant is seen by retroillumination in Fig. 1.519. The coloboma of the retina and choroid is seen in Fig. 1.520. Final vision is 20/25. These cases demonstrate that it is feasible to perform extracapsular surgery and place the lens in the capsule bag.

HETEROCHROMIC IRIDOCYCLITIS

Eyes with heterochromic iridocyclitis respond well to cataract extraction, in my experience, contrary to some reports in the literature. It is not unusual to observe a diminution or even complete disappearance of the typically white ker-

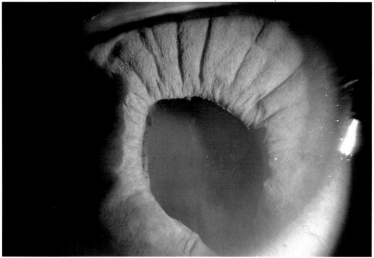

FIG. 1.512

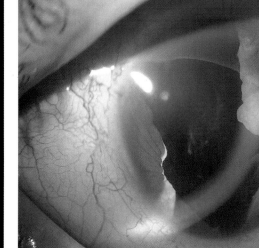

FIG. 1.513

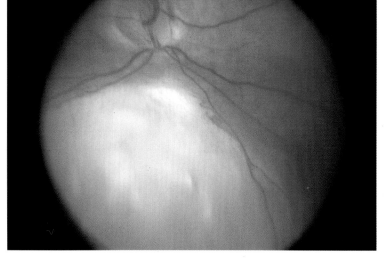

FIG. 1.514

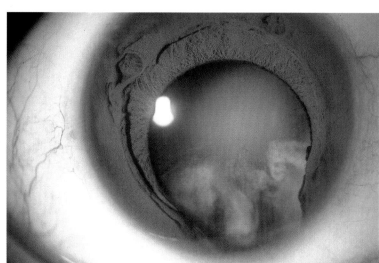

FIG. 1.515

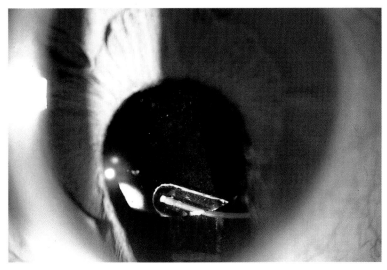

FIG. 1.516

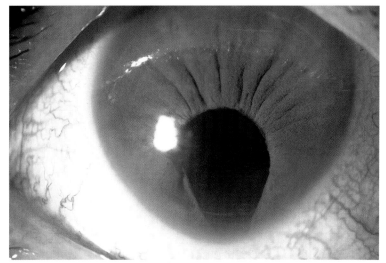

FIG. 1.517

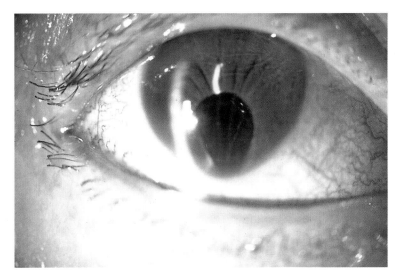

FIG. 1.518

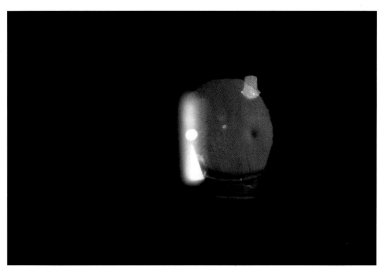

FIG. 1.519

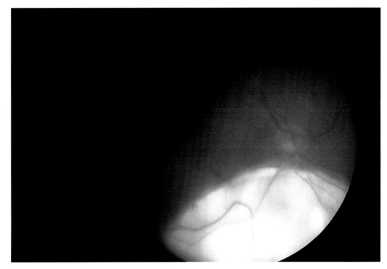

FIG. 1.520

atic precipitates after cataract extraction. The iris is usually atrophic (Fig. 1.521) and should be handled gently during the surgery. The changes in the iris appear to be of a degenerative, rather than inflammatory, origin. The appearance of the cataract in a patient with heterochromic iridocyclitis is shown in Fig. 1.522.

ASTEROID HYALOSIS

Occasionally one sees eyes with cataracts and asteroid hyalosis. The oval, brilliant white bodies of varying size adhere to the framework of the vitreous and may be so prolific as to block a view of the fundus. They consist chiefly of calcium soap. A postmortem specimen of an eye with asteroid hyalosis is seen in Fig. 1.523. In spite of their presence in the vitreous, they rarely cause much disturbance of vision. An example is seen after an intracapsular cataract extraction in Fig. 1.524.

▽ Lens Extraction in Special Situations: Heterochromic Iridocyclitis

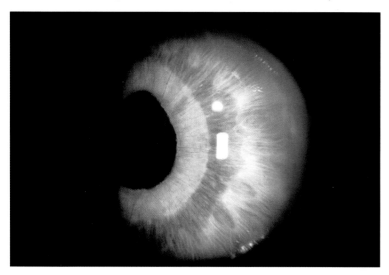

FIG. 1.521

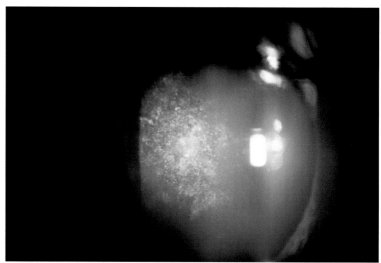

FIG. 1.522

▽ Lens Extraction in Special Situations: Asteroid Hyalosis

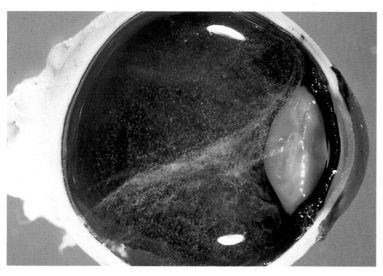

FIG. 1.523

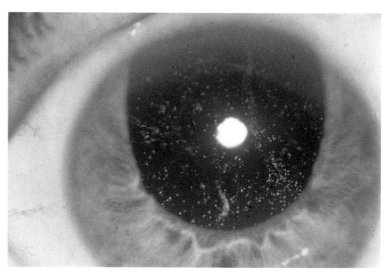

FIG. 1.524

Picture credits for this chapter are as follows: Figs. 1.209 to 1.229 courtesy of J. Elliot Blaydes, Jr., MD; Figs. 1.241 to 1.243, 1.254, 1.290, 1.312, 1.326 to 1.329, and 1.331 courtesy of W.R. Green, MD; Fig. 1.244 courtesy of McDonnell PJ, Green WR, Champion R: Pathologic changes in pseudophakia. Semin Ophthalmol 1986;1:80–103; Figs. 1.245, 1.319, and 1.325 courtesy of McDonnell PJ, Green WR, Maumenee AE, Iliff WJ: Pathology of intraocular lenses in 33 eyes examined postmortem. Ophthalmology 1983;90:386–403; Fig. 1.246 courtesy of McDonnell PJ, Champion R, Green WR: Location and composition of haptics of posterior chamber intraocular lenses. Histopathologic studies of postmortem eyes. Ophthalmology 1987;94:136–142; Figs. 1.247, 1.322, 1.330, and 1.332 courtesy of Champion R. McDonnell PJ, Green WR: Intraocular lenses. Histopathologic characteristics of a large series of autopsy lenses. Surv Ophthalmol 1985;30:1–32; Figs. 1.311 and 1.383 to 1.386 courtesy of David Apple, MD; Figs. 1.369, 1.370, 1.371, 1.373, 1.374, 1.388 to 1.391, 1.401, 1.404 (courtesy of E. Hersh), 1.406, 1.407, 1.411 to 1.413, 1.417, 1.419, 1.422, 1.423, 1.427 to 1.433, 1.440, 1.444 to 1.448, 1.452, 1.455, and 1.457 to 1.461 from Jaffe NS: Cataract Surgery and Its Complications, ed 4. St. Louis, The C.V. Mosby Co., 1984. (Figs. 1.401 and 1.411 courtesy of P.R. McDonald, MD); (Figs. 1.417 and 1.422 courtesy of P.H.Y. Chee, MD); (Fig. 1.429 courtesy of P. Henkind, MD); (Figs. 1.460 and 1.461 courtesy of R. Kirsch, MD); Fig. 1.405 courtesy of E. Hersh, MD; Fig. 1.438 courtesy of A.J. Kroll, MD; Fig. 1.439 adapted from and Fig. 1.440 courtesy of J.R. Wolter, MD (J Pediatr Ophthalmol 1969;6:153–156); Fig. 1.452 courtesy of Hogan MJ, Zimmerman LE: Ophthalmic Pathology: An Atlas and Textbook, ed 2. Philadelphia, W.B. Saunders Co., 1962; Figs. 1.512 to 1.516 and 1.518 from Jaffe NS, Clayman HM: Cataract extraction in eyes with congenital colobomata. J Cat Refr Surg 1987;13:54–58; Figs. 1.248, 1.309, 1.387, 1.392 to 1.396, 1.398, and 1.399 from Jaffe NS: in Caldwell DR (ed): Cataracts, Transactions of the New Orleans Academy of Ophthalmology. New York, Raven Press, 1988; Figs. 1.397 and 1.400 from Roussel TJ, Culbertson WW, Jaffe NS: Chronic postoperative endophthalmitis associated with Propionibacterium acnes. Arch Ophthalmol 1987;105:1199–1201; Figs. 1.414 to 1.416 courtesy of Bruner WE, Michels RG, Stark WJ, Maumenee AE: Management of epithelial cysts of the anterior chamber. Ophthal Surg 1981;12:279–285; Fig. 1.437 courtesy of D.D. Donaldson, MD (Arch Ophthalmol 1969;82:339–343 © AMA).

Acknowledgment: I am indebted to Fernando G. Gonzalez, RPB, FPBA, of the Bascom Palmer Eye Institute and Frederick G. Karrenberg, MD, of my staff for many of the photographs in this chapter.

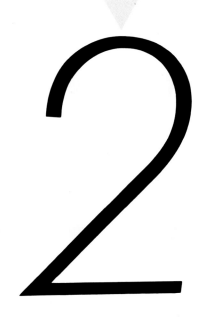

TECHNIQUES IN CORNEAL TRANSPLANTATION

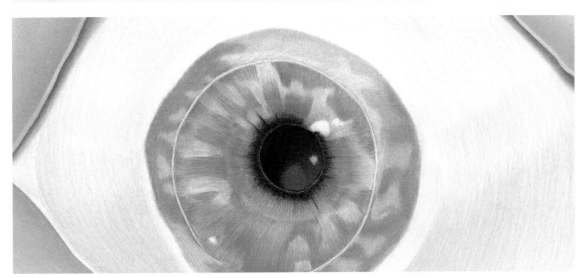

Roger H. S. Langston, MD, CM, FACS

The intent of this chapter is to review the current state of the art of corneal transplantation, with emphasis on surgical technique. It reflects both my personal preferences and contemporary surgical standards. As such, it may have value both to experienced surgeons and neophytes.

PATIENT SELECTION

Corneal transplantation may be indicated to improve vision, to relieve pain, to maintain the structural integrity of the eye, and occasionally to arrest or control an infectious process. Prior to surgery, a thorough discussion of the options, expectations, and risks is, of course, in order. It is a complicated subject but a few points are appropriate to bear in mind in all cases.

Transplanting corneal tissue into a hostile environment almost guarantees failure. Dry eyes, lid deformities, uncontrolled glaucoma, active infections, etc., should be controlled if at all possible prior to surgery. Active anterior segment inflammation substantially increases the risk of graft rejection, secondary glaucoma, persistent epithelial defects, and graft failure. It is preferable to wait until inflammation has been quiet for some months before undertaking surgery.

Morphologic factors, particularly corneal vascularization, also play a role in graft success. While superficial vascularization alone usually plays an insignificant role, deep vascularization in more than two quadrants has been associated with a graft failure rate of 50%.

The primary cause of graft failure is rejection of the donor tissue by the patient's immune system. While corneal graft "reactions" can often be controlled, they do require prompt care. Good liaison with the patient and family is critical. Several studies show that the prognosis for corneal transplants in children and in the socioeconomically deprived is limited because of increased graft reactions in the former group and difficulties in providing appropriate postoperative care in both groups. These issues should be faced frankly prior to surgery.

The average astigmatism following penetrating keratoplasty is approximately 4.00 diopters (and often is higher). As likely as not, this will be at an oblique axis. All patients, especially those whose other eye is without significant refractive error, should be counseled about the expectations for spectacles, contact lenses, or further refractive surgery.

Graft clarity and good vision are not synonymous. Figure 2.1 gives some rough estimates of the success of surgery based both on my experience and on reports in the literature.

The difference between the percentage of patients with clear grafts and the percentage with good vision is largely due to the fact that patients with a history of anterior segment inflammation tend to have secondary damage to the lens, retina, and optic nerve, and to have age-related disease.

In summary, the technical success of corneal transplantation falls short of the visual outcome. In selecting and counseling patients, it is the visual results and postoperative care that should be focused on at least as much as the events in the operating room.

DONOR TISSUE

The selection of donor tissue is the responsibility of the surgeon as well as the eye bank. The Eye Bank Association of America has issued guidelines aimed at minimizing the risk of transmitting disease and of primary graft failure. If at all possible, it is wise to use the services of a competent eye bank to evaluate the donor and the donor tissue prior to use—both for medical and legal reasons.

Although there are no data to show that donor age correlates with graft survival, most surgeons use tissue from older donors for older patients and avoid using tissue from donors over the age of 65 years. Specular microscopy of donor tissue has certainly allowed more confidence in using older tissue. Donor tissue should also be evaluated for the presence of guttata or other endothelial changes, for scars and opacities, and for the condition of the epithelium.

No firm guidelines have been established for a maximum allowable time between death and the use of tissue. The intervals between death, cooling, enucleation, preservation, and use should be as brief as possible in order to minimize the damage to the donor tissue. Most surgeons use whole globes up to 24 hours from the time of death and tissue in MK medium up to 48 hours. The use of K-Sol and CSM solution has pushed the time several days further, but exactly how long tissue can be kept in storage is still not entirely clear. Organ culture techniques extend the interval to months.

Most corneal transplantation is performed without regard to tissue matching. The available evidence suggests that if the recipient has not previously rejected the graft, and if the recipient cornea is not heavily vascularized, matching with respect to the HLA or ABO blood grouping systems does not improve results. Ongoing collaborative studies in the United States and overseas will probably show an advantage to HLA matching in high-risk patients over the next several years, especially if all surgeons make an effort to support these studies.

Frozen tissue can be used for lamellar keratoplasty though fresh tissue is easier to dissect and may ultimately be clearer.

INSTRUMENTATION

In addition to a set of anterior segment surgical knives, scissors, and forceps, corneal surgery requires trephines, cutting blocks, corneal dissectors, and a few other instruments. Corneal trephines must be sharp. In this respect, disposable trephines have an advantage. My preference is the Hessburg-Barron suction trephine (Fig. 2.2) for use on the recipient and disposable trephines and a reliable mechanical punch (e.g., Bourne punch, Fig. 2.3) for use on the donor tissue. It is important that the mechanical punch have little

ESTIMATES OF SUCCESS OF CORNEAL TRANSPLANTATION OPERATIONS BASED ON CORNEAL DISEASE BEING TREATED

CORNEAL DISEASE	GRAFT CLARITY	VISION 20/40 OR BETTER
Keratoconus	90%–98%	70%–95%
Fuchs' dystrophy triple procedure	80%–90%	70%–90%
Aphakic bullous keratoplasty	65%–90%	35%–68%
Pseudophakic bullous keratoplasty	80%–95%	16%–78%
Herpetic keratitis	67%–86%	50%–80%
Alkali burns	0%–50%	0%–30%

FIG. 2.1

Instrumentation

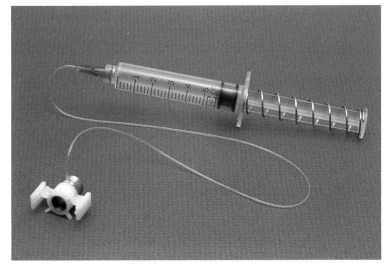

FIG. 2.2

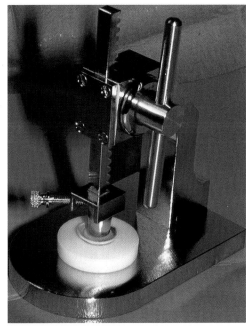

FIG. 2.3

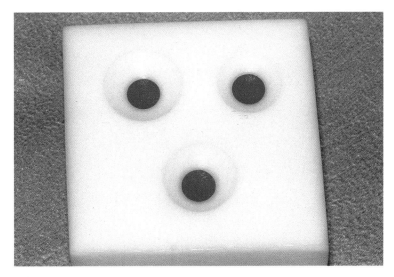

FIG. 2.4

or no play in it and allow for proper centration of the trephine on the donor button. Cutting blocks with wells of various radii (e.g., Brightbill block, Fig. 2.4) avoid distortion of the donor button. A hole in the base of the block will help drain fluid and prevent slippage of the donor button during trephination.

Stabilization of the host eye during trephination is important to ensure an even cut. If a Flieringa or other ring is used, a pair of Flieringa-Legrand fixation forceps is useful. A Thornton fixation ring is also occasionally helpful for stabilizing the globe during trephination. Figure 2.5 shows, from left to right, Flieringa rings, Flieringa-LeGrand fixation forceps, and a Thornton fixation ring. If the suction trephine is used, no additional stabilization is needed.

Scissors for completing the corneal incision should be kept very sharp and have narrow blades to minimize trauma to the iris and lens. Some surgeons find Vannas scissors or mini-Westcott scissors more satisfactory than scissors designed specifically for excising corneal tissue (Fig. 2.6, left to right).

No special forceps are needed for corneal transplantation provided that fine tooth forceps for picking up the tissue and smooth forceps for handling 10-0 or 11-0 nylon are available.

Lamellar keratoplasty can be performed with a #66 Beaver blade, a Paufique knife, or a similar instrument, but I prefer a Desmarres dissector (Fig. 2.7, left to right). An artificial anterior chamber (Fig. 2.8) makes using a corneoscleral donor segment for lamellar keratoplasty a great deal easier. Without it, it is best to use whole globes.

PREOPERATIVE PREPARATION

Corneal transplantation is often performed outside routine office hours, at nights and on weekends, when the usual hospital personnel may not be available. Hence, it is wise to anticipate administrative and logistic difficulties and to deal with them before the day of surgery. It can be useful to have all procedures and equipment specified in a written protocol for admitting officers, residents, nurses, etc. Similarly, it is important for the patient and family to be practically and psychologically prepared for the experience of the surgery prior to being called in.

Donor tissue should be evaluated as carefully as possible by the eye bank and by the surgeon prior to calling the patient in for surgery, as indicated earlier. Otherwise, the patient may have to be sent home at the last minute when the tissue is found to be unsatisfactory.

Generally, a preoperative routine of medication similar to that employed in cataract surgery is appropriate. Consider the following:

NPO prior to surgery
Prophylactic topical antibiotics
Mild preoperative sedation
Miotics, to protect the lens, in patients who will remain phakic

Mydriatics, to facilitate removal of the lens and/or vitreous, in patients who are or will be aphakic

No special efforts are necessary in prepping and draping. A separate table for preparing the donor button is necessary and its position should allow for the use of a microscope if needed.

Local anesthesia is adequate for corneal transplantation and has the value of being entirely in the hands of the surgeon. This may be an advantage if the available anesthesiologist is not familiar with ophthalmic surgery. A routine penetrating keratoplasty takes less than one hour and even the most complicated cases are feasible under local anesthetic with the use of longer-acting agents such as Marcaine. General anesthesia is appropriate for children. An important adjunct to the retrobulbar block is the use of the Honan compressor, or a similar device, to reduce the vitreous and orbital volume prior to surgery.

PREPARATION OF DONOR TISSUE

Donor tissue should be maintained at about 4°C until just prior to use. It can be kept in an ice bath in the operating room. No special warming procedures are necessary. The donor button should be prepared prior to trephining the host button.

The donor tissue, and materials coming in contact with it, should not be considered to be perfectly sterile. Hence, the instruments for obtaining and preparing the donor tissue at the back table should not be used on the patient. For medicolegal reasons, and in order to facilitate antibiotic selection should infection occur postoperatively, a sample of the donor tissue should be placed in culture medium and sent to the lab at the time of surgery.

Whole Globe Donor Tissue
The donor eye is often rather soft. In order to facilitate trephining, the pressure must be raised. This can be achieved by injecting saline into the vitreous through the optic nerve with a 30-gauge needle (Fig. 2.9). Wrapping the globe with gauze will facilitate handling the tissue and can also be used to adjust the intraocular pressure (Fig. 2.10).

Loose donor epithelium should be removed with a moistened sponge and the tissue further cleansed with a normal saline solution. Some surgeons also bathe the eye in antibiotic solution. This should be rinsed off with saline solution prior to trephination.

Trephination of the donor button can be accomplished with the Hessburg-Barron trephine or with a hand-held or motorized trephine. It is critical that the blade is sharp and, in this respect, disposable blades often have an advantage. The blade should be checked to be sure it has a good edge and is free of polishing compounds and oil prior to use.

The donor cornea should be sponged dry prior to trephination in order to diminish the tendency for the trephine to skid when pressure is applied.

Since it is not possible to know the keratometer (K) readings or visual axis of the donor tissue, centration of the tre-

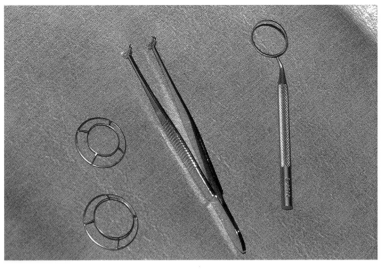

FIG. 2.5

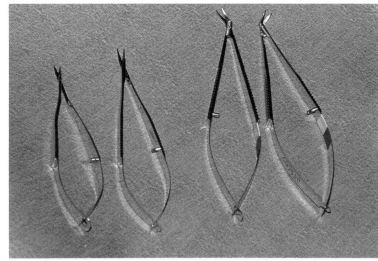

FIG. 2.6

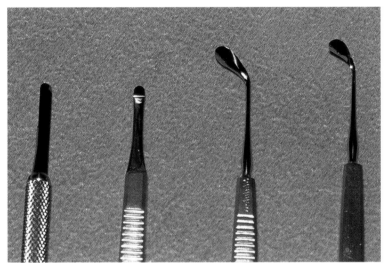

FIG. 2.7

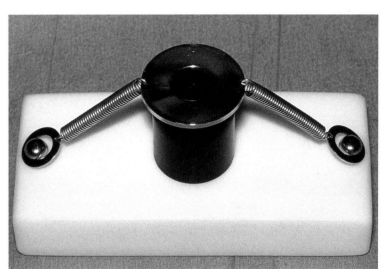

FIG. 2.8

Preoperative Preparation of Whole Globe Donor Tissue

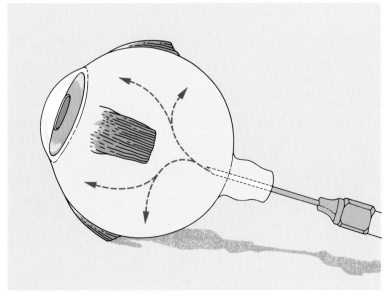

FIG. 2.9

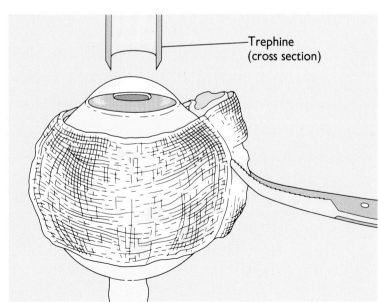

Trephine
(cross section)

FIG. 2.10

phine is best performed simply on an anatomic basis. Vertical positioning of the trephine is critical to avoid beveling of the incision (Fig. 2.11) and subsequent problems with astigmatism and wound healing. If tissue is obtained from the whole globe by trephining from the epithelial surface, trephination should be stopped as soon as the anterior chamber is entered and excision of the button completed with fine scissors, taking care not to strip Descemet's membrane and the endothelium from the button. Use of the operating microscope is helpful. The donor button is then placed in a moist chamber until it is to be used on the patient.

Corneoscleral Segment Donor Tissue

If the donor tissue is in the form of a corneoscleral segment, either preserved in MK or a similar medium, or excised at the time of surgery, the donor button can be punched from the endothelial side.

The tissue should be punched against a Teflon or other plastic block with a rounded well that is similar in curvature to the corneal tissue. It is wise to have several blocks of different curvatures in order to match the donor cornea. Centration and vertical positioning of the trephine are important (Fig. 2.12).

A very sharp trephine blade is critical. Again, if disposable blades are used, they should be checked to be sure they are clean of oil or polishing compounds and checked for defects in the edge. Regardless of whether the button is punched by hand or with a mechanical press, it is imperative that the disposable blade be properly seated in the trephine (Fig. 2.12). Otherwise, the donor button may be irregularly cut or crushed and be unusable. Once obtained, the tissue should be placed in a moist chamber until it is transferred to the patient.

SELECTION OF DONOR AND HOST TREPHINE DIAMETERS

Generally speaking, the size of the host button to be excised is that which is necessary to remove the abnormal tissue and create a clear central cornea. Usually, this will be a button of between 7 and 8.5 mm in diameter. If the button is too small, scarring from the incision and sutures may interfere with vision, and if it is too large, the tissue may approach the limbus closely enough to increase the risk of graft rejection. If the patient's endothelium is healthy, a relatively small button can be used. If the patient's endothelium is defective, there is an advantage to using a larger button as it will allow transplantation of a greater population of endothelial cells.

There are some occasions in which disparity of host and donor button size is advisable. If the donor button is punched from the endothelial surface, it is wise to use a 0.2-to-0.5-mm larger button than is used to trephine the patient due to the disparity in the posterior corneal dimensions when different trephination techniques are utilized. A heavily scarred cornea tends to be quite flat and, under these circumstances, a larger donor than host button, generally by 0.5 to 1 mm, is useful in order to maintain the anterior chamber relationships and to decrease the postkeratoplasty refractive error. Relative myopia can be induced by using substantially larger donor than host buttons or by using tissue from infants, although the refractive results are not entirely predictable.

SCLERAL SUPPORT RING

A Flieringa or similar fixation ring (Fig. 2.13) can be used to support the sclera in young aphakic patients or other patients with low scleral rigidity and an absent or damaged

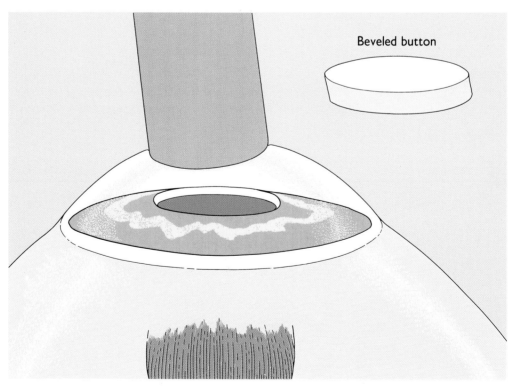

Beveled button

FIG. 2.11

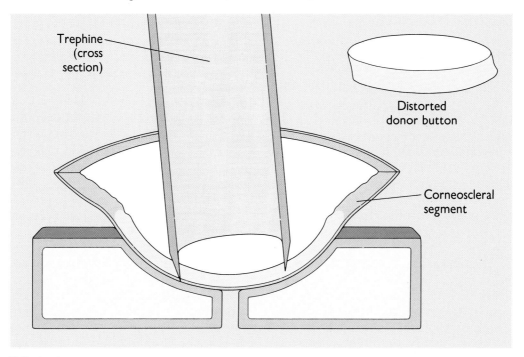

Trephine (cross section)

Distorted donor button

Corneoscleral segment

FIG. 2.12

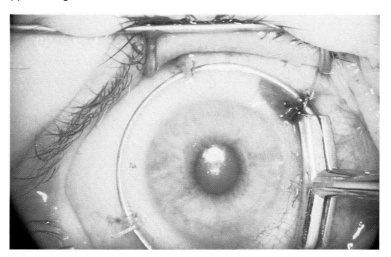

FIG. 2.13

lens–iris diaphragm. It is not necessary on routine phakic patients and usually not needed in aphakic patients over 50 years of age. The ring is secured by sutures placed through the superficial sclera and looped around the fixation rim. It is possible to distort the corneoscleral architecture in the placement of a scleral support ring. This can result in severe postoperative astigmatism. Distortion can be minimized by careful suturing and by not pulling up the sutures too tightly. Since two points can lie on any circle larger than the distance between them, the ring position can be adjusted so as to avoid distortion after placing the first two sutures. Subsequent sutures may be very carefully placed and definitely not pulled tight. The first two sutures should be placed close to the point at which the ring will be grasped for fixation with the Flieringa-LeGrand or other forceps.

HOST TREPHINATION

If a suction trephine is not used, the patient's eye should be fixed with forceps, either directly applied or applied to a fixation ring. Care must be taken not to distort the globe since it may result in high postoperative astigmatism. Trephination is ordinarily carried just to the point of entry of the anterior chamber or close to it, the depth being ascertained by judgment based on experience, by setting the obdurator in the trephine, or by seeing a gush of aqueous when the anterior chamber is entered. Cutting is best accomplished by rotating the trephine blade in one direction rather than oscillating back and forth, which may lead to irregular incisions.

If a suction trephine is used, this alone will usually suffice for fixation of the patient's eye. Care should be taken not to exert excessive pressure with the suction device since it may distort the tissue and lead to irregular cuts. With the present design of the Hessburg-Barron trephine, there is a distinct tendency for a wider posterior cut to occur when the plunger of the suction syringe is completely depressed (Figs. 2.14 and 2.15). About 3 cc of depression is appropriate in order to minimize this effect. If the cornea is heavily scarred, its surface may be too irregular for the suction trephine to hold. In this case, placement of a viscoelastic material on the surface may help.

Excision of the host button can be completed with fine scissors. If the anterior chamber has not been entered with the trephine, it can be entered with a sharp knife in the base of the trephine incision, taking care not to damage the iris and making a large enough incision so that the scissors can enter without risk of stripping Descemet's membrane. The tissue should be stabilized with forceps, taking care not to lift or pull on the tissue as it is cut, in order to minimize the chances of posterior beveling of the host cornea (Fig. 2.16). The scissors should be held so that the blades cut vertically (Figs. 2.17 and 2.18).

The host button should not be sent directly to pathology. Rather, it should be put in saline in case something happens to the donor tissue and the host button has to be replaced.

Any lip of the host tissue should be trimmed with fine scissors after the host button has been removed (Fig. 2.19).

Preoperative Preparation: Host Trephination

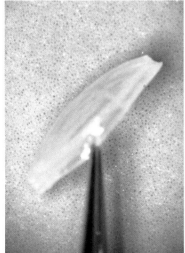

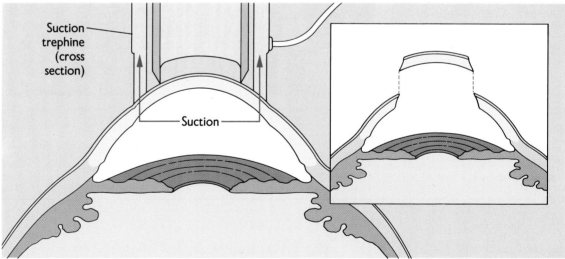

FIG. 2.14   FIG. 2.15

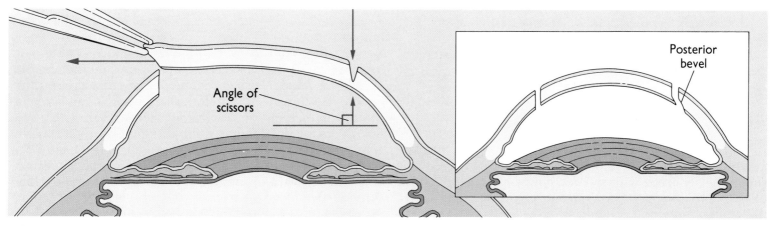

FIG. 2.16

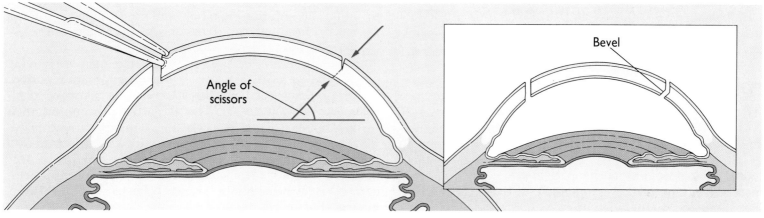

FIG. 2.17

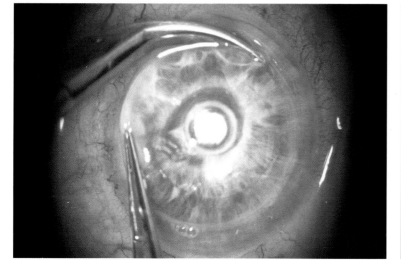

FIG. 2.18

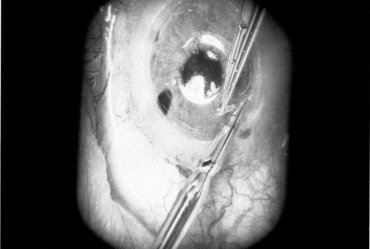

FIG. 2.19

An irregularly beveled incision induces astigmatism (Fig. 2.20).

Peripheral iridotomies may be useful if much postoperative inflammation is anticipated.

APHAKIC KERATOPLASTY

In aphakic patients, the vitreous often prolapses into the anterior chamber when the host button is removed. It should be removed with a vitrectomy unit or by placing a cannula into the posterior portion of the vitreous cavity under direct observation and aspirating liquid vitreous until the iris falls well back. Any residual formed vitreous in the anterior chamber can be removed with cellulose sponges and scissors, and the anterior chamber angle well irrigated with balanced salt solution (Fig. 2.21). Incision of iridocorneal adhesions or other repair of the iris and so forth can be accomplished at this point.

PLACEMENT OF DONOR TISSUE

After the anterior chamber architecture has been restored, if this was necessary, the donor button can be brought to the patient. It should be irrigated gently to remove any lint or other particulate matter that otherwise might inadvertently be placed inside the patient's eye. A viscoelastic material may be placed temporarily in the anterior chamber, if needed, to maintain it or to diminish bleeding, or as a safety factor, especially in pseudophakic eyes. The donor button should be sutured in place with "cardinal" interrupted sutures in the most atraumatic fashion possible so as to minimize damage to the endothelium while the anterior chamber is relatively shallow (and perhaps to decrease postoperative astigmatism). Modern sharp needles can easily be placed directly underneath fixation forceps (Fig. 2.22). This will decrease the tendency for the graft to rotate as the sutures are placed and may improve alignment. After the placement of four sutures, the anterior chamber can usually be reformed with air and/or a balanced salt solution. The surgeon should take care not to overinflate the eye since overinflation may force the iris and/or the vitreous into the wound. If a running suture is to be placed, four to eight cardinal sutures, which may or may not be subsequently removed, are helpful in order to stabilize the tissue and maintain the anterior chamber while the running suture is placed. Suture depth in excess of 50% of the corneal thickness appears to improve apposition.

A running suture has the advantage of being more quickly placed and requires less care in the postoperative period. Interrupted sutures have the advantage of allowing selective removal (Fig. 2.23). This is particularly important if healing appears likely to occur more rapidly in one quadrant than another, e.g., in a patient with a vascularized corneal bed. A combination of running and interrupted sutures may allow earlier removal of selected interrupted sutures, earlier visual rehabilitation, and, perhaps, less final astigmatism (Fig. 2.24).

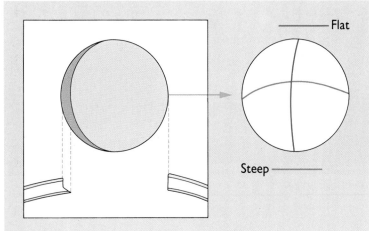
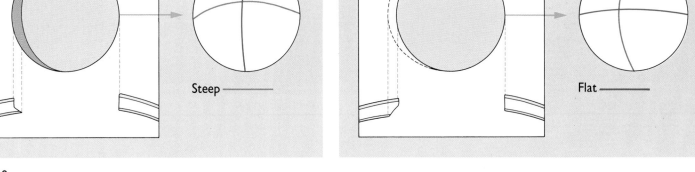

FIG. 2.20

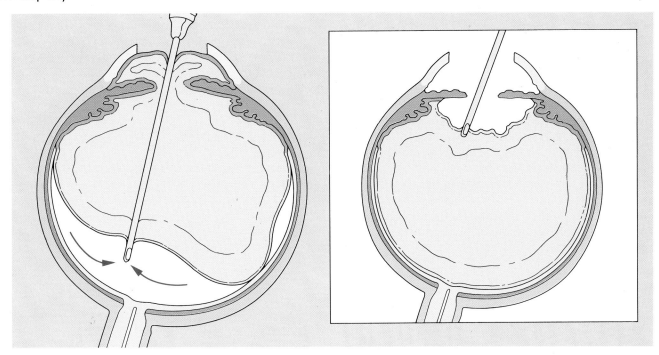

FIG. 2.21

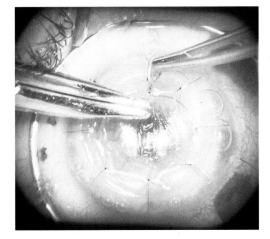

FIG. 2.22

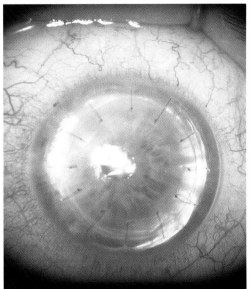

FIG. 2.23

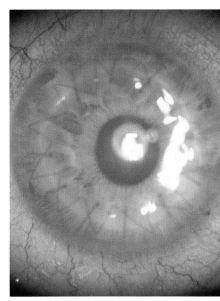

FIG. 2.24

The running suture should be pulled up, either in a single- or two-handed technique, until it is adequately tight. Judging the appropriate tension is a matter of surgical judgment. Sutures that are too tight tend to retard healing and may flatten the central cornea enough to lead to epithelial healing problems, especially in a patient with dry eye or previous inflammatory disease. If sutures are too loose, they may lead to partial wound dehiscence or frank wound leak, both of which will require subsequent repair. Care must be taken not to kink or crush the suture, especially 10-0 or 11-0 nylon, with the tying forceps since this predisposes to suture breakage (Fig. 2.25).

If knots are not cut short and buried (Fig. 2.26), either in the host or donor tissue, there will be increased postoperative inflammation, tendency to vascularization, and epithelial defects, though this tendency can be diminished by placing a soft contact lens postoperatively.

RE-FORMATION OF THE ANTERIOR CHAMBER

Following completion of suturing, air in the anterior chamber can be replaced with balanced salt solution, bringing the intraocular pressure up to normal. The wound should be inspected to be sure that it is water-tight. A slight oozing down the suture tracks is acceptable. Leaking through the wound margin should be repaired prior to termination of the procedure.

A running suture can be adjusted to minimize astigmatism, though permanent astigmatism is due more to cutting technique than suture placement.

DRESSINGS AND MEDICATIONS

The operated eye should be protected with a patch and shield for the first night at least. No special medications are required in a noncomplicated case. Consider the use of subconjunctival antibiotics and a steroid/antibiotic ointment topically as a matter of routine for prophylactic value. Cycloplegics may be of value in an inflamed eye and miotics in a patient with a lens implant present. If substantial postoperative inflammation is anticipated, subconjunctival steroids can be given; experience shows that the operated eye will tolerate topical steroids as frequently as every hour starting immediately after the surgery.

LAMELLAR KERATOPLASTY

Lamellar keratoplasty is rarely indicated in modern ophthalmology because of the relatively poor visual acuity in the early postoperative period, compared with penetrating keratoplasty, and because of substantial risk of late interface opacification. Nonetheless, it may be appropriate in patients with normal endothelium but high risk of immune reactions, in the management of recurrent pterygium, or for tectonic purposes in patients with peripheral or generalized corneal thinning.

Since there is a risk of perforation in a deep lamellar dissection with consequent need to convert to a penetrating keratoplasty, the donor button is not cut until the host bed has been prepared. Trephination of the host button should be performed carefully to the depth appropriate to encompass the pathology, at least 30% of the corneal thickness. Very careful dissection in a single plane is imperative in order to create a clear interface and decrease the risk of either perforation or of later scarring or vascularization of the interface. This can be done with a variety of knives. "Super sharp" blades are often more difficult to keep in a single interlamellar plane than are standard blades. The dissection can be carried out with the button held in its normal anatomical position (Figs. 2.27A and 2.28), or by retracting the superficial corneal tissue and dissecting in the whitish area at the base of the cleft (Figs. 2.27B and 2.29). I prefer a combination of these techniques. In either case, the blade

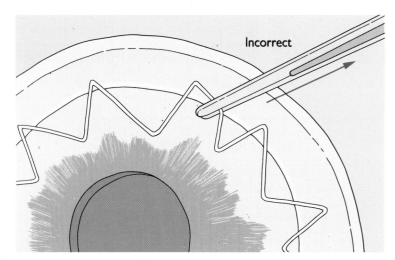

FIG. 2.25

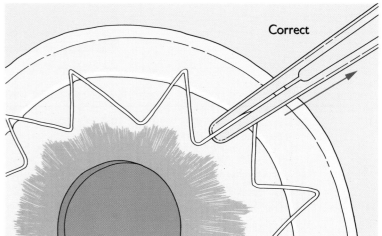

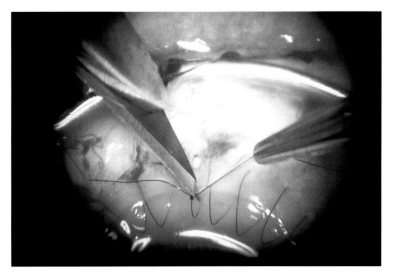

FIG. 2.26

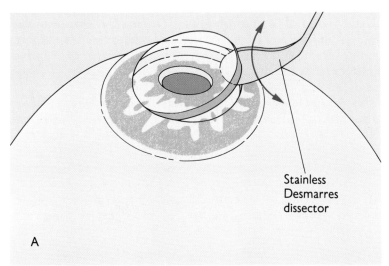
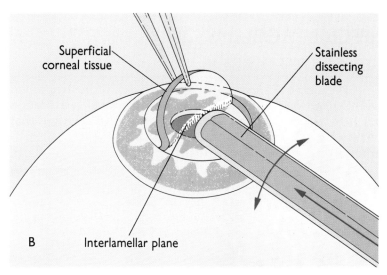

A

Stainless
Desmarres
dissector

B

Superficial
corneal tissue

Stainless
dissecting
blade

Interlamellar plane

FIG. 2.27

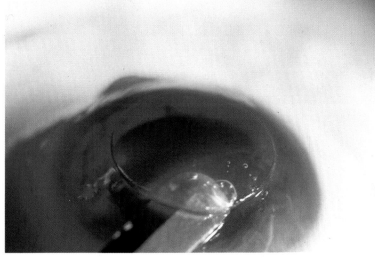
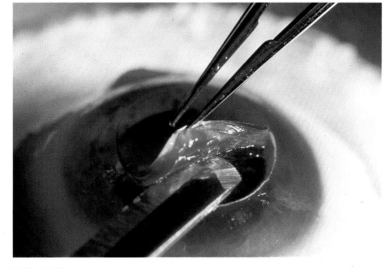

FIG. 2.28

FIG. 2.29

should be held in the plane of the corneal lamellae. The peripheral cornea should be undermined a millimeter or so in order to facilitate tight closure of the wound between host and donor.

Donor tissue is ordinarily obtained in much the same fashion as the host button is removed, though plano-"lenticules" are now becoming available commercially. All endothelium should be removed if a full-thickness button is used and care must be taken to keep the epithelium out of the interface. The interface should be irrigated thoroughly to remove debris before placing the donor button. The donor button ordinarily should be approximately 0.5 to 1.0 mm oversized. Either interrupted or running sutures can be used. The former have the distinct advantage of selective and early removal to decrease the risk of vascularization of the interface. If only corneoscleral donor tissue is available, the artificial anterior chamber allows cutting partial-thickness donor buttons (Fig. 2.30). Without it, it is extremely difficult to obtain a good donor button unless a whole globe is used.

SPECIAL PROBLEMS
PERFORATED CORNEAS

A cornea with a descemetocele can usually be trephined with a suction trephine. However, a corneal perforation leads to a relatively soft and unstable anterior segment that makes accurate trephination difficult, even with this instrument. If the perforation is small, a paracentesis incision can be used to inject air or a viscoelastic material in order to raise the intraocular pressure and stabilize the anterior segment (Fig. 2.31). Larger perforations may be temporarily closed with cyanoacrylate adhesives, if available, or a small piece of donor cornea followed by an injection of air or viscoelastic material (Fig. 2.32).

A small perforation (Fig. 2.33) is amenable to repair by lamellar keratoplasty (Fig. 2.34). With a large perforation, aqueous tends to collect in the interface.

COMBINED PROCEDURES

Intracapsular or extracapsular cataract extraction combined with penetrating keratoplasty presents no unusual problems. In younger patients, a Flieringa or similar ring should be considered, especially if intracapsular cataract extraction is anticipated. With intracapsular extraction, an extra pair of hands may be necessary to retract the iris since the pupil often comes down during excision of the host button (Figs. 2.35 and 2.36). With extracapsular extraction, there may be some difficulty in stripping all of the peripheral cortex since the iris and anterior capsule tend to collapse onto the posterior capsule. Higher flow of irrigating solution or cautious use of viscoelastic material to open the capsular bag can be helpful. Most styles of posterior chamber lenses are readily placed through a 7.5-mm or larger corneal incision. Viscoelastic material is almost always necessary to place the implant in the bag. It should be available to keep the donor endothelium away from the implant during the initial wound closure if the anterior chamber will not hold air or balanced salt solution.

Anterior chamber lenses are best placed in the vertical or horizontal meridians since they may induce some astigmatism, especially if the corneal suturing is tight, and it is easier for the patient to deal with a regular than an oblique astigmatism. Implant power selection may require using the K readings from the opposite eye if they cannot be obtained for the operated eye. With time, the surgeon may also be able to develop a "fudge factor" to adjust for his own technique.

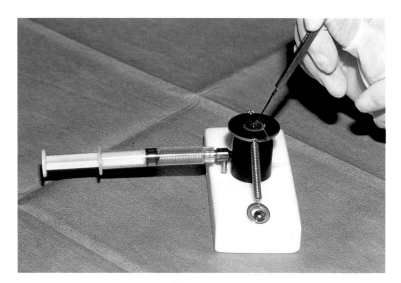

FIG. 2.30

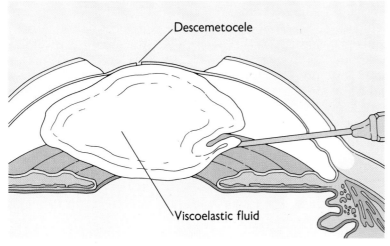

FIG. 2.31

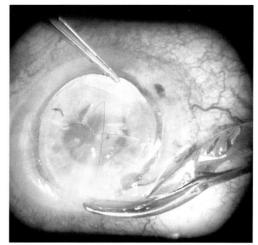

FIG. 2.32

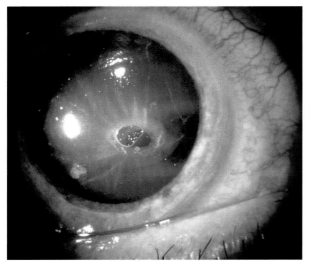

FIG. 2.33

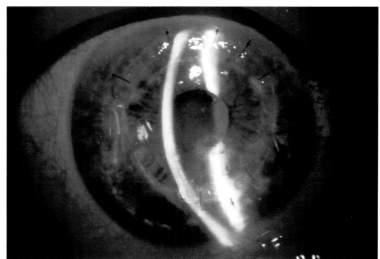

FIG. 2.34

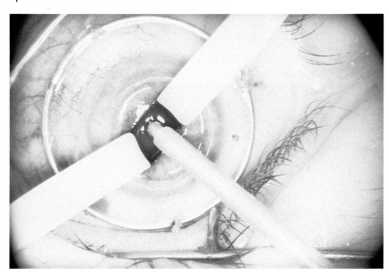

FIG. 2.35

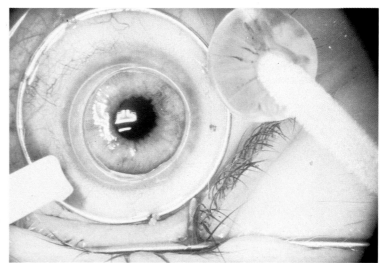

FIG. 2.36

CORNEOSCLERAL GRAFTS

Corneoscleral grafts required for trauma, ulceration, tumors, epithelial downgrowth, etc., may have to be partially or completely hand-cut. If donor sclera is included, care must be taken to clean off uveal, conjunctival, and episcleral tissue in order to reduce the risk of infection. Apposition of scleral edges must be exact since sclera does not swell in the same fashion as corneal tissue and wound leakage can be a problem. Corneoscleral grafts tend to induce some astigmatism, often an irregular astigmatism, which makes it difficult to fit contact lenses later. Interrupted sutures are preferable in corneoscleral grafts since the rate of healing often varies at different portions of the wound. Because corneoscleral grafts have a high incidence of graft rejection, it is best if they can be kept out of the visual axis and involve a minimum of host cornea. Figures 2.37 to 2.39 show a penetrating keratoscleroplasty for an epithelial cyst.

POSTOPERATIVE COMPLICATIONS

A comprehensive consideration of postoperative complications is beyond the scope of this book. However, several important complications have been included to close the chapter.

Primary Donor Failure

With current eye bank techniques, it is unlikely that tissue will fail to survive the transplantation process. However, if the donor button is severely edematous on the first postoperative day and does not clear during the next five or six days (Fig. 2.40), there is no advantage to waiting any longer to repeat the graft, except to control excessive inflammation, glaucoma, or other problems that might compromise the results of the repeat graft. If surgery is repeated within several months, it is generally easy simply to lift out the failed graft after removing the sutures and replace it with a new donor button of the same size.

Wound Leaks

A positive Seidel test is occasionally seen for a day or two after surgery at one or more suture tracks in the host tissue. It should not require treatment other than patching if the anterior chamber is deep and the intraocular pressure is normal. Persistent leaks or leaks through the wound margin should be repaired with additional sutures to decrease the risk of endophthalmitis, epithelial downgrowth, glaucoma, and graft failure. This can be performed under topical anesthesia. A wound leak that leads to anterior synechiae should

be carefully repaired with restoration of the anterior chamber architecture since it may contribute to progressive angle closure and irreversible glaucoma.

Wound dehiscences usually occur after suture removal. I have seen this occur when the suture was removed as long as 3 years after surgery. This happens in part because of posterior beveling or other imperfections in the wound and in part because the surgeon cannot tell absolutely when the wound is adequately healed. Some clues exist, however: a suture that is loose is not contributing to wound strength and can and should be removed since it tends to excite inflammation, melting, microabscess formation, and vascularization. A wound that is compact and scarred or vascularized is probably healed. If the margins of the donor and host are edematous, the wound is probably not healed. Generally, I am reluctant, except in children, to remove running sutures before 6 months. Interrupted sutures can be removed selectively as the wound appears to heal. Interrupted sutures and loose sutures tend to lead to more rapid wound healing than running sutures and tight sutures.

Epithelial Defects

If epithelial defects are seen on the first postoperative day, the eye should be patched, or a soft lens applied, and topical medications minimized if possible in order to promote epithelial healing. This is especially true in eyes with herpetic disease, burns, or dry eye states since these types are prone to develop defects that persist for weeks and months if epithelial healing cannot be accomplished within a week or so of surgery.

Rejection

Graft rejection is the major cause of graft failure. Although rejection episodes are not entirely preventable, their prompt recognition and treatment can limit endothelial damage. It is important for the patient to recognize the symptoms of graft reaction and to have prompt access to his surgeon. Appropriately treated, grafts can survive a rejection episode and continue to be clear for many years.

Any episode of anterior segment inflammation accompanied by increasing graft edema should be considered to be a rejection episode and treated as such. Generally, so should any anterior uveitis. However, the hallmark of endothelial graft rejection is the endothelial rejection line with sectorial graft edema (Fig. 2.41). Diffuse endothelial rejection (Fig. 2.42) also can occur, often with keratic precipitates on the endothelium. No matter how edematous the cornea appears, the episode should always be treated as if

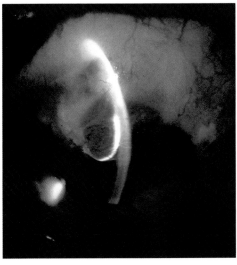

FIG. 2.37

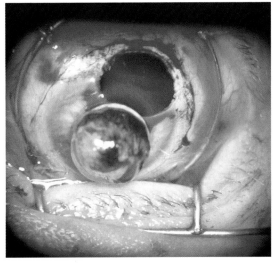

FIG. 2.38

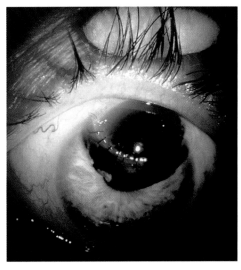

FIG. 2.39

Special Problems: Primary Donor Failure

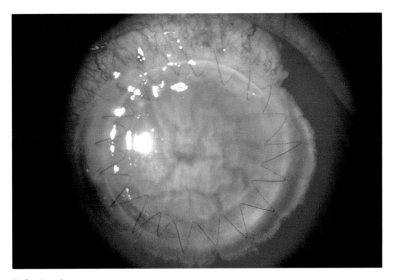

FIG. 2.40

Special Problems: Rejection

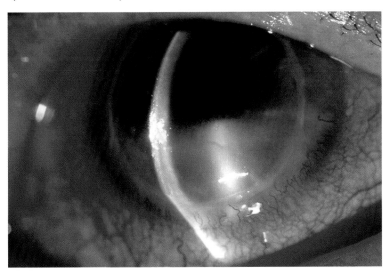

FIG. 2.41

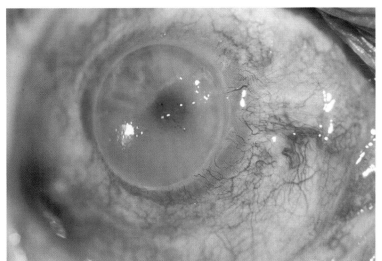

FIG. 2.42

it were reversible. Figure 2.43 shows the same eye as Fig. 2.42 after 2 weeks of treatment. I administer corticosteroid drops hourly while the patient is awake for at least a week before tapering, reserve depot steroids for those patients who cannot be relied upon to take their drops regularly, and rarely administer systemic steroids.

Epithelial rejection episodes (Fig. 2.44) are less serious since they do not lead to graft failure. This is true of the "subepithelial infiltrates" (stromal rejection, Fig. 2.45) that can easily be overlooked if the graft is not examined with oblique and diffuse illumination. Epithelial rejection lines and subepithelial infiltrates may be harbingers of an endothelial rejection episode, however. I treat both of these reactions with lower-dose steroids, usually one drop four times daily and tapering, and follow the patient closely.

Astigmatism

Until the sutures are removed, they will induce some astigmatism. In smaller grafts, this may be irregular enough in the center of the cornea to affect spectacle acuity. Once the sutures have been removed, the corneal topography will generally stabilize in 3 to 6 weeks and the final prescription can be given. If the patient cannot be adequately corrected with spectacles or a contact lens, refractive surgery should be considered to modify the shape of the cornea. The use of a corneoscope, which creates a topographical map of the cornea (Fig. 2.46), is especially useful in visualizing which areas of the graft are steep or flat. A placido disk is almost as useful. A keratometer has limited value.

Currently, the major approaches to modifying graft astigmatism include relaxing incisions, with or without compression sutures, wedge resections, and modifications of the Ruiz procedure.

In my experience, relaxing incisions are effective and allow for future modification. Hence, they should be tried first. A diamond knife incision to 80% of the corneal thickness (as measured by a pachymeter), just inside the wound, extending one to two hours on either side of the steep meridian at each end, gives 4.00 to 8.00 D of flattening in that meridian (Fig. 2.47).

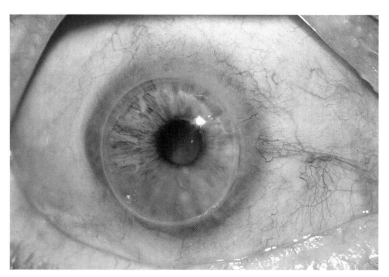

FIG. 2.43

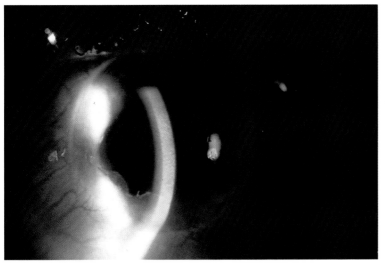

FIG. 2.44

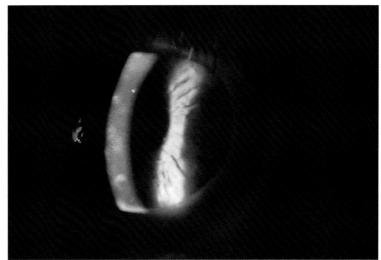

FIG. 2.45

Special Problems: Astigmatism

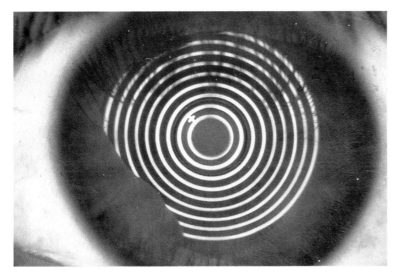

FIG. 2.46

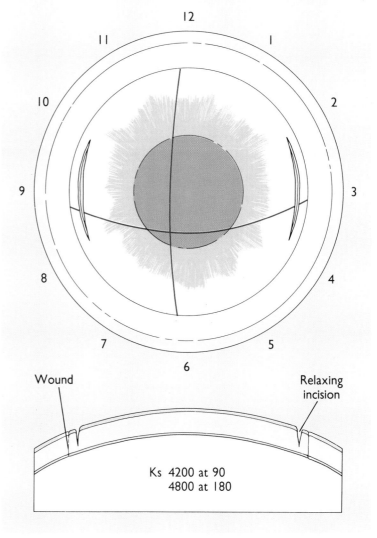

Wound

Relaxing incision

Ks 4200 at 90
4800 at 180

FIG. 2.47

If there is a big posterior lip in the donor tissue in that meridian, the effect may be much less, even nil. Under these circumstances, and in general, the effect of the relaxing incisions can be augmented by compression sutures in the opposite meridian. I prefer 9-0 nylon for this and tight sutures overcorrecting by about 100% since the effect tends to biodegrade.

Wedge resections can correct more astigmatism but are more difficult to perform and easily lead to overcorrections. They can induce some myopia. Wedge resections must be performed in the operating room with retrobulbar or general anesthesia, whereas relaxing incisions and augmentation sutures can be performed in the office or minor operating room, respectively.

For wedge resections, I excise a 3 o'clock, 80% depth, crescentic wedge using a diamond blade and Vannas scissors. The wedge is about 1 mm wide at the center, in the flattest meridian, and closed with 10-0 nylon. The incision is placed in the wound scar and the wedge then excised from the inside edge. Perforation is not a serious problem since the new incision is closed with sutures anyway. I generally reserve this procedure for cases where there is

clearly excess host tissue in the form of a posterior lip. The effect achieved is variable but keratometric monitoring with a 6.00-to-8.00-D overcorrection seems satisfactory (Fig. 2.48).

The Ruiz procedure, or trapezoidal procedure, is especially useful in patients who have induced myopia since it leads to flattening in two meridians. The amount of flattening depends primarily on how closely the semiradial incisions approach the visual axis and can be increased by paired tangential incisions. Although the results are variable, the overall effect of the semiradial incisions, performed at 80% of the central corneal thickness, appears to be approximately 4.50 D in the meridian of the incisions and 3.50 D at 90° for a 3-mm optical zone and 3.00 and 1.00 D, respectively, for a 5-mm optical zone. A single pair of tangential incisions done 5 mm apart roughly doubles the effect. The semiradial incisions are ordinarily made two clock hours apart (Fig. 2.49).

In summary, the results of refractive surgery following penetrating keratoplasty are quite variable and attention to detail during the initial keratoplasty is consequently well worthwhile.

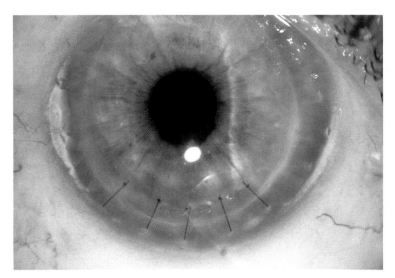

FIG. 2.48

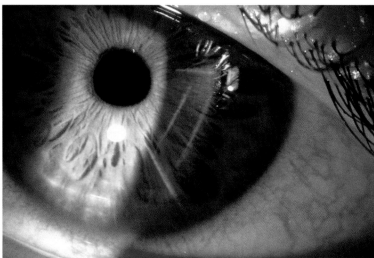

FIG. 2.49

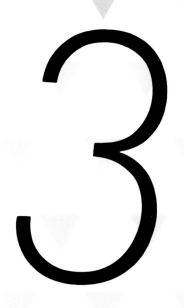

SURGERY FOR GLAUCOMA AND RELATED CONDITIONS

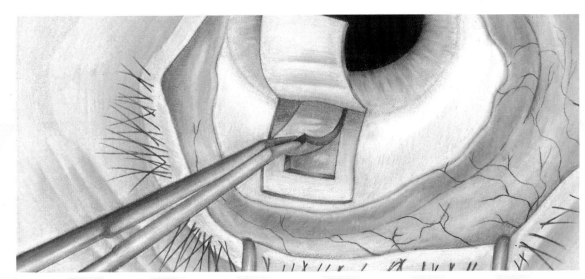

George Nardin, MD

Thom J. Zimmerman, MD, PhD

Recent advances in the fields of biochemistry, pharmacology, physiology, and physics have brought a better understanding of surgical procedures to treat glaucoma and related conditions. In the wake of the advances have come a variety of new pharmacologic agents, new lenses, new devices and new surgical instruments. Despite the many new tools available, the approach to management of the glaucoma patient has remained fairly constant. The management of angle closure glaucoma is still primarily surgical, though laser treatment has largely supplanted conventional surgical intervention. Congenital glaucoma, likewise, remains a disease treated by surgical intervention. Open angle glaucoma is treated medically in this country unless medical therapy is proven ineffective in arresting progression of the disease. When this occurs, we resort to laser surgery and eventually to conventional surgery if laser and medical management do not control the disease.

PRIMARY AND SECONDARY OPEN ANGLE AND CHRONIC ANGLE CLOSURE GLAUCOMAS

PENETRATING TRABECULECTOMY

When a patient with primary or secondary open angle glaucoma or chronic angle closure glaucoma has poorly controlled pressure, progressive visual field loss, and optic nerve damage on maximally tolerated medical therapy, and an argon laser trabeculoplasty has failed to lower adequately the intraocular pressure, a trabeculectomy is felt to be the surgical procedure of choice. To perform a penetrating trabeculectomy, a fornix-based conjunctival flap is fashioned for approximately the superior 180° (Fig. 3.1). This flap is bluntly dissected back from the limbus using round-tipped Westcott scissors. The superonasal and superotemporal quadrants are opened using blunt section with the Westcott scissors posterior to the equator of the globe (Fig. 3.2). When this is done, light cautery is applied to achieve hemostasis. The remaining tags of Tenon's capsule are removed from the episclera.

A superonasal or superotemporal site is usually selected for performing the trabeculectomy. A 5 by 5-mm superficial scleral flap is fashioned of about 20% scleral thickness and hinged 1 mm onto clear cornea (Figs. 3.3 and 3.4). When this is done, a microsharp blade or a diamond tip blade is used to cut a 2 by 4-mm block beginning at the base of the superficial scleral flap and extending posteriorly 2 mm into the trabecular meshwork then extending along the limbus approximately 4 mm (Fig. 3.5). The block is completely excised, leaving an unobstructed fistula into the anterior chamber (Fig. 3.6). When this is completed, the iris is grasped through the trabeculectomy site and pulled through it. A large peripheral iridectomy is fashioned, tak-

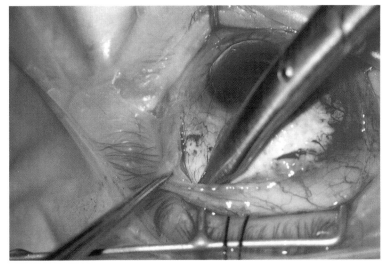

FIG. 3.1

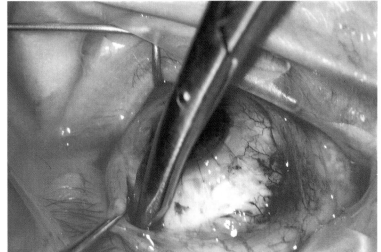

FIG. 3.2

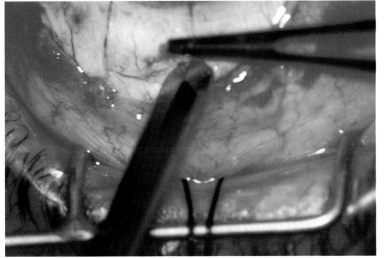

FIG. 3.3

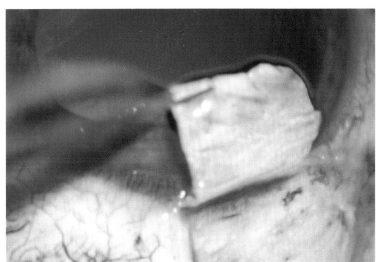

FIG. 3.4

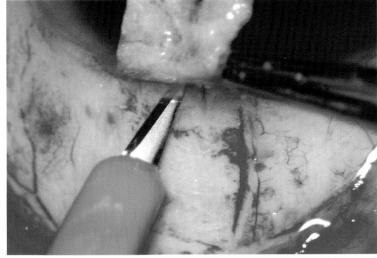

FIG. 3.5

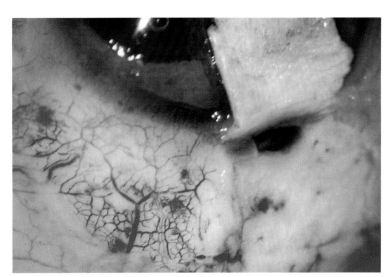

FIG. 3.6

ing care not to entrap ciliary processes (Figs. 3.7 and 3.8). Should ciliary processes be excised at this time, extensive bleeding will occur.

On completing the iridectomy, the iris is replaced in the eye. The superficial scleral flap is put back into position and tacked into place with 10-0 nylon sutures (Fig. 3.9). This is done loosely so as not to create corneal astigmatism or to seal the trabeculectomy site. The conjunctiva is then brought down over the trabeculectomy and tacked at approximately the 9 and 3 o'clock positions. This too must not be sutured too tightly or the site of the trabeculectomy may develop rapid fibrosis and lead to failure. At the end, the anterior chamber may be reformed as necessary by injecting balanced salt solution through a paracentesis site.

NONPENETRATING TRABECULECTOMY

The first steps in performing a nonpenetrating trabeculectomy are similar to those performed in a standard penetrating trabeculectomy. First, a 180° conjunctival peritomy is fashioned superiorly and dissected back from the limbus and both superonasal and superotemporal quadrants are opened. Hemostasis is again achieved using very light cautery, taking care not to scorch the scleral bed. The superonasal or superotemporal site is selected and a 5 by 5-mm superficial scleral flap is outlined using a No. 69 or 64 beaver blade (Fig. 3.10). When this is done, a flap of approximately 20% thickness is dissected forward and hinged into clear cornea (Fig. 3.11). This superficial flap is then folded back onto the cornea and a 4 by 4-mm deep scleral block is outlined extending from the very base of the superficial flap posteriorly about 4 mm. It is dissected with a 15° microsharp blade (Fig. 3.12) or a diamond-tip blade. This incision is carried down in scratch fashion to a depth just superficial to the choroid and ciliary body.

The posterior portion of the wound is grasped and a flap is created and carried forward at the depth just superficial to the ciliary body/choroid. As the flap is brought forward, the first recognizable anatomical landmark will be the scleral spur, where the fairly random orientation of the

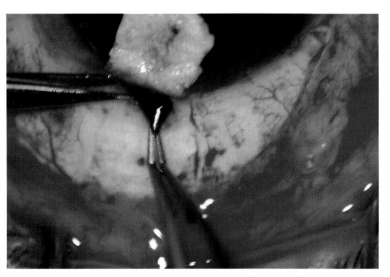

FIG. 3.7

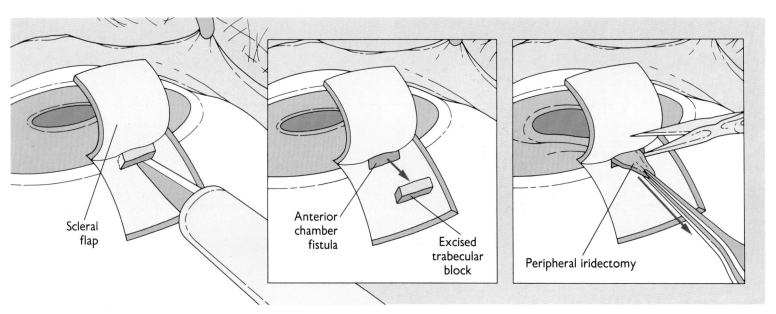

Scleral flap

Anterior chamber fistula

Excised trabecular block

Peripheral iridectomy

FIG. 3.8

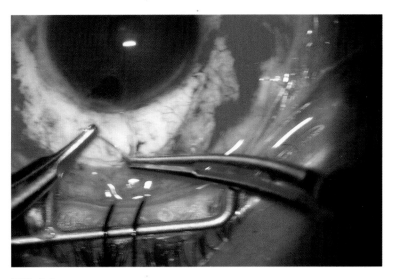

FIG. 3.9

Nonpenetrating Trabeculectomy

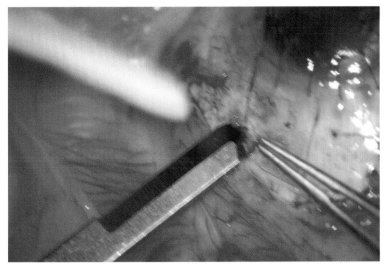

FIG. 3.10

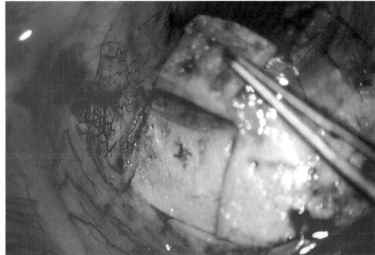

FIG. 3.11

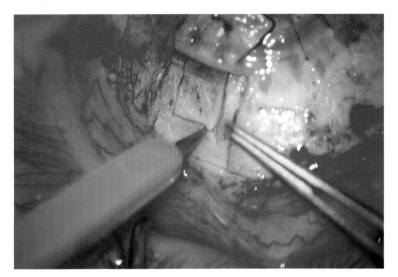

FIG. 3.12

scleral fibers will begin to take on a circumferential appearance (Fig. 3.13). In this region, sections of the margins of the flap will transect Schlemm's canal and a small amount of oozing of blood may be noted from the cut ends of Schlemm's canal. Beyond this point, the dissection of the flap is carried into the cornea by peeling the corneal lamellae apart (Fig. 3.14). As the dissection is carried over the trabecular meshwork, the percolation of aqueous fluid through the remaining thin layer of uveal trabecular meshwork will be noted. Without pulling excessively on this deep scleral flap, it is dissected forward to the base of the superficial flap and then amputated using Vannas scissors, taking care not to leave a large stump (Fig. 3.15).

At this point, aqueous fluid should be noted to percolate continuously through the trabecular meshwork, which can be recognized as a fine diaphenous membrane. In most cases this can be accomplished without total collapse of the anterior chamber. At this point, the superficial scleral flap is brought over the deep bed and tacked with two interrupted 10-0 nylon sutures (Fig. 3.16). The conjunctiva is then returned to the limbus and tacked at approximately the 3 and 9 o'clock positions with 8-0 Vicryl sutures. Twenty milligrams of Garamycin and 2 mg of Decadron are injected into the sub-Tenon's space of the lower fornix, taking care not to exert pressure on the globe.

POSTERIOR LIP SCLERECTOMY

When an unguarded filtering procedure is desirable in the surgical management of glaucoma, a posterior lip sclerectomy may be done. This may be done as a procedure by itself or in conjunction with cataract surgery. When doing this as a procedure by itself, a limbal-based conjunctival flap is fashioned by incising the conjunctiva approximately 5 to 6 mm posterior to the limbus along its superior 160°. The conjunctiva and Tenon's capsule are dissected cleanly to the limbus, with care being taken to prevent any buttonholing of these tissues. When the flap is brought to the anterior limbus, a No. 64 or 69 beaver blade is used to scrape free any remaining Tenon's tags. A paracentesis is done using a No. 75 microsharp blade at the temporal limbus. A midlimbal incision approximately 3 to 4 mm in length is made (Fig. 3.17). The posterior lip of this wound is grasped using 0.12-mm toothed forceps. A scleral punch (Holth), a microsharp blade, a pair of Vannas scissors, or a diamond-tip blade is then used to remove an approximately 1.5-to-2-mm full-thickness bite from the posterior scleral lip (Fig. 3.18).

When this is accomplished the wound is released and the sclerectomy site is examined to ensure that a full-thickness ostium into the anterior chamber has been made (Fig. 3.19). An iridectomy is fashioned at the site using a pair of toothed forceps and Vannas scisssors (Fig. 3.20). If the

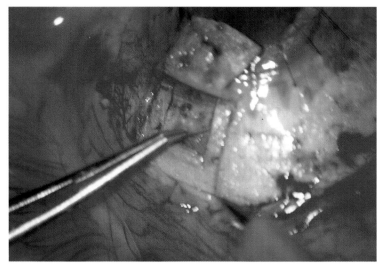

FIG. 3.13

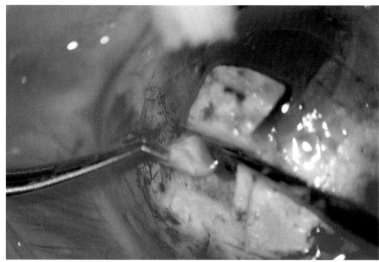

FIG. 3.14

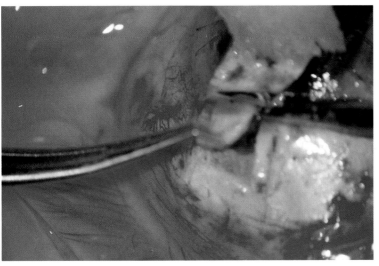

FIG. 3.15

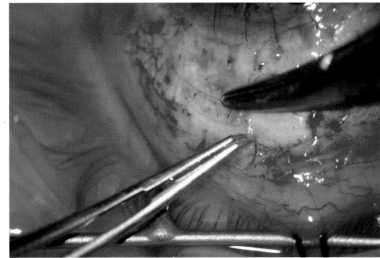

FIG. 3.16

Posterior Lip Sclerectomy

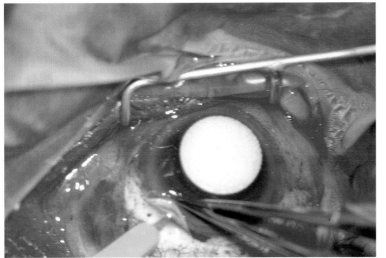

FIG. 3.17

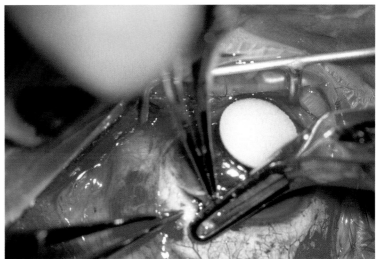

FIG. 3.18

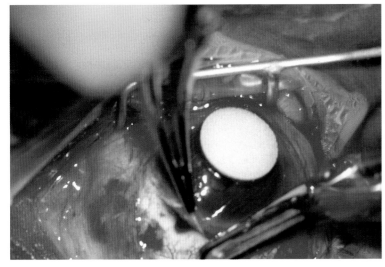

FIG. 3.19

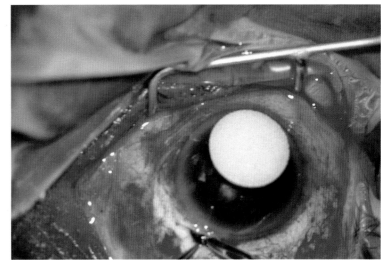

FIG. 3.20

wound tends to gape, a 10-0 nylon suture is used to approximate the wound without closing the sclerectomy site. Following this, the conjunctiva is carefully sutured in watertight fashion along its entire length using an 8-0 Vicryl suture (Fig. 3.21). The anterior chamber is reformed using balanced salt solution injected through the paracentesis site. At this point, an obvious bleb should be present.

The eye should be patched and shielded to prevent inadvertent application of pressure to the globe. A frequent complication of this procedure is persistent oozing of blood from the sclerectomy site. Moderate cautery may be applied to the sclerectomy site to curtail hemorrhaging. Application of cautery may be used to enlarge the sclerectomy site to improve aqueous outflow. Occasionally, because of the positioning of the initial incision, not enough tissue is able to be removed from the posterior lip of the wound to create an adequate opening. When this occurs, a small portion of the anterior lip may be removed to enlarge the filtration site. When this is done, extreme care must be taken not to buttonhole the conjunctiva at its limbal insertion.

When a posterior lip sclerectomy is to be done in conjunction with cataract surgery, a fornix-based conjunctival flap is fashioned for approximately 180° superiorly as is done for standard cataract surgery. A midlimbal groove is then fashioned. A paracentesis is performed using a No. 75 microsharp blade at the temporal limbus. An anterior capsulotomy is fashioned, the lens nucleus delivered, the cortex aspirated, and the lens implant inserted as is done in routine extracapsular surgery. A site is selected for the location of the sclerectomy and a Holth punch is used to remove a bite from the posterior wound margin. The cataract wound is then resutured with 10-0 nylon sutures, being careful to leave the sclerectomy site patent. A peripheral iridectomy is done at this region, and the conjunctiva is brought down over the sclerectomy site and resutured at approximately the 9 and 3 o'clock positions. When this is complete, the anterior chamber is reformed if necessary using balanced salt solution injected through the paracentesis site.

CILIARY BODY DESTRUCTIVE PROCEDURES

Ciliary body destructive procedures are a group of procedures used to control intraocular pressure and are usually employed as a last resort in certain types of intractable glaucoma. Typically, they are used in absolute glaucoma with uncontrolled pressures and a painful eye, in neovascular glaucoma when other procedures have failed, in aphakic glaucoma, and in other sorts of secondary glaucomas that have not been controlled by standard medical or surgical therapy. All of these procedures have in common the goal of destruction of the ciliary body and secondarily decreasing aqueous production, thereby lowering intraocular pressure.

CYCLODIATHERMY

Cyclodiathermy may be done by one of two means, either penetrating or nonpenetrating. In penetrating cyclodiathermy, the conjunctiva is incised approximately 5 mm posterior to the limbus and parallel to it. The conjunctiva is dissected free along 180° of the limbus down to the level of the episclera. The sclera is dried and a penetrating diathermy electrode is applied to the sclera along an arc approximately 5 to 6 mm from the limbus. About 15 applications are applied in two rows about 2 mm apart. The conjunctiva is then closed using a running 8-0 Vicryl suture. A variation of this procedure is to use a 1-mm electrode applied directly through the conjunctiva with no incisions made. The diathermy applications are spaced approximately 4 to 5 mm from the limbus in a fashioned cover of approximately 180° as well. Each probe application is kept in contact with the globe for approximately 10 s.

CYCLOCRYOTHERAPY

Because of the extreme destructive nature of cyclodiathermy to both the conjunctiva and sclera in addition to the desired effect on the ciliary body, this procedure has been largely supplanted by cyclocryotherapy. A retinal cryoprobe with a temperature of −80°C is applied in approximately six confluent applications for approximately 180° over the region of the ciliary body approximately 4 to 5 mm posterior to the limbus (Figs. 3.22 and 3.23). The application time is 1 to 1½ minutes. Care should be taken to avoid application over the site of the rectus muscle insertions.

ANGLE CLOSURE GLAUCOMA
SURGICAL PERIPHERAL IRIDECTOMY

In recent years, the availability of argon and Neodymium-YAG lasers has largely supplanted the need for surgical intervention in the presence of narrow angle, acute angle closure, or chronic angle closure glaucoma. Despite this, the need for surgical peripheral iridectomy occasionally still arises.

To perform this procedure, the patient is anesthetized (with a retrobulbar anesthetic and lid block) as for other types of intraocular surgery. A fixation suture is put into place after a lid speculum is inserted. After a small conjunctival peritomy is formed, a 2-to-3-mm limbal incision is fashioned using a microsharp surgical blade. Light pressure is applied to the posterior margin of the incision in an attempt to allow aqueous out of the wound and to wash the iris to the incision. This allows easy grasping of the iris tissue without reaching into the anterior chamber. If this cannot be accomplished, curved Colibri-type forceps is inserted through the incision and the iris is delicately grasped at approximately the junction between the outer one-quarter of the iris and the inner three-quarters. Care must be taken not to grasp or damage underlying zonules, vitreous, or lens capsules. A small knuckle of the iris is brought to the wound

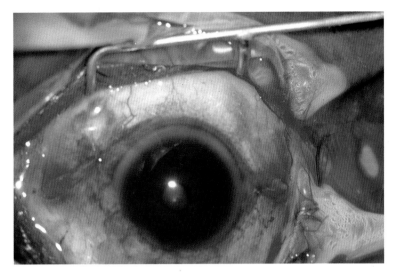

FIG. 3.21

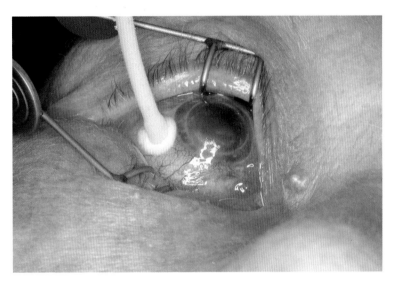

FIG. 3.22

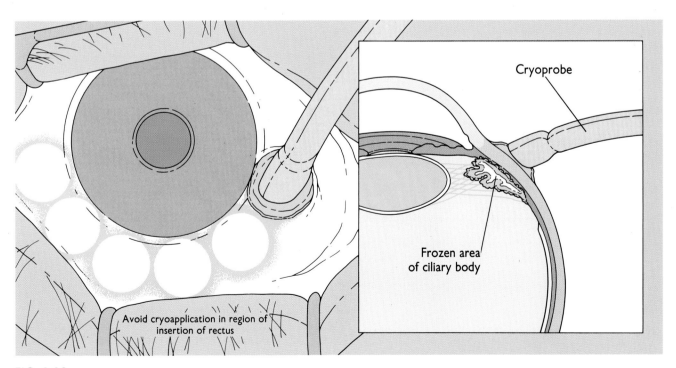

Cryoprobe

Frozen area
of ciliary body

Avoid cryoapplication in region of
insertion of rectus

FIG. 3.23

and out (Fig. 3.24A). Iridectomy scissors (Vannas) are then used to excise a full-thickness portion of the peripheral iris (Fig. 3.24B). Excising a portion of the iris centrally runs the risk of damaging the lens capsule; an excision too peripheral risks damaging the greater vascular circle of the iris. When the iridectomy is completed, balanced salt solution is used to irrigate the iris back into the eye (Fig. 3.24C). The resumption of a round pupil to its proper position is a helpful indicator that the iris tissue is not still incarcerated in the wound. When this is done, the corneal incision is sutured with one or two interrupted 10-0 nylon sutures.

SURGICAL IRIDOTOMY

A surgical iridotomy is carried out in much the same manner as the surgical iridectomy. Again, an approximately 2-to-3-mm limbal incision is fashioned after anesthesia of the globe is achieved and the conjunctiva is taken down. Light pressure is applied to the posterior margin of the incision in an attempt to allow aqueous out of the wound and to wash the iris to the incisions. This allows easy grasping of the iris tissue without reaching into the anterior chamber. If this cannot be accomplished, curved Colibri forceps is inserted through the incision and the iris is delicately grasped at approximately the junction between the outer one-quarter of the iris and the inner three-quarters. The grasped knuckle of peripheral iris is brought to the wound and out. The iridectomy scissors are then used to incise the iris, making one incision perpendicular to the limbus, thereby creating an iridotomy without excision of iris tissue (Fig. 3.25). When this is done, the iris is manipulated back into the anterior chamber using balanced salt solution and again the limbal incision is sutured closed using 10-0 nylon sutures.

CONGENITAL GLAUCOMA

Congenital glaucoma is a disease entirely different from adult-onset glaucoma. Because of the maldevelopment of the anterior chamber angle and the trabecular meshwork, this disease is poorly responsive to standard glaucoma med-

ical therapy. Rarely are agents that reduce the rate of aqueous secretion and that improve aqueous outflow effective in long-term management. Surgical intervention is the treatment of choice for this disease.

GONIOTOMY

Goniotomy is a technically difficult procedure, requiring both an accomplished surgeon and a facile assistant. To perform this procedure, a corneal contact lens allowing direct visualization of the angle structures (Koeppe-type lens), a suspended slit-lamp biomicroscope, and a goniotomy knife (Barkan or Maumenee type) are required. The pupil is made as miotic as possible using pilocarpine; the corneal contact lens is placed on the eye using Healon as a coupling agent (Fig. 3.26A). Balanced salt solution may be used if Healon is unavailable. If the cornea is edematous or hazy due to elevated intraocular pressure, the epithelium may be denuded for better visualization. The assistant surgeon fixates the globe using toothed forceps at approximately the 12 and 6 o'clock limbi. The surgeon uses one hand to control the position of the contact lens and the assistant then rotates the eye to the appropriate position to allow the surgeon maximal visualization of the angle.

The goniotomy knife is used to enter the anterior chamber at the limbus in an oblique direction approximately 1 mm anterior to the limbus (Fig. 3.26B and C). The penetration into the anterior chamber is usually done from the temporal aspect of the eye. Healon may be used to maintain the anterior chamber. The knife is passed carefully across the anterior chamber under direct visualization and the point of the blade is inserted just posterior to Schwalbe's line (Fig. 3.27A). The blade is then moved in the counterclockwise position for approximately one-third of the circumference of the anterior chamber, the blade being inserted only superficially into the angle tissue (Fig. 3.27B). After a counterclockwise sweep of the blade is fashioned, a clockwise sweep over approximately the same distance is performed (Fig. 3.27C). When the angle incision is completed, the knife is withdrawn, avoiding the iris and lens tissue.

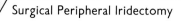
Surgical Peripheral Iridectomy

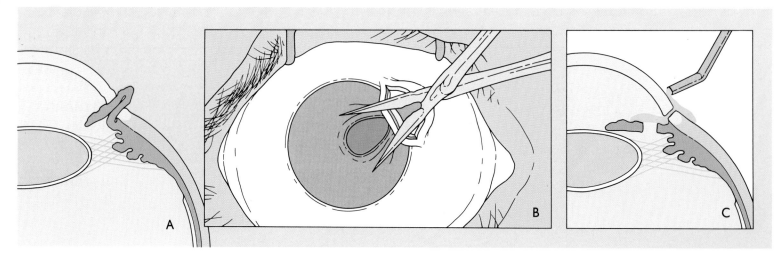

A   B   C

FIG. 3.24

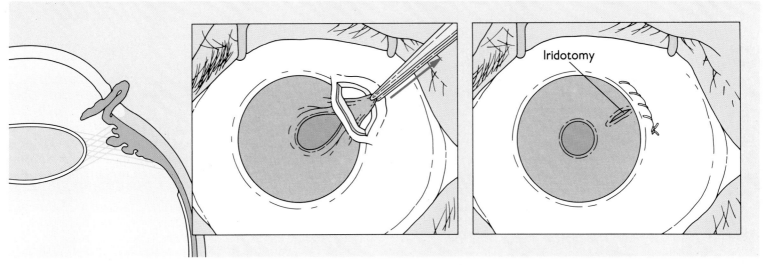

FIG. 3.25

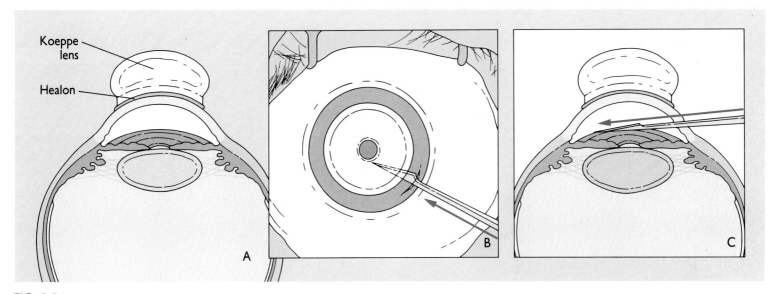

FIG. 3.26

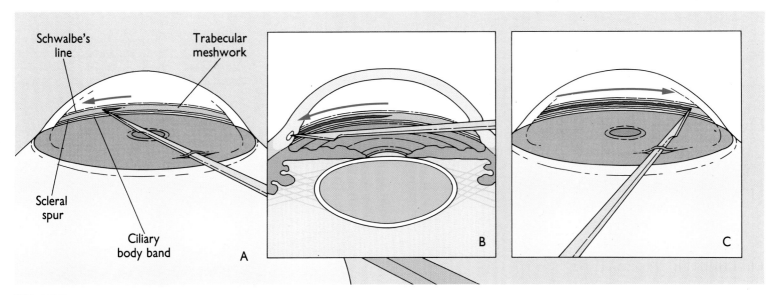

FIG. 3.27

An alternative method for performing goniotomy uses slightly different instrumentation. Here 4-0 silk sutures are placed in the superior and inferior recti for stabilization of the globe. A Swan-Jacobson lens (Fig. 3.28) is used in conjunction with the standard operating microscope for visualization. The microscope is brought into place and the Swan-Jacobson lens placed on the cornea. While visualizing the angle through the operating microscope, a Maumenee goniotomy knife cannula attached to an irrigating handpiece (Fig. 3.29) is inserted through the temporal limbus (Fig. 3.30A). At the same time, the assistant fixates the globe with superior and inferior recti stay sutures. The irrigating cannula is attached to the handpiece and irrigation is provided by BSS through a syringe controlled by the assistant. The surgeon, holding the contact lens in one hand and the Maumenee goniotomy handpiece in the other, inserts the blade into the nasal trabecular meshwork (Fig. 3.30B). Under visualization through the operating microscope, the meshwork is incised in a counterclockwise fashion as far as possible. The goniotomy blade is then rotated in the opposite direction as far as it can be visualized (Fig. 3.30C). While this is being done the assistant maintains the chamber with a slow gentle irrigation of BSS through the cannula. When the goniotomy is completed, the knife is removed from the anterior chamber and 10-0 nylon suture is put through the wound to seal it.

GONIOPUNCTURE

The technique for performing goniopuncture is somewhat similar to that used for goniotomy. The Tenon's capsule and conjunctiva are ballooned up in the 6 o'clock region using an injection of balanced salt solution in the sub-Tenon's space. (Fig. 3.31A). When this is done, a modified goniotomy knife (Scheie) is used to penetrate the cornea at the temporal limbus. The knife is passed across the anterior chamber to the inferior angle. The knife is pushed through the trabecular meshwork to the sub-Tenon's space in a plane parallel to the iris and then withdrawn back into the anterior chamber angle at right angles to the direction in which it was initially inserted (Fig. 3.31B and C). Care must be taken not to insert the knife too far posteriorly or it will inadvertently lacerate the ciliary body and cause extensive bleeding. Additionally, when manipulating the blade across

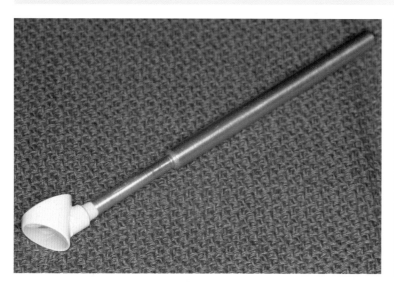

FIG. 3.28

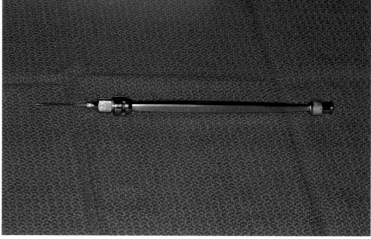

FIG. 3.29

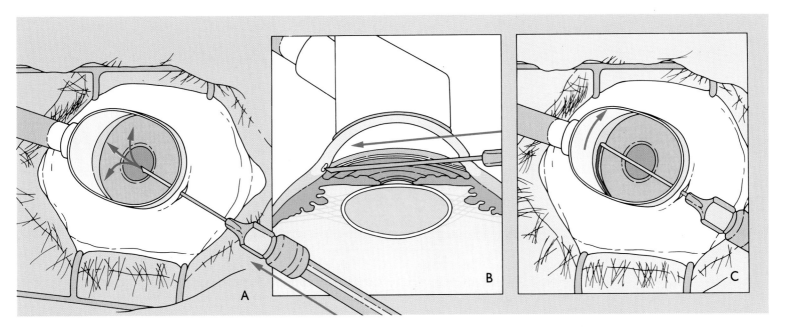

FIG. 3.30

Goniopuncture

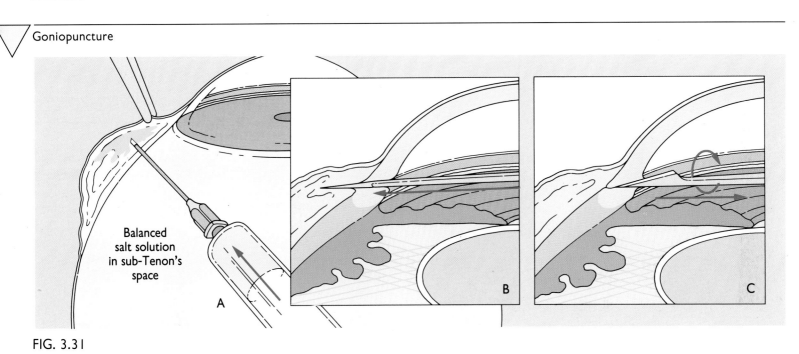

Balanced
salt solution
in sub-Tenon's
space

FIG. 3.31

the anterior chamber, care must be taken not to cause collapse of the anterior chamber, causing damage to the intraocular tissues. Healon may be used to prevent this. Because of its low success rate and technical difficulty, this procedure has been largely abandoned for others.

TRABECULOTOMY AND/OR TRABECULECTOMY

Trabeculotomy may be performed instead of goniotomy or goniopuncture for the treatment of congenital glaucoma. Because of its relative safety in comparison to goniotomy, many people prefer trabeculotomy. To perform this procedure, a 5 by 5-mm superficial scleral flap is fashioned and hinged onto the cornea similar to the superficial square flap made in a penetrating trabeculectomy (Fig. 3.32A). When this is done, a 3 by 3-mm deep lamellar scleral block is dissected down to the level just superficial to the ciliary body (Fig. 3.32B and C). The dissection plane in this scleral block is carried forward over Schwalbe's line, over the scleral spur, and into the clear cornea. The deep flap is left in place at this time to tamponade leakage of aqueous from the anterior chamber. This should allow adequate exposure of the cut ends of Schlemm's canal. Often, a small amount of blood will reflux from these ends.

A right-hand trabeculotome (Harms or McPherson) is introduced into the cut end of Schlemm's canal on the right-hand side of the incision and inserted to its full extent into Schlemm's canal (Fig. 3.33A). When this is done, the external guide of the trabeculotome is grasped with a pair of heavy forceps. In a carefully controlled fashion, the trabeculotome is rotated toward the anterior chamber until the distal tip of the internal arm of the trabeculotome is seen to rupture the trabecular meshwork into the anterior chamber (Fig. 3.33B and C). When this is done, the trabeculotome is maintained in this position and withdrawn from Schlemm's canal in such a manner that the remainder of the trabecular meshwork is opened all the way back to the site of insertion of the instrument. Next, the left-handed trabeculotome is inserted into Schlemm's canal in a manner similar to the right and again the trabecular meshwork is ruptured and opened back to the site of insertion. If a trabeculectomy is felt to be needed, the deep lamellar block is excised at this point and the underlying trabecular meshwork removed (Fig. 3.34A and B). A peripheral iridectomy is made, and the superficial scleral flap is tacked down using 10-0 nylon sutures (Fig. 3.34C). Finally, the conjunctiva is brought down over the operation site and sutured with 8-0 Vicryl sutures.

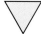

Trabeculotomy and/or Trabeculectomy

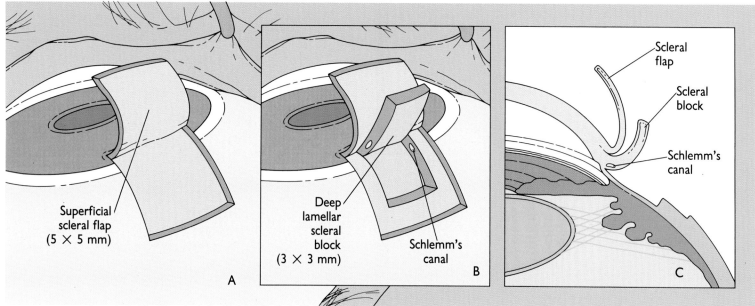

FIG. 3.32

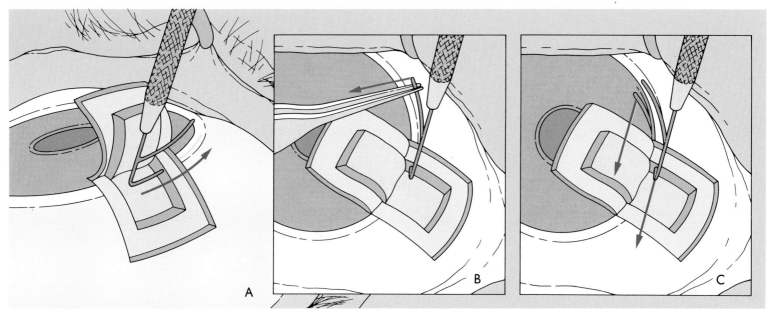

FIG. 3.33

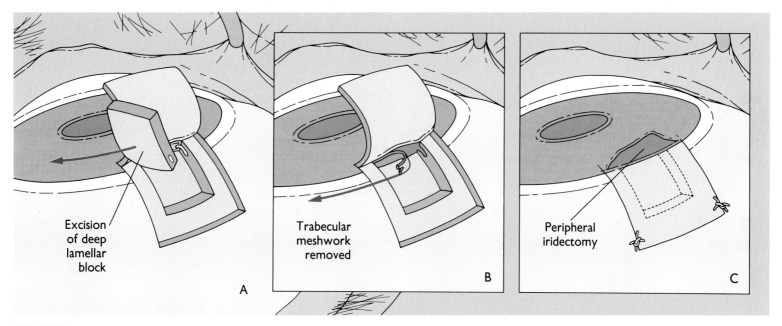

Excision
of deep
lamellar
block

Trabecular
meshwork
removed

Peripheral
iridectomy

A   B   C

FIG. 3.34

RELATED CONDITIONS

REPAIR OF CYCLODIALYSIS

A rare complication of anterior segment surgery is the development of cyclodialysis. Postoperatively, the eye may demonstrate prolonged and profound hypotony. Gonioscopic examination will usually reveal a patent cyclodialysis cleft. Because many of these clefts will spontaneously seal themselves, it is best to observe without intervention for several months. When hypotony persists and macular edema develops, intervention becomes necessary. If a cyclodialysis cleft is small and the margins are able to be visualized gonioscopically, the argon laser may be applied to the margins in an attempt to seal the cleft from the rest of the suprachoroidal space. This allows the reabsorption of fluid from the suprachoroidal space and reattachment of the ciliary body and will often restore normal intraocular pressure. If sequestering the cyclodialysis cleft from the remainder of the suprachoroidal space cannot be achieved using laser therapy, confluent applications of cyclocryotherapy along the margins may accomplish closure of the cleft.

If neither of these procedures is successful at restoring normal intraocular pressure, closure of the cleft may be attempted surgically. For this procedure, retrobulbar anesthesia is administered. The conjunctiva is dissected from the limbus, forming a fornix-based flap at the site of the cyclodialysis (Fig. 3.35). The margins of the cyclodialysis are identified by gonioscopy through the operating microscope and marked with a marking pen (Fig. 3.36). When the sclera overlying the site of the cyclodialysis is freed of conjunctiva and Tenon's capsule and hemostasis has been achieved, a dog-ear-type sclerotomy is made over the central zone of the cyclodialysis (Fig. 3.37). Fluid is drained from the sclerotomy site through the dog-ear flap, after which cautery is introduced and used to cauterize lightly the periphery of the cyclodialysis cleft in an attempt to seal the margins (Figs. 3.38 and 3.39). When this is done, the sclerotomy flap is closed with 9-0 nylon interrupted sutures. The conjunctiva is returned to its location at the limbus and suture. Postoperatively, the patient is followed for several weeks for resorption of the suprachoroidal fluid and resumption of normal intraocular pressure.

▽ Repair of Cyclodialysis

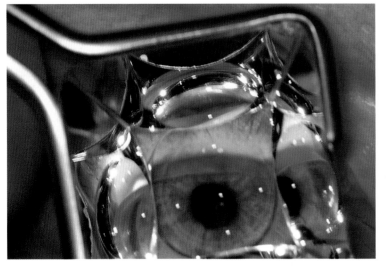

FIG. 3.35

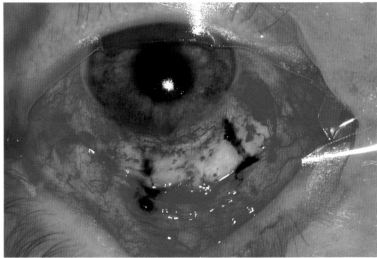

FIG. 3.36

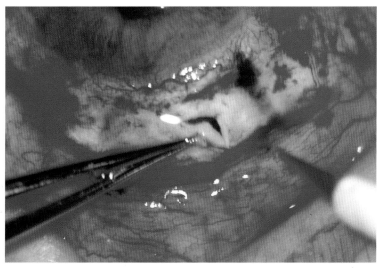

FIG. 3.37

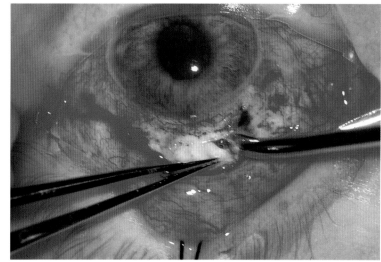

FIG. 3.38

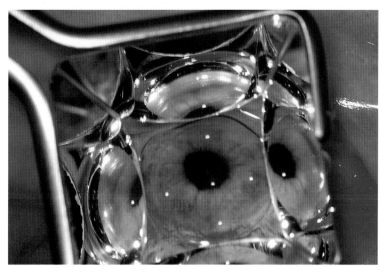

FIG. 3.39

SURGERY OF THE RETINA AND VITREOUS

4

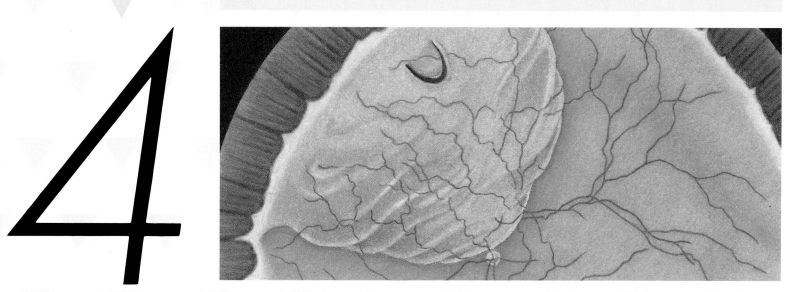

H. MacKenzie Freeman, MD

The surgical management of the more common vitreoretinal disorders, including retinal breaks without detachment, retinal detachments of varying degrees of severity, and spontaneous and traumatic vitreous hemorrhage, are dealt with in this chapter. Surgical procedures of varying degrees of complexity, from a simple outpatient pneumatic retinopexy to retinectomy for severe proliferative vitreoretinopathy, will be described to provide an overview, though not all-inclusive, of the modalities of treatment currently available.

MANAGEMENT OF RETINAL BREAKS WITHOUT RETINAL DETACHMENT

The management of retinal breaks without retinal detachment is a very common problem because retinal breaks occur in approximately 7.8% of the United States population, or approximately 16 million people. The incidence of retinal detachment is about 1:9,000 persons per year; it is therefore obvious that all retinal breaks do not require treatment.

CONSIDERATIONS

In deciding whether prophylactic treatment is advisable, the factors that should be considered are listed in Fig. 4.1. They are discussed in detail below.

Characteristics of Retinal Break

Characteristics of the retinal break are important factors in deciding whether treatment is indicated. Peripheral retinal breaks may be classified into three types: retinal tears, retinal dialyses, and retinal holes (Fig. 4.2). Each of these retinal breaks has a different predisposition to causing a retinal detachment.

In most cases a *retinal tear* forms at the site of an abnormal isolated vitreoretinal adhesion or along an irregularity in the posterior vitreous base (Fig. 4.2A). As the vitreous gel undergoes liquefaction and collapse, a posterior vitreous detachment develops that extends anteriorly to exert traction on this adhesion, resulting in the formation of a retinal tear. Following vitreous detachment, fluid vitreous comes in contact with the retinal tear to promote the development of a retinal detachment. For these reasons, retinal tears show the greatest predisposition to retinal detachment, and I treat all prophylactically.

A *retinal dialysis* is a retinal break that occurs at the ora serrata (Fig. 4.2B). The most common type of dialysis occurs in young males in the inferotemporal quadrant. A traumatic form of dialysis develops superior nasally after blunt ocular trauma or inferior temporally after direct trauma to that quadrant. Retinal detachments caused by a dialysis tend to progress slowly and pose less of an immediate threat to the macula; nonetheless they ultimately cause retinal detachments and therefore prophylactic treatment is indicated.

A *retinal hole* is the retinal break least likely to cause a retinal detachment and therefore rarely requires treatment. Retinal holes are not caused by traction but are usually the result of an atrophic process, probably an underlying vascular insufficiency. A retinal hole is round or oval shaped, varying in size from pinpoint to 1.5 disk diameters (DD).

Lattice degeneration occurs in approximately 6.4% of eyes of the general population, affecting both sexes equally. This degeneration has a propensity for bilaterality. It occurs as oval or spindle-shaped areas of retinal thinning, 0.5 to 1.5 DD wide, varying in length from 2 DD to an entire quadrant. Lattice lesions extend parallel to the ora serrata and are located between the ora serrata and the equator. White interlacing lines of sheathed or occluded vessels are frequently seen within the lattice. Most forms of lattice degeneration are benign and nonprogressive, with only 1% of eyes developing retinal detachment. The benign form occurs near the ora serrata and is usually located in the inferotemporal quadrant. It is not associated with vitreoretinal traction and therefore requires no treatment. A less common form of degeneration is progressive, especially in highly myopic eyes or in patients with Wagner's syndrome.

Retinal tears develop along the posterior margin or at the ends of the lattice as a result of traction from vitreous membranes (Fig. 4.2C). Treatment of the retinal tears should be undertaken without delay because retinal detachments tend to develop rapidly in these eyes.

Retinal holes develop in approximately 23% of eyes with lattice degeneration. The holes are usually small, are round or oval-shaped, and are located within or adjacent to the lattice lesions (Fig. 4.2D). Retinal holes are much less likely to cause retinal detachment than retinal tears; however, if there is a history of retinal detachment in the family or the fellow eye, I tend to treat these eyes.

The larger and the greater the number of retinal breaks, the stronger and the more urgent are the indications for treatment. Retinal detachment resulting from retinal breaks located superiorly, temporally, and especially posterior temporally pose a greater threat to the macula than those located nasally, anteriorly, and inferiorly.

Other Significant Ocular Findings

Retinal breaks present in eyes with high myopia, vitreous hemorrhage, and retinopathy of prematurity have a greater predisposition for retinal detachment. Treatment is indicated when retinal breaks occur in eyes with a developing cataract because the ability to visualize an early detachment decreases as the lens becomes more cataractous.

Retinal breaks found in patients with such systemic syndromes as Marfan's syndrome, Wagner's syndrome, Ehlers-Danlos syndrome, and atopic dermatitis should be treated because of the poor prognosis associated with retinal detachments that tend to develop in these connective tissue diseases.

FACTORS TO BE CONSIDERED IN PROPHYLACTIC TREATMENT OF RETINAL BREAKS

Characteristics of retinal breaks
    Type
    Size
    Number
    Location

Associated ocular pathology
    Lattice degeneration
    High myopia
    Vitreous hemorrhage
    Retinopathy of prematurity
    Cataract

Retinal breaks or a history of retinal detachment in fellow eye

Family history of retinal detachment

Systemic syndromes predisposing to retinal detachment

FIG. 4.1

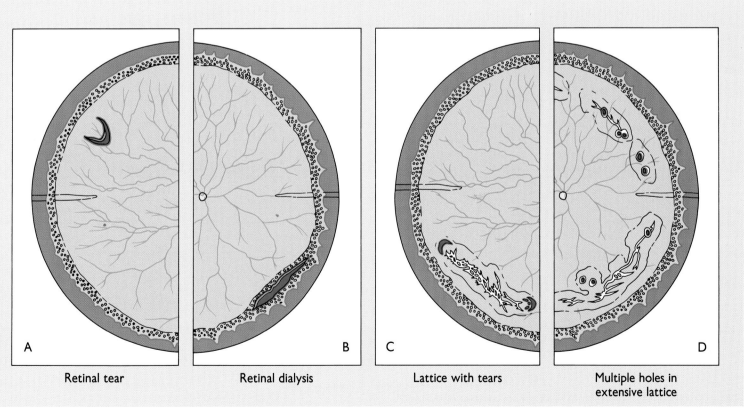

A	B	C	D
Retinal tear	Retinal dialysis	Lattice with tears	Multiple holes in extensive lattice

FIG. 4.2

SELECTION OF TREATMENT MODALITY

Retinal breaks without detachment can be treated with photocoagulation, cryopexy, or scleral buckling. Cryopexy is preferable for the treatment of retinal breaks located anterior to the equator (Fig. 4.3A). I prefer photocoagulation to cryopexy for lesions located in the region of or posterior to the equator because it can be done without a conjunctival incision that would be required for cryopexy (Fig. 4.3B). Scleral buckling is used for large retinal tears, retinal tears associated with vitreous hemorrhage, and in eyes with severe vitreous traction as evidenced by multiple or recurrent retinal tears.

A thorough preoperative workup including measurement of visual acuity and visual field as well as slitlamp and complete fundus examination is very important. Quite often the surgeon is dealing with an eye with 20/20 vision; therefore, thorough examination and documentation is vital in the event of a retinal detachment or medicolegal action. The patient should be explicitly informed of the complications of treatment and that retinal detachment may develop in spite of treatment. The steps of the proposed treatment should be described to the patient, and the patient should be asked if there are additional questions before the informed consent form is signed. A statement that the patient said he or she understood and had no further questions should be recorded in the chart.

A patient with a retinal break or detachment must be thoroughly examined with scleral depression and indirect ophthalmoscopy. This detailed search for additional retinal breaks is best done with the patient in the supine position. The examination is done using a +20.00 D lens and, if the pupil is small or the media is hazy, a +27.00 D lens is helpful. The +14.00 D lens is used to study fine details. The fundus chart is held on a clipboard resting on the patient's chest with the chart oriented upside down so that 12 o'clock on the chart is toward the patient's feet and 6 o'clock is toward the chin. As the observer sees the inverted image of the fundus through the indirect ophthalmoscope, he simply records on the chart what he sees, as he sees it. The color code used to represent fundus details is given in Fig. 4.4.

Biomicroscopy of the posterior segment is important in evaluating vitreoretinal relationships, vitreous, and preretinal membranes and for examining suspicious areas of the fundus with high magnification. The Goldmann 3-mirror contact lens is particularly suited for studying retinal breaks or detachments. The slit beam of the slit lamp microscope can be particularly helpful in detecting or confirming a retinal break that appears as a discontinuity of the beam.

Cryopexy

Transconjunctival cryoapplications are used in the prophylactic treatment of retinal dialysis, anterior retinal holes surrounded by a localized retinal detachment, retinal holes in multiple areas of lattice degeneration, and small anterior retinal tears (Fig. 4.5). Visualization and treatment of reti-

---

Retinal Breaks Without Retinal Detachment: Selection of Treatment Modality

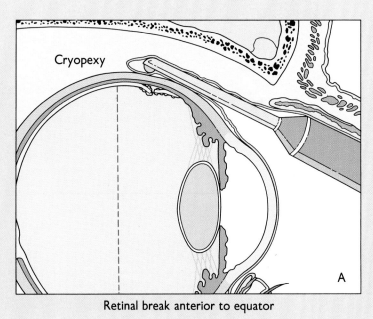

Retinal break anterior to equator

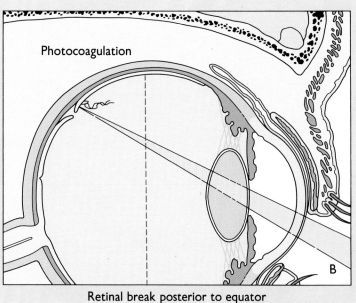

Retinal break posterior to equator

FIG. 4.3

FUNDUS CHART COLOR CODE

COLOR	FUNDUS DETAILS
Blue	Detached retina and retinal veins
Red	Attached retina and retinal arteries, and hemorrhage in retina
Red lined with blue	Retinal breaks
Black	Retinal pigmentation and choroidal pigmentation seen through attached retina
Brown	Choroidal pigmentation seen through detached retina
Green	Opacities in the media, including vitreous hemorrhage
Yellow	Choroidal exudation and macular edema

FIG. 4.4

Retinal Breaks Without Retinal Detachment: Cryopexy and Photocoagulation

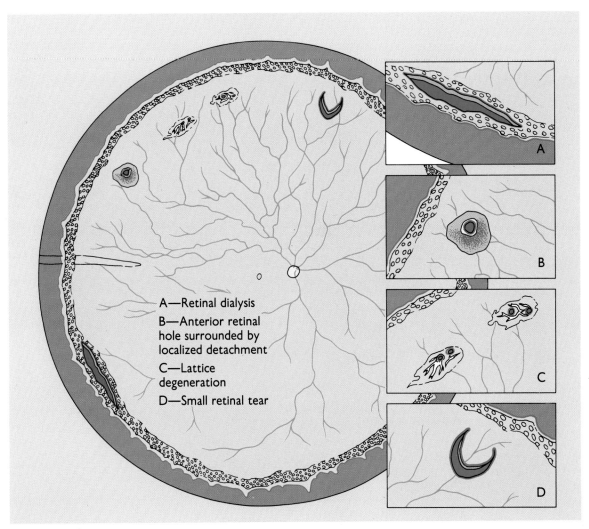

A—Retinal dialysis
B—Anterior retinal hole surrounded by localized detachment
C—Lattice degeneration
D—Small retinal tear

FIG. 4.5

nal breaks near the ora serrata is easier using indirect ophthalmoscopy and scleral depression with the cryoprobe than using photocoagulation through the mirror of a Goldmann 3-mirror lens.

When beginning cryotreatment or photocoagulation, the pupil is maximally dilated with 10% phenylephrine hydrochloride and 1% cyclopentolate instilled every 5 minutes three times one-half hour prior to treatment. After topical anesthesia is achieved with 0.5% proparacaine hydrochloride, the conjunctiva is tented up using a smooth Bishop Harmon forceps. Using a 30-gauge needle on a tuberculin syringe, 0.1–0.2 cc of 1% xylocaine is injected under the conjunctiva in the quadrant of the retinal break (Fig 4.6). The needle tip is directed tangentially so that it is visible.

While the patient maintains fixation by gazing at his or her outstretched thumb, cryoapplications are applied under observation with the indirect ophthalmoscope and a 20.00-D aspheric condensing lens (Fig. 4.7). A small retinal tear is surrounded by contiguous cryoapplications (Fig. 4.8A). When treating retinal breaks in lattice degeneration, cryoapplications are placed surrounding the lesion in a thicker area of the retina, where a stronger chorioretinal adhesion will develop.

Photocoagulation

When using photocoagulation to treat a retinal tear, topical anesthetic of 0.5% proparacaine hydrochloride is instilled prior to placement of the Goldmann 3-mirror contact lens.

A spot size of 500 μm and an application time of 0.2 s of argon laser are used. The power intensity is arrived at by starting at a low level and gradually increasing the power until a yellow-white burn is obtained. Four to five rows of laser applications are applied around the retinal tear (Fig. 4.8B). Four rows of photocoagulation applications are made in a more healthy retina surrounding the lattice degeneration (Fig. 4.8C).

After cryopexy or photocoagulation, a mild oral analgesic is given to the patient in the event of pain en route home. A patch is placed over the eye and the patient is instructed to remove it after 12 hours. Patients who have had cryopexy are told that the eye may be red and the conjunctiva slightly swollen and that they may experience a foreign body sensation for a few days. If extensive cryoapplications have been made or the iris may have been burned by photocoagulation, a topical corticosteroid and a short-acting cycloplegic are prescribed for five days.

The patient is reexamined 2 weeks later, at which time pigmentation should be seen in the treated areas. If adequate treatment is noted, the patient is reexamined at 2 months and then every 6–12 months, depending on the nature of the underlying pathology.

Scleral Buckling

Scleral buckling will reduce vitreous traction and therefore offers the best long-term prognosis in eyes with severe traction that has caused large or multiple retinal tears (Figs. 4.9

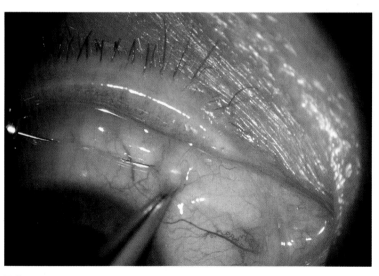

FIG. 4.6

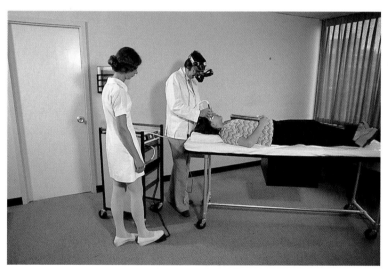

FIG. 4.7

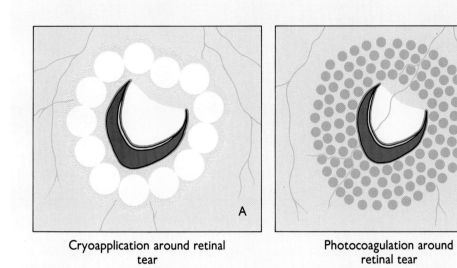
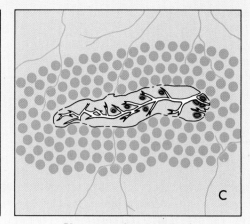

Cryoapplication around retinal tear	Photocoagulation around retinal tear	Photocoagulation around lattice degeneration
A	B	C

FIG. 4.8

Retinal Breaks Without Retinal Detachment: Scleral Buckling

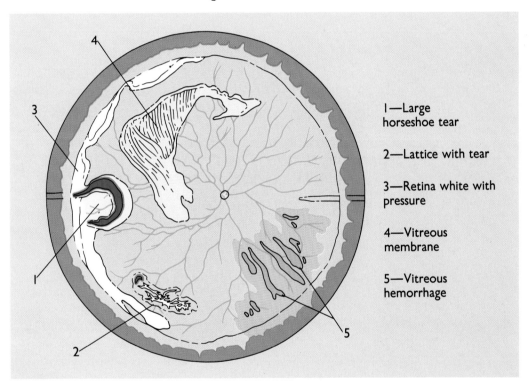

1—Large horseshoe tear

2—Lattice with tear

3—Retina white with pressure

4—Vitreous membrane

5—Vitreous hemorrhage

FIG. 4.9

and 4.10). The use of an encircling element provides permanent indentation and reduces the incidence of implant extrusion (Fig. 4.11). The techniques of episcleral and intrascleral buckling are discussed in the section on management of primary retinal detachment.

Vitreous hemorrhage may be the result of traction, which causes the retina to tear across a blood vessel. A substantial amount of vitreous hemorrhage may cause condensation of the vitreous gel and increased traction. Unless traction to the blood vessel is relieved, vitreous hemorrhage may recur.

When a substantial amount of vitreous hemorrhage is present, I perform a scleral buckling in order to seal the retinal tear, relieve the traction, and prevent recurrence of vitreous hemorrhage. To promote clearing of the vitreous hemorrhage, which will make possible a search for additional retinal tears, a two-to-three-day trial of bed rest with the head of the bed elevated 45° and with binocular patching is done prior to scleral buckling surgery.

MANAGEMENT OF PRIMARY RETINAL DETACHMENT

PNEUMATIC RETINOPEXY WITHOUT CONJUNCTIVAL INCISION

Hilton et al. have defined the indications for pneumatic retinopexy to be the occurrence of a retinal detachment with one retinal break or group of breaks that is no larger than one clock hour and is located in the superior eight hours of the fundus. Contraindications include grades C or D proliferative vitreoretinopathy, mental incompetence, or severe glaucoma. I advocate scleral buckling in most primary retinal detachments and use pneumatic retinopexy primarily in patients in whom severe systemic illness precludes general anesthesia, or in whom debilitation or lack of cooperation would hamper surgery under local anesthesia.

Figure 4.12 shows a temporal retinal detachment with a superior temporal retinal tear extending less than one hour of the clock. Preoperative preparation includes the admin-

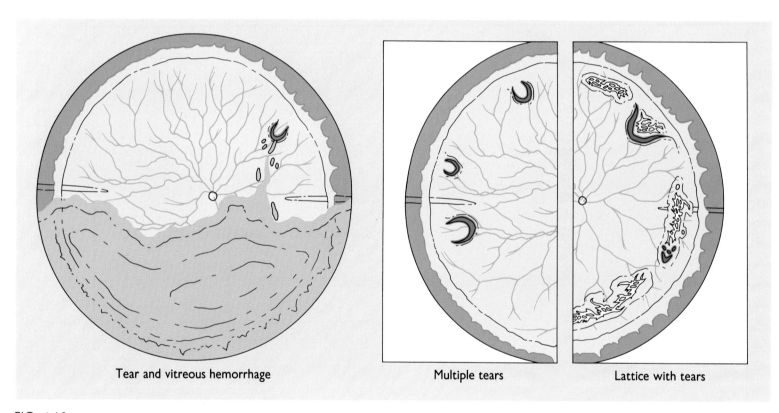

Tear and vitreous hemorrhage   Multiple tears   Lattice with tears

FIG. 4.10

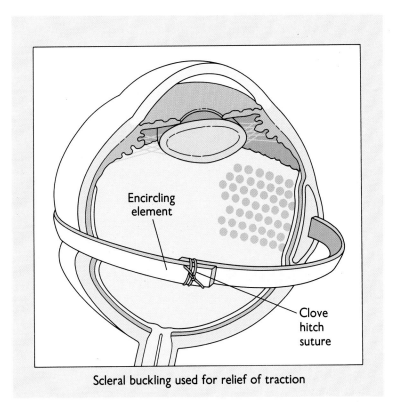

Scleral buckling used for relief of traction

FIG. 4.11

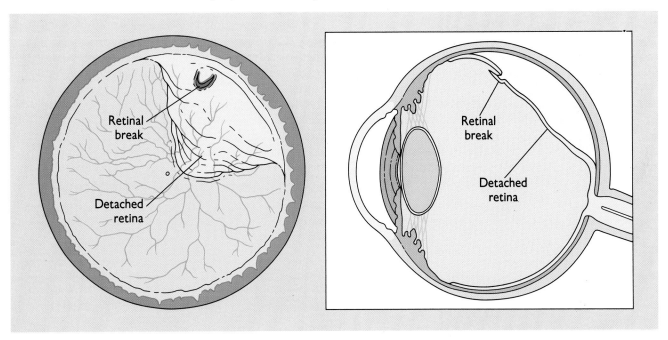

FIG. 4.12

istration of topical Gentamycin hourly for five hours pre-operatively. The pupil is maximally dilated using Ocufen instilled every five minutes three times for three dosages. Retrobulbar anesthesia is given using 1% Xylocaine.

The retinal break is treated with two rows of contiguous cryoapplications applied under indirect ophthalmoscopic control. Intraocular pressure is lowered to near zero with intermittent indentations of the sclera using the cryoprobe. A wire lid speculum is inserted and the conjunctiva and cornea are treated with three drops of povidone–iodine solution prepared with equal parts of povidone–iodine solution and balanced salt solution. After three minutes, the pars plana injection site is dried with a sterile cotton stick applicator. Three tenths of a milliliter of perfluoropropane gas is drawn through a millipore filter into a tuberculin syringe through a ½-inch, 30-gauge needle. The patient's head is positioned so that the injection site is uppermost and the injection is made 0.4 mm posterior to the limbus (Fig. 4.13). As the needle is withdrawn from the eye, the needle tract is immediately covered with a sterile cotton stick applicator to prevent loss of gas.

The head is then rotated to move the gas bubble away from the injection site and the cotton applicator is then removed. The central artery is examined with indirect ophthalmoscopy and the intraocular pressure is measured 5 and 10 minutes after the injection. If the central artery is closed and does not begin to pulsate within four minutes, a paracentesis of the anterior chamber or aspiration of gas or fluid from the vitreous cavity is performed.

If ophthalmoscopy reveals multiple gas bubbles are present that might pass subretinally, a thump is applied to the uppermost part of the globe using a cotton stick applicator in order to promote the coalescence of bubbles into a single bubble. This thump is performed by flexing a cotton-tipped applicator and then releasing its tip to strike firmly the pars plana (Fig. 4.14). Topical antibiotic is instilled and the eye is patched.

Postoperatively, the patient is instructed to position the head so that the retinal break is uppermost for 16 hours a day for five days (Fig. 4.15A). With proper positioning so that the retinal break is tamponaded by the gas bubble (Fig. 4.15B), the retina is usually reattached by the first postoperative day. The intraocular tension is measured at ½, 1, 6, and 24 hours postoperatively. Topical steroid drops are prescribed three times a day. Follow-up examinations are at 1, 2, 4, 8, and 16 days. The patient is allowed to return to work 2 weeks after surgery.

If multiple gas bubbles are present in the vitreous cavity following pneumatic retinopexy, some bubbles may pass subretinally. A moderate or large amount of subretinal gas will produce a bullous detachment with the retina dragged toward the position of the gas bubbles. With the patient in the supine position, the retina will be moved toward the lens (Fig. 4.16). The detached retina overlying the gas bubbles has a pearly opalescent appearance, the result of light reflected from the subretinal gas bubbles. A small bubble of subretinal gas may be difficult to diagnose, especially when viewed through a large gas bubble in the vitreous cavity, and thus may escape detection as the cause of a persistent retinal detachment.

Management of subretinal gas should start with positioning the patient's head to allow the subretinal gas to pass into the vitreous cavity. If multiple bubbles are present and positioning fails to deliver the bubbles through the retinal break, an attempt is made to form one subretinal bubble using the thump technique previously described. If the subretinal bubble exits through the retinal break, another "thump" is done to coalesce this bubble with the bubble in the vitreous cavity.

If the subretinal gas cannot be removed by positioning and the retinal break remains open, surgery is indicated. If the subretinal bubble is small or can be positioned away from the retinal break, a scleral buckle is made to close the retinal break. If the bubble is large, it may be evacuated during the drainage of subretinal fluid. Vitrectomy for the purpose of subretinal gas removal and gas–fluid exchange can be hazardous because the retina may be pulled toward the lens. Insertion of the infusion cannula, vitrectomy probe, extrusion needle, or endoilluminator through this displaced retina may produce a large retinal break. This can

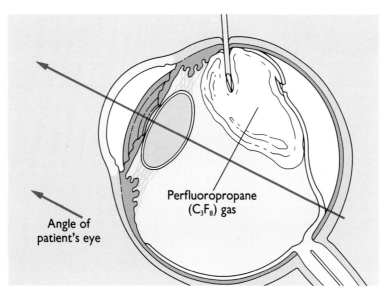

Perfluoropropane (C₃F₈) gas

Angle of patient's eye

FIG. 4.13

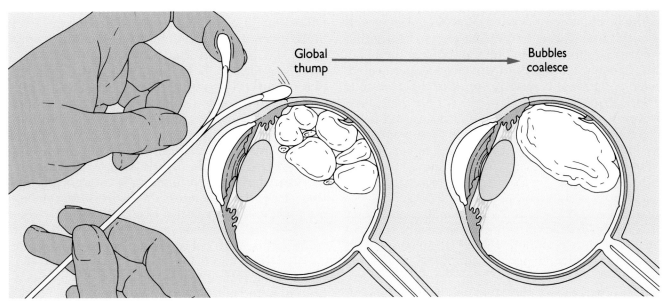

Global thump → Bubbles coalesce

FIG. 4.14

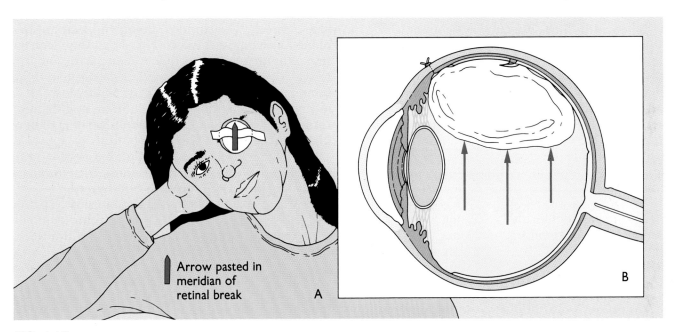

Arrow pasted in meridian of retinal break

A

B

FIG. 4.15

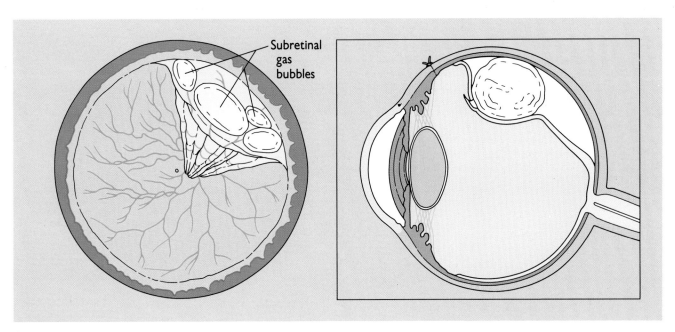

Subretinal gas bubbles

FIG. 4.16

be avoided by positioning the eye to allow the intravitreous gas to rise to the area where the instrument is to be inserted and thus move the subretinal bubbles away from the penetration site. A complete air–fluid exchange is performed, during which an attempt is made to remove the subretinal gas using the extrusion needle.

A controversy exists regarding the indications and desirability of pneumatic retinopexy. Until a larger series of cases with longer follow-up by a greater number of surgeons is reported this controversy will continue.

SEGMENTAL EPISCLERAL BUCKLE

Use of a segmental episcleral buckle is especially effective for a retinal tear in a quadratic retinal detachment (Fig. 4.17). In such cases, drainage of subretinal fluid may be unnecessary.

When retinal detachment threatens the macula, binocular patching and bed rest are instituted, and the patient's head is positioned to impede the extension of the detachment to avoid involvement of the macula. Preoperative cultures are taken and then topical Gentamycin 0.3% is instilled three times the evening prior to surgery and three times ½ hour preoperatively. Cephazolin is given 1 g IV preoperatively and 1 g during the operation.

Maximum pupillary dilatation is generally obtained by administration of a combination of 0.3% scopolamine hydrobromide and 10% phenylephrine hydrochloride. In older patients, the scopolamine is replaced by 1% cyclopentolate hydrochloride (Cyclogyl). If drops are ineffective, a subconjunctival injection of 0.2 mL of the following mixture may be tried:

Phenylephrine hydrochloride	50 mg
Homatropine hydrobromide	25 mg
Procaine hydrochloride	25 mg
Distilled water	1 mL

Dilatation is maintained with four dosages of ibuprofen 0.3% given every 15 minutes for one hour preoperatively.

The lid is tented away from the globe with a cotton-tipped applicator. Lid sutures of 4-0 black silk are placed 2 mm from the lid margin through the tarsal plate. The lids are retracted using a wire speculum. The conjunctiva and Tenon's capsule are grasped near the limbus with toothed Bishop Harmon forceps and a limbal peritomy is made using curved iris scissors. Radial relaxing conjunctival incisions 8 mm long are made slightly below the nasal horizontal meridian and above it temporally to prevent symblepharon (Fig. 4.18). Using a muscle hook to retract the muscle tendon, bridle sutures of 4-0 black silk are placed around the insertion of the rectus muscles (Fig. 4.19). The arms of the bridle sutures are cut approximately 4 inches in length.

After the sclera is inspected for thin areas, the posterior edge of the retinal tear is localized. The surgeon positions himself in the meridian opposite the retinal break and localizes the break using a 20.00-DD aspheric lens and an indirect ophthalmoscope mounted on a mobile stand. The assistant positions the Arruga retractor in the meridian of the retinal break. The surgeon directs the assistant to move the blunt localizing electrode (Fig. 4.20, the electrode at bottom of figure) so that its indentation corresponds to the posterior edge of the retinal break. The surgeon then instructs the assistant to make a mark by depressing the diathermy switch. While visualized with indirect ophthalmoscopy, the retinal tear is surrounded by two rows of confluent cryoapplications using a probe temperature of approximately − 80°C. The goal of the application is an orange-red color of the choroid. After each application, the surgeon holds the probe steady until the iceball has thawed.

Suturing is done with 5-0 Dacron using a spatulated needle with a quarter-circle bite. Scleral bites should be deep and long so they do not erode through the sclera postoperatively. The needle should be introduced very slowly into the sclera until the proper depth is reached and then

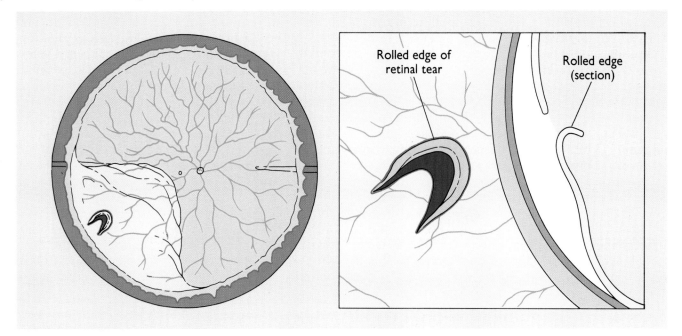

FIG. 4.17

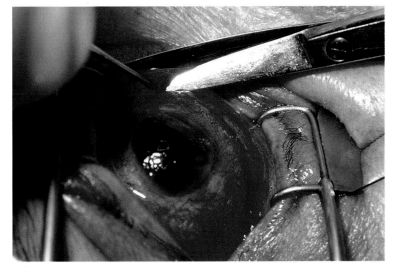

FIG. 4.18

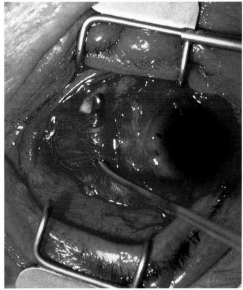

FIG. 4.19

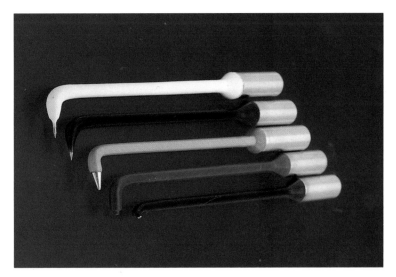

FIG. 4.20

pushed carefully along the scleral lamellae. The intrascleral course should be as long as possible, i.e., a minimum of 3 mm, thus reducing the risk of the suture pulling out (Fig. 4.21A). The desired depth is ½ to ⅔ scleral thickness. Vortex veins and ampulla should be carefully avoided. A mattress-type suture is used to straddle the sponge.

The amount of separation of the arms of the suture depends on the width of the implant selected. A good rule is to place the sutures 1½ times the width of the implant. For a 4-mm implant, sutures are placed 6 mm apart and for a 5-mm implant 7.5 mm apart. A 5-mm sponge adequately closes a 3-mm-wide break. A 7.5-mm sponge closes breaks 5 to 6 mm in width.

The hydrogel sponge is placed under the mattress sutures (Fig. 4.21B). The sponge material should be kept in an antibiotic solution and not removed from it until used. A variety of widths and shapes are available (Fig. 4.22). The assistant indents the sponge into the sclera using a cotton swab and the sutures are pulled up using forceps (Fig. 4.21C). The

sutures are tightened and tied with a slip knot. Patency of the ophthalmic artery is checked by ophthalmoscopy. After tying a suture it may be necessary to wait a few minutes for the intraocular pressure to decline before another suture is tied. Intravenous acetazolamide may be used to lower intraocular pressure. If the retinal break is closed by the indentation of the sponge, subretinal fluid is not drained.

Indirect ophthalmoscopy at the end of the operation reveals that the retinal tear is closed and well situated on the indentation produced by the sponge (Fig. 4.23). Providing there is no preretinal organization, the subretinal fluid should be absorbed spontaneously within a few days.

The conjunctiva is sutured to the episclera at the limbal end of the radial relaxing incision using 6-0 Vicryl. An interrupted suture is place posteriorly to it (Fig. 4.24).

If the sponge is located too far anteriorly, is too large, or is inadequately covered by Tenon's capsule, it may erode through Tenon's capsule or the conjunctiva to become secondarily infected (Fig. 4.25). The eye becomes painful,

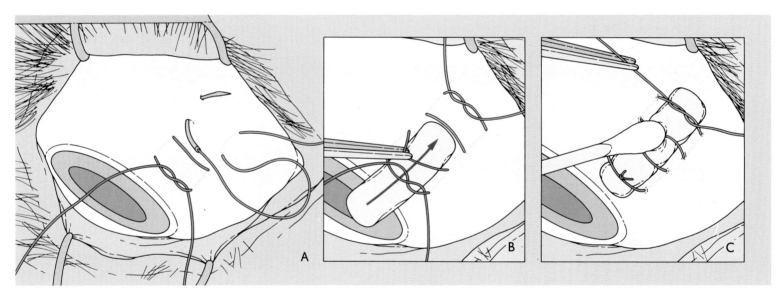

FIG. 4.21

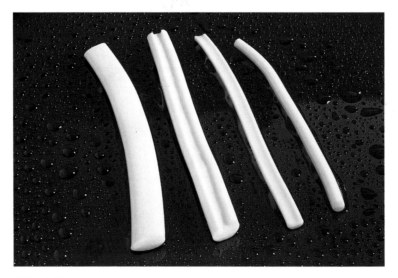

FIG. 4.22

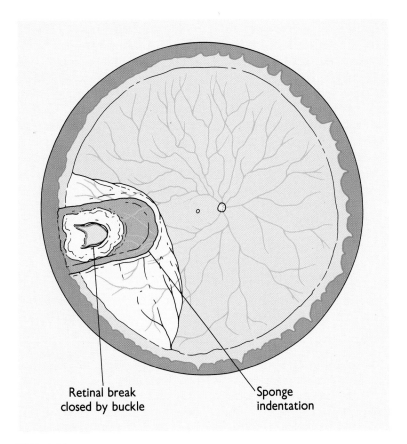

Retinal break
closed by buckle

Sponge
indentation

FIG. 4.23

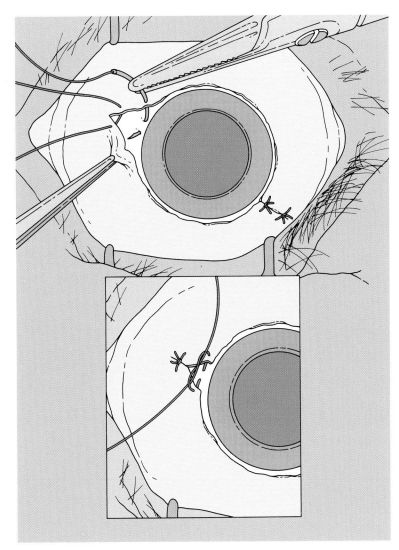

FIG. 4.24

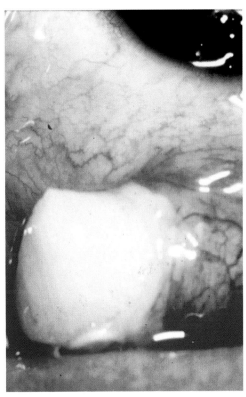

FIG. 4.25

infected, and may have a purulent discharge from a fistula tract in the conjunctiva. Topical or systemic antibiotics will not eradicate this infection; the sponge and sutures must be removed. To do this, using sharp curved iris scissors, the conjunctiva and Tenon's capsule are cut to expose the entire sponge. A traction suture of 4-0 silk is inserted through the tendon of the inferior rectus muscle to improve the exposure of the sponge and sutures. The sutures are cut and removed, then the sponge is gently extracted and sent for culture. The area is irrigated with an antibiotic solution. Tenon's capsule and the conjunctiva are closed in separate layers.

SCLERAL UNDERMINING, SCLERAL BUCKLING, AND EXTERNAL DRAINAGE OF SUBRETINAL FLUID

I prefer scleral undermining for retinal detachments with marked vitreous base condensation manifested by multiple retinal tears in two or more quadrants. Scleral undermining permits the use of diathermy, which is less apt than cryoapplications to produce dispersion of pigment epithelial cells through the multiple tears that would increase the risk of proliferative vitreoretinopathy. Burying an anteriorly placed implant under scleral flaps results in less tendency for implant erosion than by placing an episcleral sponge.

Figure 4.26 shows a total bullous retinal detachment with lattice degeneration and multiple medium-sized retinal tears located along the posterior margin of the vitreous base. The retinal breaks are localized with indirect ophthalmoscopy and localizing marks are made at the posterior edge of the small retinal tears. The anterior horns and posterior margin of the largest retinal tear are localized in order to determine the width of the scleral buckle. The distance from the limbus to the posterior edge of the tear is measured using an Amsler marker (Fig. 4.27A). This information helps to determine the location of the circumferential incision for the lamellar scleral undermining that will straddle these marks.

Using a scarifier, an incision is made through ⅔ of the thickness of the sclera. A radial incision is made 6 mm lateral to the retinal break (Fig. 4.27B,C). In order to avoid cutting too deeply, the flap is placed on tension using toothed Bishop Harmon forceps and the undermining follows a tissue plane in the sclera to produce a scleral flap of uniform thickness (Fig. 4.29). The posterior and anterior flaps of the undermining are dissected so that the undermining will extend 4.5 mm posterior, 3 mm anterior, and 6 mm lateral to the retinal breaks (Fig. 4.27C).

A blunt diathermy electrode (Fig. 4.20, middle electrode) is used to place diathermy applications approximately 1.5 mm apart in the scleral undermining (Figs.

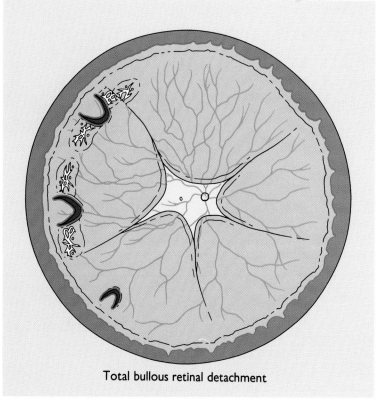

Total bullous retinal detachment

FIG. 4.26

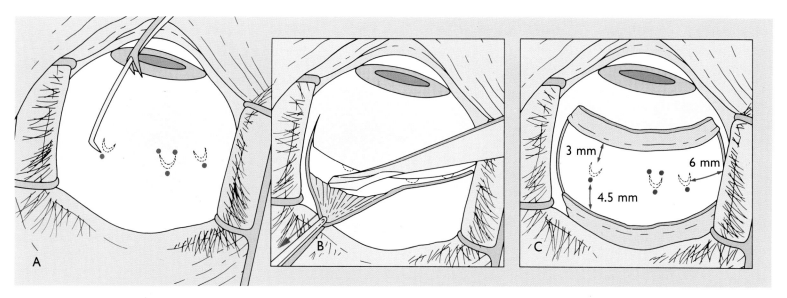

FIG. 4.27

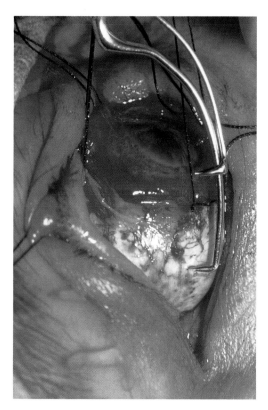

FIG. 4.28

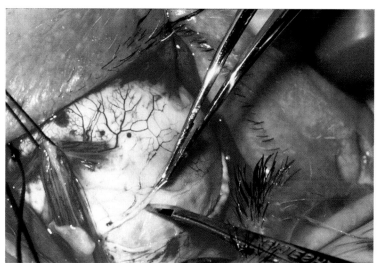

FIG. 4.29

4.30A and 4.31). Applications are made with slight pressure on sclera that has been dried with a cotton-tipped applicator. If the retina is attached, a yellow-orange colored diathermy retinal burn is desirable. If the retina is slightly elevated, gentle pressure with the blunt conical electrode may produce the desired gray retinal burn. If no mark is visible on the retina, a diathermy setting that will produce a slight charring of the sclera is used.

The long posterior ciliary artery and nerve are visualized by transillumination in order to avoid diathermizing them. The operating room is darkened and a hand-held transilluminator is applied to the cornea near the limbus in the meridian opposite the vessel and nerve to be transilluminated. The artery appears as a thin red line; the nerve is lined by two parallel lines that represent the pigmented epineurium (Fig. 4.30B).

Mattress sutures of 5-0 polyester are placed through the anterior and posterior flaps of the scleral undermining, 2 mm apart and 2 mm from the edge of the scleral flap. A suture is placed in the meridian of the larger tears so that if it is necessary to support them with an additional radial implant, the suture will identify that meridian (Fig. 4.30C). In order to produce an adequate indentation of the scleral undermining, an implant must be selected or trimmed so that it will be approximately 2 to 3 mm narrower and 2 to 3 mm shorter than the lamellar scleral undermining. Implants that are too large fail to produce a good indentation. In order to prevent the implant from eroding through the sclera, sharp edges of solid silicone rubber implants should be trimmed.

The ends of the encircling element are beveled to facilitate their passage under the sutures. After rinsing the implant and encircling element in a solution of polymixin B, they are inserted beneath the mattress sutures using a smooth Bishop Harmon forceps (Figs. 4.32 and 4.33). The ends of the encircling element are joined using a clove hitch suture of 5-0 polyester. The clove hitch is then threaded around both ends of the encircling element and tied with a temporary slipknot.

It is important to localize the site for drainage of subretinal fluid just prior to making the sclerotomy rather than to rely entirely on the preoperative fundus drawing. The implant is moved aside and the meridian along which there is an abundance of subretinal fluid is localized with indirect ophthalmoscopy using indentation with a cotton-tipped applicator (Fig. 4.34). A 4-0 black silk suture is placed around the implant so that it can be retracted by the assistant to expose the meridian selected for drainage of subretinal fluid. This meridian is examined using a hand-held transilluminator in order to place the sclerotomy in an area near the meridian that appears devoid of large choroidal blood vessels (Fig. 4.34, inset). This area is marked using a gentian violet pen. Using the scarifier, a 3-to-4-mm radial sclerotomy is made through the mark. It is important that the sclerotomy incision be perpendicular because a shelved incision tends to close as the eye softens during the drainage of subretinal fluid. Using the blunt conical electrode, diathermy is applied to the margin of the sclerotomy to make it gape enough to expose a knuckle of choroid that can be

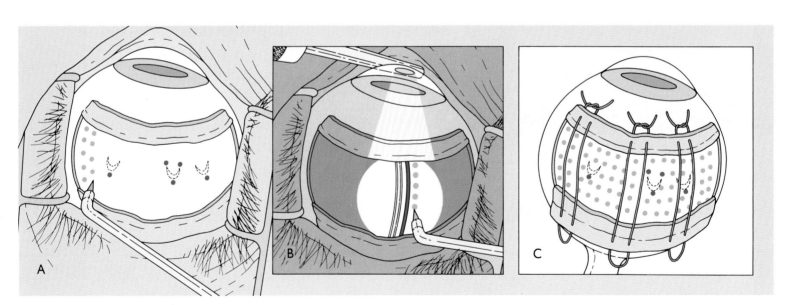

FIG. 4.30

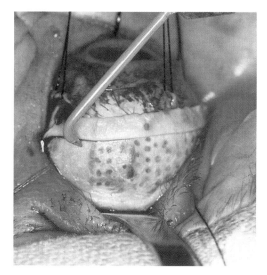

FIG. 4.31

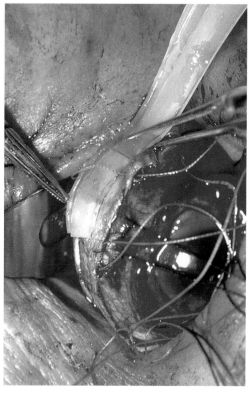

FIG. 4.32

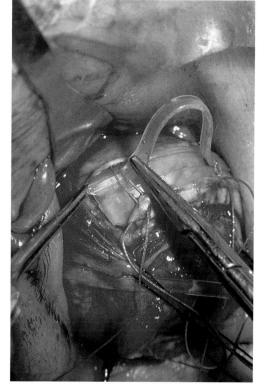

FIG. 4.33

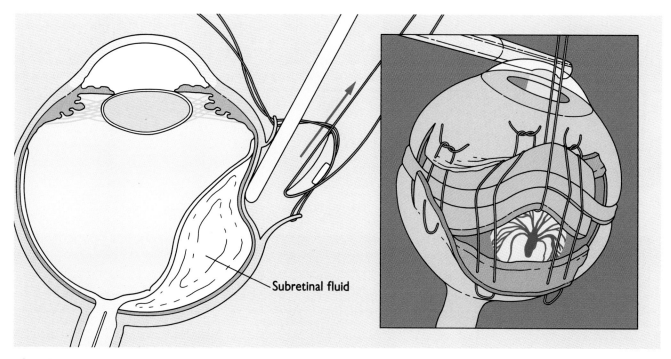

Subretinal fluid

FIG. 4.34

examined by transillumination (Fig. 4.35A). Figure 4.36 shows drainage of subretinal fluid through a sclerotomy posterior to the scleral buckle. With a diathermy current less than that used on the sclera, multiple confluent applications are applied with a blunt conical electrode over the exposed choroid to obliterate small choroidal tributaries not evident by transillumination (Fig. 4.35B). The diathermized choroid is then reexamined by transillumination and additional diathermy is applied if any blood vessels appear patent.

A sharp diathermy electrode (see Fig. 4.20, top) is used to perforate the choroid. Subretinal fluid is allowed to drain spontaneously (Fig. 4.35C); only when the globe becomes hypotonous is pressure applied distal from the sclerotomy. After most of the subretinal fluid has been drained, flecks of pigment may appear in the escaping fluid. When sub-retinal fluid ceases to drain, the mattress sutures over the implant are tightened and tied with a slipknot (Fig. 4.37). Ophthalmoscopy is performed to determine if any subretinal fluid remains and if the retinal breaks are flat on the scleral buckle. If ophthalmoscopy reveals an excessively high buckle with radial folds extending over it, the mattress sutures are loosened and saline is injected into the vitreous cavity. Injection is made through the pars plana in phakic eyes and through the limbus in aphakic or pseudophakic eyes. When the desired buckling effect is obtained, implant that extends beyond the undermining is trimmed (Fig. 4.38).

After the encircling element has been tightened slightly to relieve hypotony, the clove hitch is permanently tied and anchoring sutures of 5-0 polyester are placed in each quadrant outside the buckle (Figs. 4.39 and 4.40). Indirect

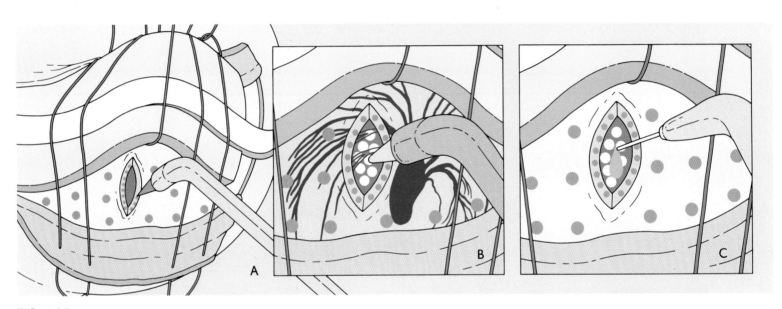

FIG. 4.35

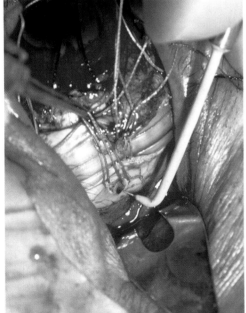

FIG. 4.36

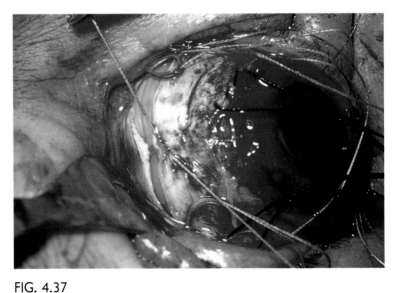

FIG. 4.37

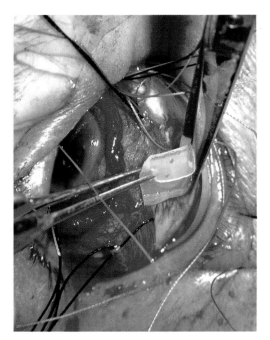

FIG. 4.38

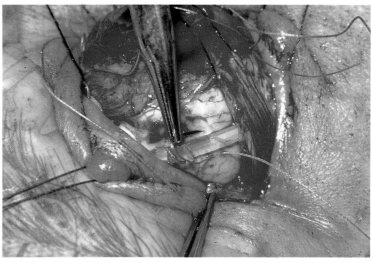

FIG. 4.39

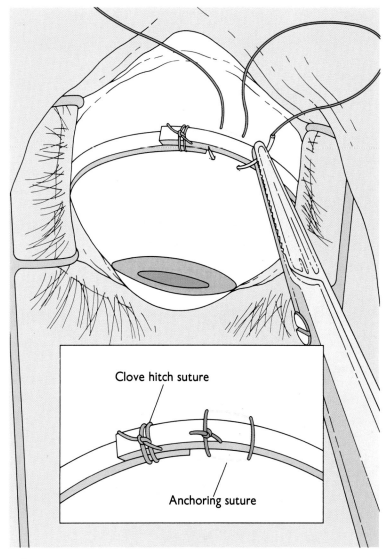

Clove hitch suture

Anchoring suture

FIG. 4.40

ophthalmoscopy is performed to determine if the ophthalmic artery is patent (Fig. 4.41). Intraocular tension is measured with a Schiotz tonometer. A desired pressure of 15 mm Hg is obtained by varying the tension of the encircling element or the mattress sutures or by injecting saline. The conjunctiva is closed with four interrupted sutures of 6-0 plain catgut. Polysporin ointment is placed in the inferior cul de sac and along the lid margins before a patch and shield are applied.

COMPLICATIONS DURING SURGERY

Fishmouthing Retinal Break With Meridional Fold
Following the drainage of subretinal fluid and tightening of the mattress sutures of the scleral undermining, ophthalmoscopy may reveal that a retinal tear gapes open (fishmouths) and a fold extends from the tear posteriorly over the scleral buckle (Fig. 4.42). In some eyes the gaping retinal break may be closed and the meridional fold flattened by lowering the buckle and injecting a balanced salt solu-

tion enriched with bicarbonate, dextrose, and glutathione (BSS Plus solution) into the eye. The injection is made through the pars plana in phakic eyes and through the limbus in aphakic eyes. The mattress sutures of the scleral flaps are loosened. The phakic eye is steadied by grasping the tendon of the superior rectus muscle with the Bishop Harmon forceps while BSS Plus solution is injected through a short 30-gauge needle inserted superior temporally 4.00 mm from the limbus.

A meridional implant is placed under the retinal tear if it cannot be closed with a BSS Plus injection. A 4-0 black silk suture is used to retract the implant to expose the scleral undermining in the meridian of the fishmouthing tear (Fig. 4.43A). The undermining is extended 6 mm posteriorly and 6 to 8 mm circumferentially. Diathermy is applied in the extended undermining.

A meridional implant is cut from a hydrogel implant (Fig. 4.43B), with a wide portion at one end that will extend 4 mm posterior to the solid silicone rubber implant. The implant is placed beneath the silicone rubber implant in the

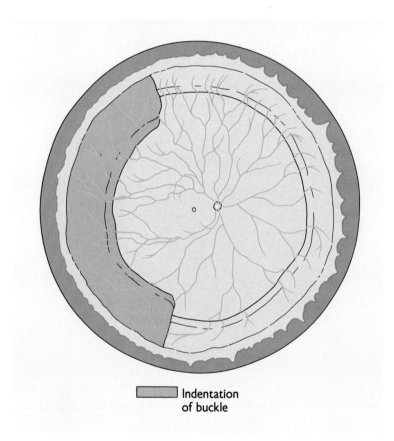

 Indentation
 of buckle

FIG. 4.41

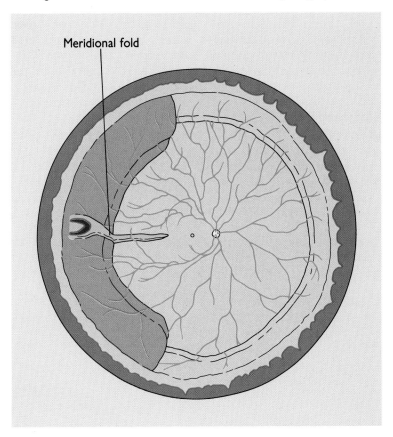

FIG. 4.42

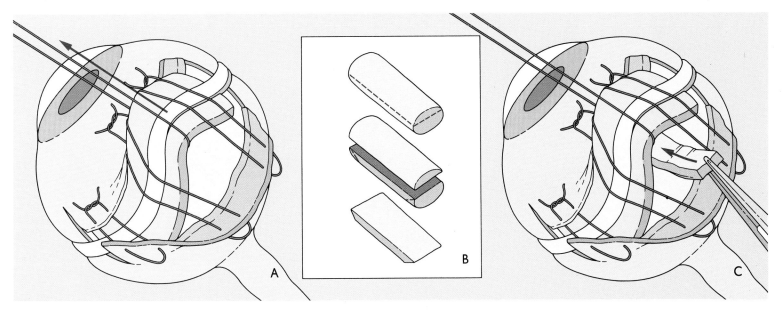

FIG. 4.43

meridian of the retinal break (Fig. 4.43C) and the mattress sutures are tightened. Figure 4.44 shows in cross section, as well as the fundus appearance of, the hydrogel implant beneath the solid silicone rubber implant. Indirect ophthalmoscopy is performed to assure that the meridional implant is in the proper position to close the break and flatten the retinal fold.

Complications of Drainage of Subretinal Fluid

Retinal Incarceration   A sudden cessation of the drainage of subretinal fluid may indicate a retinal incarceration in the perforation site. Indirect ophthalmoscopy should be performed at once before any attempts are made to promote further drainage of subretinal fluid. If the retina is incarcerated, a dimpling of the retina or retinal folds will be seen radiating from the perforation site (Fig. 4.45). If these folds do not communicate with a retinal break to prevent it from being closed, no further treatment is indicated. Any retraction or manipulation of the globe is avoided so that there will be no increase in intraocular pressure to cause the retinal incarceration to develop into a retinal hole. The incarceration site is quickly covered with the silicone implant.

Retinal Hole   Indirect ophthalmoscopy may reveal a retinal hole at the center of the retinal folds radiating from the sclerotomy site (Fig. 4.46A). Cessation of drainage of fluid may be followed by continued oozing of subretinal fluid and fluid vitreous (Fig. 4.46B). If the sclerotomy is located posterior to the scleral undermining, it is closed

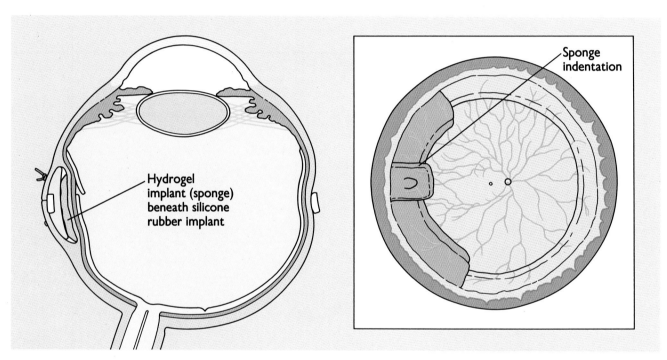

Hydrogel implant (sponge) beneath silicone rubber implant

Sponge indentation

FIG. 4.44

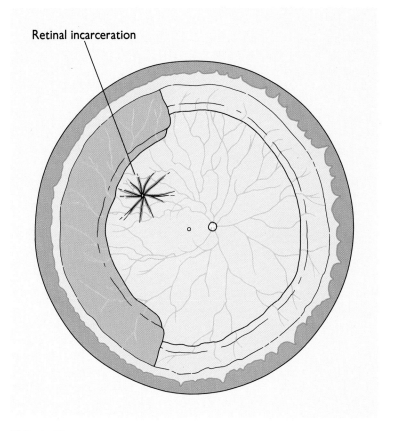

FIG. 4.45

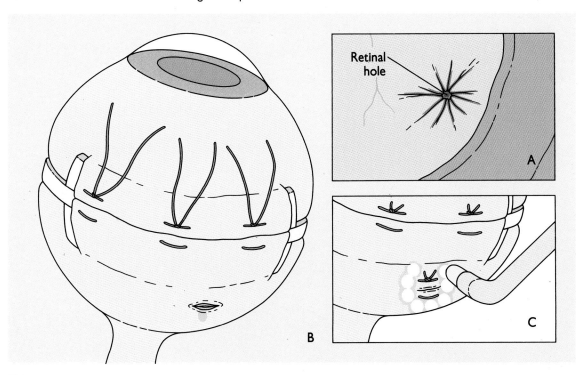

FIG. 4.46

with a mattress suture and surrounded with cryoapplications (Figs. 4.46C and 4.47). If the sclerotomy is in the scleral undermining, no cryoapplication is applied.

Iatrogenic Retinal Hole and Vitreous Loss Vitreous gel may prolapse through the iatrogenic retinal hole at the perforation site and the retinal hole may remain elevated and surrounded by radial retinal folds and detached retina (Fig. 4.48). The sclerotomy is sutured with 8-0 nylon sutures and then surrounded by cryoapplications. An episcleral hydrogel implant is sutured over the sclerotomy to produce a buckle to close the iatrogenic retinal break and flatten the radial retinal folds (see Figs 4.21 and 4.22).

POSTOPERATIVE COMPLICATIONS

Postoperative Choroidal Detachment

A postoperative choroidal detachment appears as a solid, immobile, orange-to-brown-colored elevation in the fundus (Fig. 4.49). The overlying retina may appear smooth or wrinkled because of an associated exudative retinal detachment. The choroidal elevations may be single or multilobular. Choroidal detachment may progress in an annular direction around the entire fundus periphery or may extend posteriorly to obscure the optic disk or macula. When temporal and nasal elevations extend posteriorly until they come in contact, they are termed "kissing" choroidal detachments. Most postoperative choroidal detachments subside spontaneously and require no treatment. When the choroidal elevation extends posterior to the equator and around the entire fundus periphery, resulting in shallowing of the anterior chamber, 100 mg prednisone is given daily orally for five to seven days.

Surgery is indicated when the choroidal detachment obscures the macula or disk, or in the presence of "kissing" choroidals or angle closure glaucoma. A radial sclerotomy is made 8 to 10 mm posterior to the limbus in the meridian of the most-marked choroidal elevation.

It is important to avoid profound hypotony during the drainage of subchoroidal fluid. After approximately 0.5 cc of fluid is drained, BSS Plus solution is injected through the pars plana in the phakic eye using a 30-gauge needle. In the aphakic or pseudophakic eye, constant infusion into the anterior chamber is accomplished through a bent 25-gauge needle attached to an IV infusion bottle. Care must be taken to keep the IV bottle at a level that does not produce ocular hypertension. Additional subchoroidal fluid may be released using an iris spatula inserted tangentially into the sclerotomy.

In some cases, it may be necessary to make a sclerotomy posterior to the buckle to drain all of the subchoroidal fluid. A preplaced mattress suture is placed over the sclerotomy. In such cases, the infusion bottle must be kept at a very low level to prevent retinal or choroidal incarceration.

Angle Closure Glaucoma

A peripheral choroidal detachment may elevate the ciliary body around the scleral spur, bringing the iris root against the filtration angle, to shallow or close the filtration angle (Fig. 4.50). Elevated intraocular pressure may produce corneal edema so that an early diagnosis of angle closure may be missed. Routine postoperative biomicroscopy and measurement of the intraocular pressure is important in detecting an early shallowing of the anterior chamber that may become flattened within a few days. Ophthalmoscopy may reveal a rather shallow annular choroidal evaluation (Fig. 4.50, inset).

A radial sclerotomy for the drainage of subchoroidal fluid is made 3 mm posterior to the limbus. When the intraocular tension is lowered, saline is injected to deepen the anterior chamber. Drainage of subchoroidal fluid is continued until ophthalmoscopy reveals no annular choroidal elevation. If the cornea is clear, gonioscopy is attempted to determine if the angle is open.

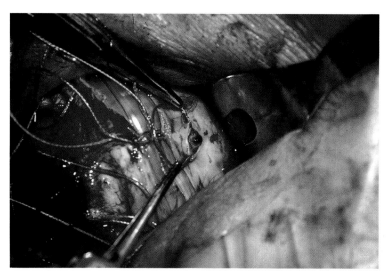

FIG. 4.47

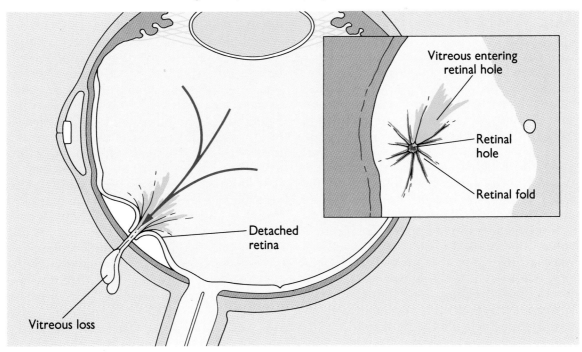

FIG. 4.48

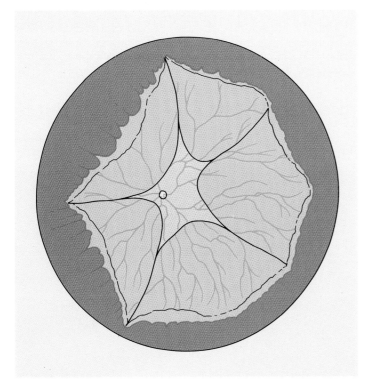

FIG. 4.49

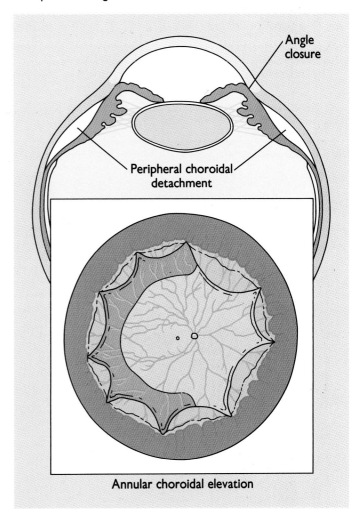

FIG. 4.50

MANAGEMENT OF CHRONIC VITREOUS HEMORRHAGE WITH VITRECTOMY

CONSIDERATIONS

Diabetic patients with bilateral vitreous hemorrhage that shows little or no tendency toward clearing are candidates for early vitrectomy. If vitreous hemorrhage is present in an only eye of a diabetic, timing of the vitrectomy will depend on the patient's visual needs and social and emotional desires.

In diabetic patients with unilateral vitreous hemorrhage and functional vision in the other eye, ultrasonography should be performed at intervals of 2 to 3 months to rule out the development of a tractional or rhegmatogenous retinal detachment. If ultrasonography indicates that a retinal detachment involves the posterior pole or a tractional detachment is encroaching upon the macula, vitrectomy should be seriously considered. If the hemorrhage fails to clear in 6 to 9 months then vitrectomy is performed. In eyes with severe iris neovascularization, early vitrectomy may be attempted to permit panretinal photocoagulation for the rubeosis iridis. Figure 4.51 shows a dense vitreous hemorrhage involving most of the vitreous cavity.

PREPARATION OF SCLEROTOMIES

Using curved iris scissors, a limbal peritomy is made extending 270° to expose the superior nasal and superior and inferior temporal quadrants (see Fig. 4.18). The conjunctiva is lifted up with Bishop Harmon forceps as Tenon's fascia and conjunctiva are undermined to the equator.

The sclerotomy for the infusion cannula is made in the inferotemporal quadrant near the inferior border of the lateral rectus muscle. Episcleral tissue over the intended site for the sclerotomy is scraped away using a scarifier. Episcleral blood vessels are coagulated with an eraser. In normal-sized eyes, the sclerotomies are made 3.5 mm from the limbus, where a mark is made with a gentian violet marking pen. The infusion cannula (Fig. 4.52, middle) is anchored to the sclera with a 6-0 Vicryl suture with a spatula needle. Scleral bites should extend to at least one-half of the depth of the sclera (Fig. 4.53). The sclerotomies are made with a microvitreal knife (MVR) (Fig. 4.54) with a blade 1.4 mm in width that produces an incision that snugly accommodates a 20-gauge instrument (see Fig. 1.121). To avoid penetrating the lens, the blade is inclined so that its point is directed toward the center of the vitreous cavity. Penetration of the sclera and vitreous cavity is done under visualization with the operating microscope.

A stiletto is rotated 180° to enlarge the width of the incision in the sclera, uvea, and vitreous base so that instruments will pass through easily. A 4-mm infusion cannula (see Fig. 4.52, middle) is used in most eyes. If the ora serrata and pars plana ciliaris are elevated, and the eye is aphakic, a longer cannula (see Fig. 4.52, top) is used. One edge of the sclerotomy is held with the colibri forceps while the cannula is inserted with a rotary motion. One loop of the suture is placed on the shoulder of the cannula while the opposite loop is pulled up and tied with a slipknot, leaving the arms of the suture 1 inch in length (Fig. 4.55). Before the infusion line is opened, it is vitally important to check that the tip of the cannula has penetrated the uvea and pars plana and entered the vitreous cavity. A scleral plug is placed in the sclerotomy in order to prevent vitreous prolapse (Fig. 4.55, inset).

▽ Chronic Vitreous Hemorrhage With Virectomy: Considerations

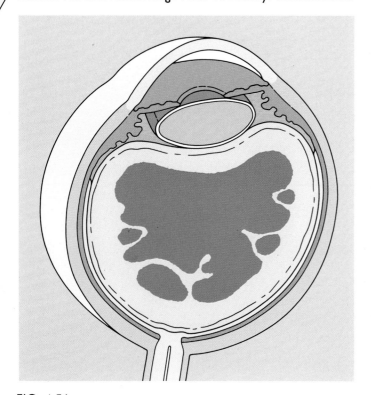

FIG. 4.51

▽ Chronic Vitreous Hemorrhage: Preparation of Sclerotomies

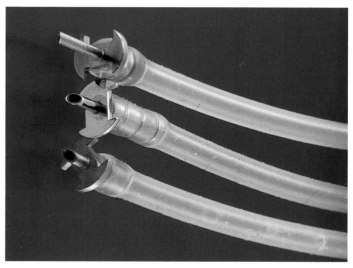

FIG. 4.52

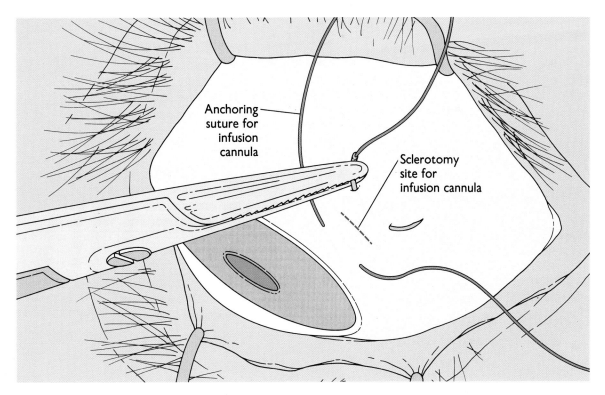

Anchoring suture for infusion cannula

Sclerotomy site for infusion cannula

FIG. 4.53

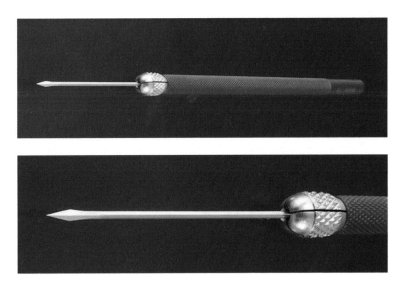

FIG. 4.54

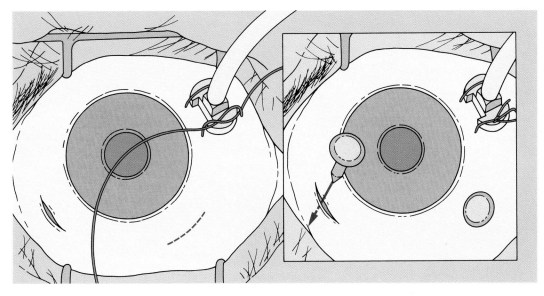

FIG. 4.55

Sclerotomies for the vitrectomy probe and endoillumi-nator are made 3.5 mm from the limbus in the 9:30 and 2:30 meridians (See Fig. 1.121). The edge of the sclerotomy is grasped with colibri forceps while the endo-illuminator or the vitrectomy probe is introduced with a rotary motion.

VITRECTOMY

An anterior vitrectomy is performed first. In order to avoid damaging the lens, the port of the vitrectomy probe is turned sidewise facing 90° from the posterior capsule of the lens. During retrolental vitrectomy, the cutting speed is increased and the suction pressure is set at a low level. A 0.1-mm air bubble is injected into the infusion line from a tuberculin syringe. This bubble will gravitate to the poste-rior surface of the lens so that it can be identified and avoided during vitrectomy. Once the retrolental space has been cleared, vitrectomy is carried out peripherally and posteriorly with visualization through a fundus contact lens (Fig. 4.56).

It is important to keep the cutting port visible at all times while performing vitrectomy. Slow deliberate movements of the vitrector with intermittent stops to assess the sur-rounding vitreous are important. While the vitrector is held still, exploration is accomplished by moving the endoillu-minator into regions to be cut. The midvitreous is removed from the midline in a widening circle until a central fluid-filled cavity is created. It is not necessary to extend the vitrectomy peripherally into the region of the vitreous base unless the vitreous hemorrhage was the result of a pene-trating injury.

REMOVAL OF SUBHYALOID BLOOD

In some eyes the vitreous is detached posteriorly and blood accumulates in the subhyaloid space (Fig. 4.57). A small hole is made in the nasal half of the condensed posterior hyaloid through which blood can be removed.

After lowering the infusion bottle to decrease the intra-ocular pressure to prevent vitreous prolapse through the sclerotomy, the vitrectomy probe is removed and replaced by the extrusion needle. With the endoilluminator moving in tandem, the extrusion needle is introduced through the hole in the posterior hyaloid (Fig. 4.58). The index finger is removed from the vent in the handle, allowing subhyaloid blood to be evacuated from the eye. The posterior hyaloid may be thickened and attached to the optic disk (Fig. 4.59). If this thickened posterior hyaloid extends to the vitreous base, it is excised using the vitrectomy probe (inset).

After the infusion bottle has been lowered, the vitrector and endoilluminator are removed from the vitreous cavity and plugs are placed in the sclerotomies in order to prevent prolapse of vitreous. The superior sclerotomies are closed with 8-0 nylon suture in a figure eight fashion and the suture ends are trimmed to the knot with a knife or Vannas scissors. The arms of the suture are freed from the shoulders of the infusion cannula, which is removed by the assistant

Chronic Vitreous Hemorrhage: Vitrectomy

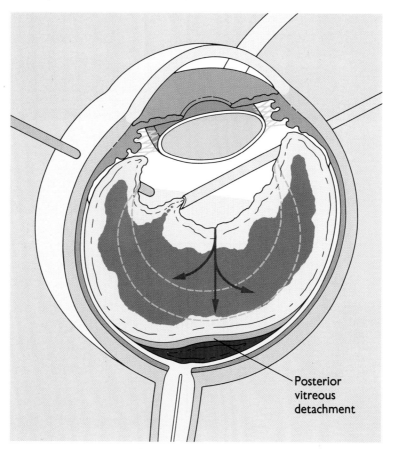

Posterior
vitreous
detachment

FIG. 4.56

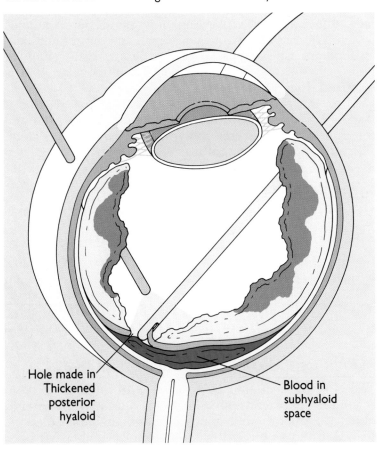

FIG. 4.57

Hole made in Thickened posterior hyaloid

Blood in subhyaloid space

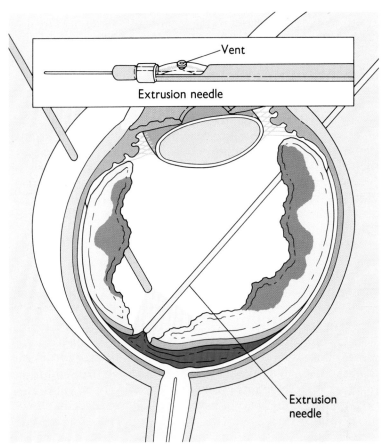

FIG. 4.58

Vent

Extrusion needle

Extrusion needle

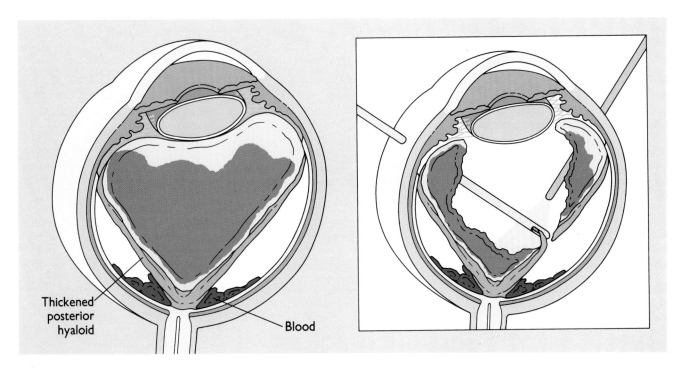

FIG. 4.59

Thickened posterior hyaloid

Blood

while the suture is tightened and then tied in a square knot. The conjunctiva is closed with interrupted sutures of 7-0 chromic gut. After obtaining a culture, Gentamycin and polymixin are injected under Tenon's capsule.

POSTOPERATIVE GAS–FLUID EXCHANGE

A postoperative gas–fluid exchange may be used to remove recurrent vitreous hemorrhage or to tamponade the retina after surgery for retinal reattachment. Removal of vitreous hemorrhage after vitrectomy permits visualization and photocoagulation if indicated. It is desirable in some cases of retinal detachment with residual preretinal traction to provide an extensive inferior internal tamponade with gas for at least two weeks during the development of the chorioretinal adhesion.

This intraocular procedure carries the risks of hyphema, ocular hypertension, flattening of the anterior chamber, and endophthalmitis. To minimize and deal with these complications, I perform the procedure in an ambulatory operating room rather than at the slitlamp in an examining room. The skin around the eye is scrubbed with a povidine–iodine solution and a small plastic eye drape is applied to the periorbital region. A preoperative culture is taken from the conjunctival cul de sac. The patient is placed in a semiprone position with the chin resting on a closed fist and supported on a Mayo stand. The gowned and gloved surgeon sits on an adjustable stool with an elbow supported on a Mayo stand. Topical 4% cocaine is applied at the limbus at the site selected for injection. To steady the globe, the conjunctiva is grasped with toothed Bishop Harmon forceps. A mixture of 20% perfluoropropane (C_3F_8) gas and air is drawn into a 6-cc syringe and attached to a short 27-gauge needle. In aphakic eyes the needle is inserted into the inferior anterior chamber. To avoid penetrating the iris, the needle is inserted into the anterior chamber parallel to the iris surface. In phakic and pseudophakic eyes, the needle is inserted through the pars plana. Small amounts of intraocular fluid are aspirated and exchanged for a small volume of 20% C_3F_8 mixture until most of the intraocular fluid is removed (Fig. 4.60).

After the fluid–gas exchange, the paracentesis site is inspected for leakage, intraocular pressure is measured, and the ophthalmic artery is examined to be sure it is patent. The aspirant is sent for culture.

MANAGEMENT OF TRAUMATIC VITREOUS HEMORRHAGE AND CORNEOSCLERAL LACERATION

Figure 4.61 shows a penetrating ocular injury resulting in a corneoscleral laceration extending posteriorly to the region of the equator. The lens has been damaged so that cortical lens material is mixed with vitreous hemorrhage. Uveal tissue and vitreous gel have prolapsed through the laceration.

REPAIR OF CORNEOSCLERAL LACERATION

The corneal laceration is repaired with interrupted 10-0 nylon sutures placed approximately 1 mm apart. In order to obtain optimal wound approximation, the first suture is placed at the limbus. After the anterior chamber has been reformed, it is vitally important to determine the posterior extent of the scleral laceration. A peritomy is performed over one quadrant and the conjunctiva is reflected using curved sharp iris scissors (Fig. 4.62A). The sclera is exposed by sharp dissection of Tenon's capsule and the conjunctiva.

Chronic Vitreous Hemorrhage: Postoperative Gas–Fluid Exchange

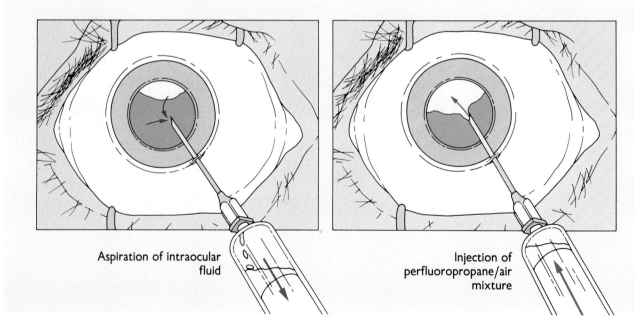

Aspiration of intraocular fluid

Injection of perfluoropropane/air mixture

FIG. 4.60

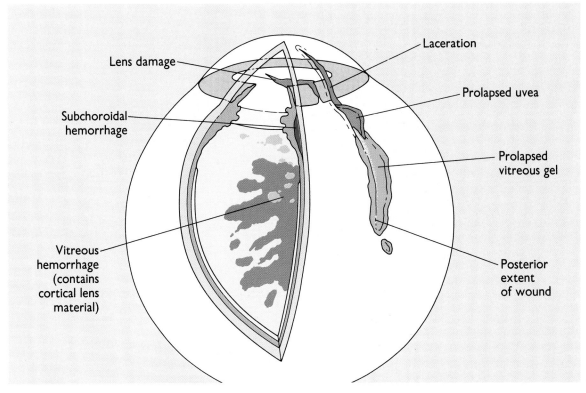

Lens damage

Laceration

Subchoroidal hemorrhage

Prolapsed uvea

Prolapsed vitreous gel

Vitreous hemorrhage (contains cortical lens material)

Posterior extent of wound

FIG. 4.61

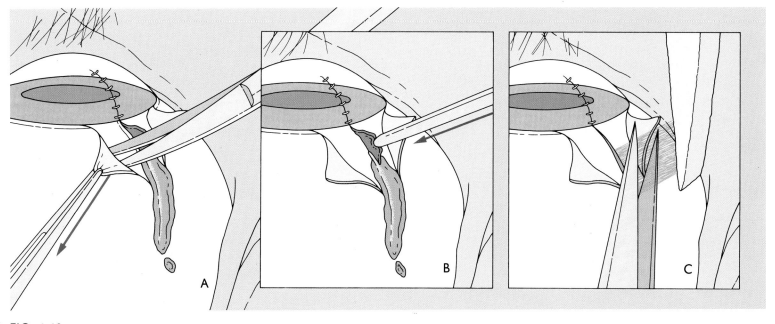

A

B

C

FIG. 4.62

If there is any indication that a second perforation may be present, the peritomy is extended around 360° to permit a more thorough exploration of the sclera.

Every effort should be made to reposit rather than excise the ciliary body or uveal tissue, which bleeds profusely when cut. Uveal tissue is reposited using a bent iris or retinal spatula (Fig. 4.62B). If the uveal tissue appears grossly contaminated, it is diathermized with underwater diathermy before and during excision. Excised tissue suspected of being retina is sent for histologic examination. Prolapsing vitreous is drawn away from the globe using a cellulose sponge so that it can be cut flush with the wound using Vannas scissors (Fig. 4.62C). The scleral wound is then closed using interrupted 8-0 nylon sutures.

The pupil is dilated with 0.1 cc of epinephrine bitartrate 1:10,000 solution injected into the anterior chamber in order to assess the extent of the damage to the lens. During lensectomy, BSS Plus solution is constantly infused into the anterior chamber using a bent 25-gauge needle inserted through a limbal incision. Lensectomy is performed with the vitrectomy probe introduced through a second incision at the limbus. In young patients the nucleus can be removed with suction and cutting. A sclerotic nucleus may require ultrasonic fragmentation. A concerted effort should be made to remove as much peripheral cortical lens material as possible by using suction with the cutting port of the vitrectomy probe directed horizontally in order to avoid traction to vitreous gel (see Chapter 1, Cataract Surgery and Intraocular Lens Implantation).

ANTERIOR VITRECTOMY VIA THE LIMBUS

An anterior vitrectomy is performed for the removal of anterior vitreous hemorrhage and cortical lens material (see Fig. 1.415). Because visualization through the cornea is usually poor, no attempt is made to remove the peripheral vitreous and vitreous base. Indirect ophthalmoscopy is performed in an attempt to assess the damage to the posterior segment. Ultrasonography is performed after three to four days to determine if the retina is attached.

VITRECTOMY

A deep vitrectomy is not performed until 5 to 10 days later, depending on the clarity of the cornea. The vitrectomy probe and endoilluminator are inserted into the vitreous cavity through sclerotomies in the pars plana. Vitrectomy is extended laterally and posteriorly to the detached posterior hyaloid (see Figs. 4.56 and 1.133 and 1.135).

Providing visualization is good, the peripheral vitreous is removed cautiously using scleral depression. Removal of the peripheral vitreous will decrease the incidence of a tractional retinal detachment and may decrease the chance of the development of anterior proliferative vitreoretinopathy.

An air–fluid exchange is then performed using the extrusion needle and endoilluminator (see Fig. 4.58). Indirect ophthalmoscopy and scleral depression are performed to determine if any traumatic or iatrogenic retinal breaks are present. Endolaser is applied around any retinal breaks and in five rows around the circumference of the fundus between the ora serrata and the equator (Fig. 4.63).

EPISCLERAL BUCKLING

In order to reduce postoperative vitreous traction from the remainder of the vitreous base, an episcleral buckling procedure is performed. A solid silicone implant 9 mm in width and an encircling band are placed around the globe, slightly anterior to the equator (Fig. 4.63, inset). Prior to removal of the infusion cannula and closure of the conjunctiva, a gas–fluid exchange is done by lavaging 50 cc of a 20% mixture of C_3F_8 gas and air through the globe.

MANAGEMENT OF PROLIFERATIVE VITREORETINOPATHY

Proliferative vitreoretinopathy (PVR) develops in 5% to 10% of rhegmatogenous retinal detachments and is the most common cause of failure of retinal detachment surgery. It is characterized by the growth of membranes on both surfaces of the detached retina and on the posterior surface of the detached vitreous gel.

The term posterior PVR is used to describe cases in which the proliferative changes are most severe in the posterior fundus. Anterior PVR describes eyes in which proliferative changes predominate in the anterior fundus and the region of the vitreous base.

POSTERIOR PROLIFERATIVE VITREORETINOPATHY

The clinical picture of PVR has been classified by the Retina Society into several categories of varying degrees of severity. Figure 4.64A and B shows severe or massive PVR (Grade D-2), which is characterized by full-thickness retinal folds in all quadrants. The retinal detachment has the appearance of a giant starfold involving the entire retina with radial spokes centered about the optic nerve head. This produces a funnel-shaped retinal detachment. Figure 4.64C shows a funnel-shaped retinal detachment in which the apex of the funnel has become closed, obscuring the optic disk.

After a limbal peritomy of the conjunctiva, bridle sutures of 4-0 black silk are placed around or through the tendons of the rectus muscles. Sites for the three sclerotomies are marked 3.5 mm posterior to the limbus in the 10:30 and 2:30 meridians and along the inferior margin of the lateral rectus muscles.

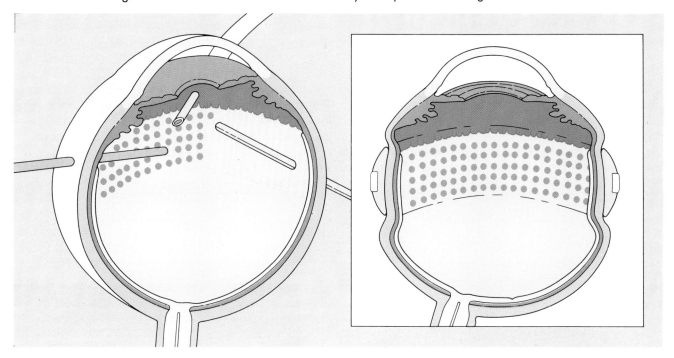

FIG. 4.63

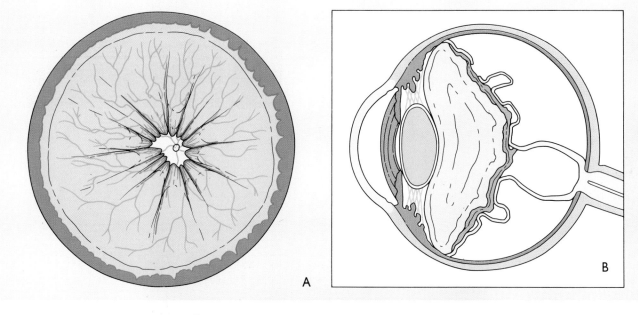

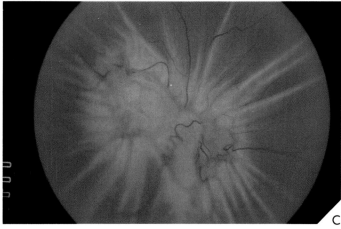

FIG. 4.64

Vitrectomy

Scleral buckling techniques are used for mild and moderate forms (Grades B, C-1, C-2) of PVR. Vitrectomy and preretinal or subretinal membrane surgery is necessary in severe forms as illustrated in Fig. 4.65. The vitrectomy probe is used to remove the vitreous gel that is condensed and retracted anteriorly to produce the funnel-shaped retinal detachment.

Membrane Peeling

It is necessary to find or isolate an edge of a preretinal membrane before it can be peeled from the retina. The membrane peeler (Fig. 4.66) is a blunt-tipped instrument designed for that purpose, the tip of which is passed between shallow retinal folds while exploring for the edge of a preretinal membrane (Fig. 4.67A). A variety of spatulas (Fig. 4.68) is used to separate preretinal membranes between deep radial retinal folds (Fig. 4.67B and C). The forked teeth of the retinal scratcher (Fig. 4.69) are ideal for separating the edge of an adherent membrane (Fig. 4.67D). Pick forceps (Fig. 4.70) are useful for both dissecting and gripping membranes with the same instrument.

Once the edge of a membrane has been separated from the retina, it is grasped with an end-gripping forceps (Fig. 4.71) designed for grasping fine structures on the surface of

---

Posterior Proliferative Vitreoretinopathy: Vitrectomy

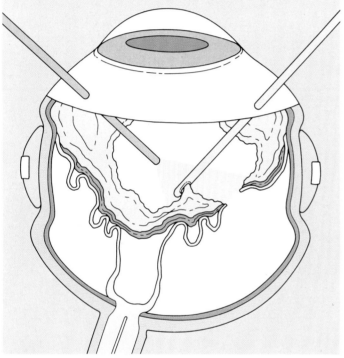

FIG. 4.65

Posterior Proliferative Vitreoretinopathy: Membrane Peeling

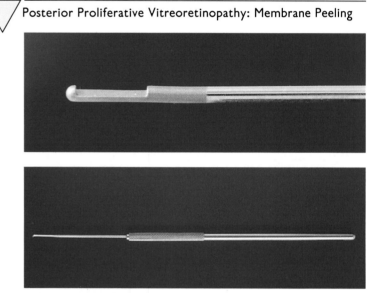

FIG. 4.66

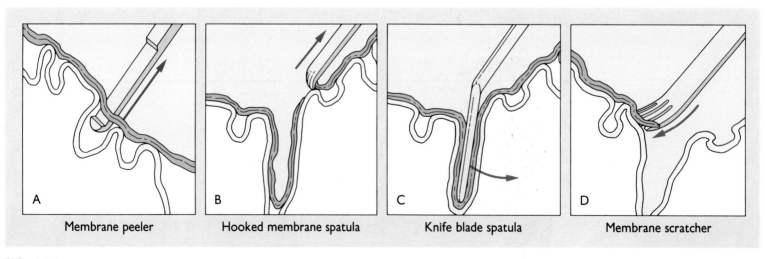

A	B	C	D
Membrane peeler	Hooked membrane spatula	Knife blade spatula	Membrane scratcher

FIG. 4.67

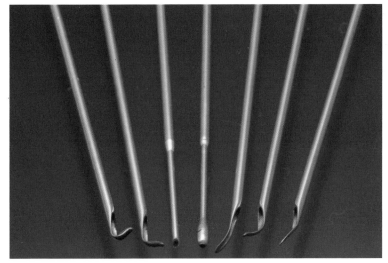

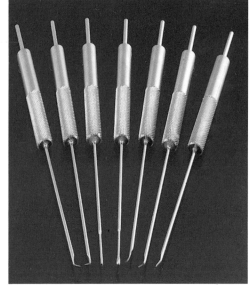

FIG. 4.68

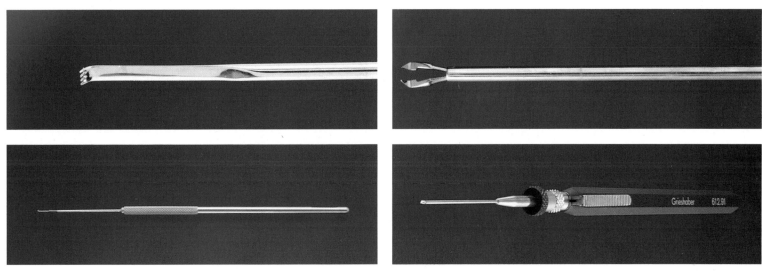

FIG. 4.69

FIG. 4.70

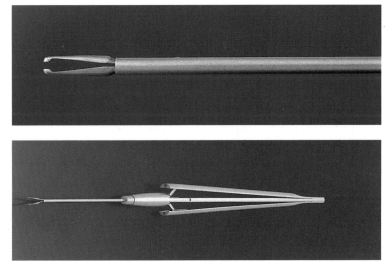

FIG. 4.71

the retina. The membrane is lifted gently in order to peel it off in a large sheet or in smaller segments (Fig. 4.72A). The separated membrane is removed with the forceps or the vitrectomy probe. If resistance is encountered when peeling a membrane, counterpressure is exerted very gently with the endoilluminator on the retina adjacent to the membrane attachment to prevent an iatrogenic retinal break (Fig. 4.72B). The endoilluminator can also be used as a probe to separate the retina from the membrane being held by the forceps. Membranes that are tightly adherent and resist peeling are resected using right-angled scissors.

Internal Drainage

Whenever possible, internal subretinal fluid is drained through a preexisting retinal break rather than by performing a retinotomy. A peripheral retinal break is marked with endodiathermy so that it will be easily visualized during and following air–fluid exchange. The tip of the cannulated subretinal aspirator (Fig. 4.73) is positioned near the retinal tear, after which the flexible cannula is advanced into the subretinal space through the retinal tear (Fig. 4.74). Subretinal fluid is forced through the vent in the handle of the instrument by air introduced into the vitreous cavity by the air pump. After reattachment of the retina has been achieved, the cannula is retracted through the retinal break.

Endolaser

The retinal breaks are surrounded with four rows of endolaser (Fig. 4.75). Five rows of endolaser are placed around 360° of the fundus on the indentation produced by the scleral buckle and encircling element (inset). Prior to closure of the conjunctiva, a gas–air exchange is performed using a 20% mixture of C_3F_8 gas and air.

ANTERIOR PROLIFERATIVE VITREORETINOPATHY

In eyes with anterior proliferative vitreoretinopathy (APVR), proliferative changes produce a membrane that extends from the peripheral retina across the vitreous base to attach to either the pars plana, the ciliary processes, or

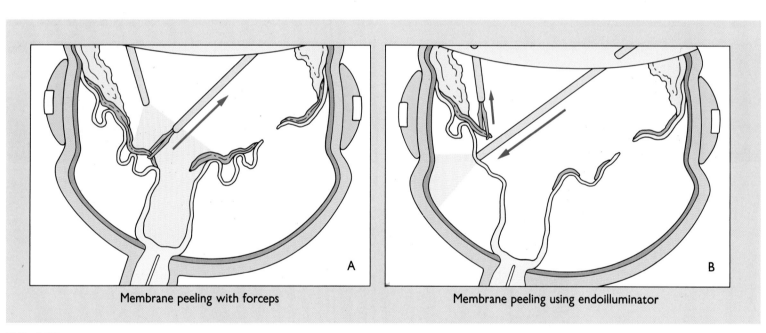

Membrane peeling with forceps

Membrane peeling using endoilluminator

FIG. 4.72

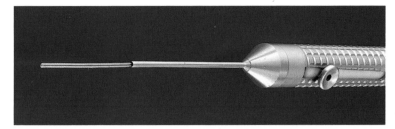

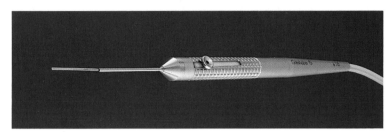

FIG. 4.73

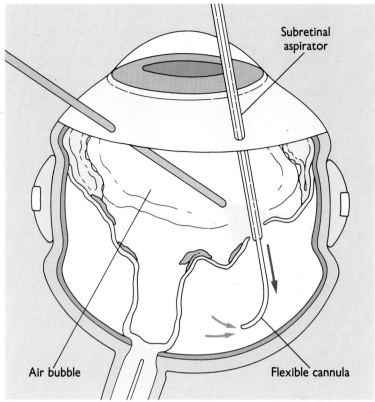

Subretinal aspirator

Air bubble

Flexible cannula

FIG. 4.74

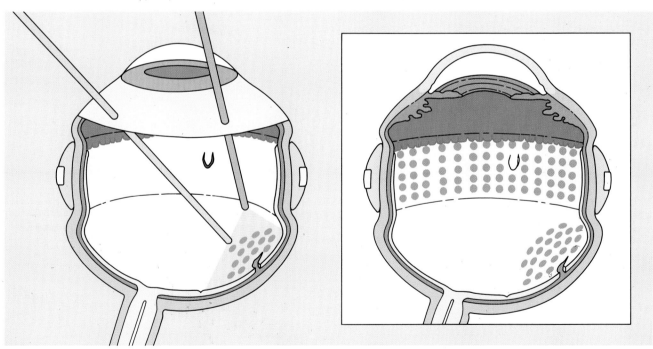

FIG. 4.75

the posterior surface of the iris (Fig. 4.76). Contraction of this anterior membrane pulls the peripheral retina anteriorly, producing a fold in the retina that runs parallel to the ora serrata. Shrinkage of the vitreous base in a circumferential direction decreases its diameter and throws the peripheral retina into accordianlike, radial retinal folds.

The anterior membrane extends from the peripheral retina across the vitreous base, which acts as a scaffold. The membrane attaches to either the pars plana ciliaris (Fig. 4.77A) or ciliary processes (Fig. 4.77B), the posterior surface of the iris (Fig. 4.77C), or the pupillary margin (Fig. 4.77D). The amount of anterior traction exerted by this membrane accounts for the anterior displacement of the circumferential fold in the peripheral retina. When a mild degree of traction is present, the fold is located midway between the ora serrata and the equator (Fig. 4.77A). With severe degrees of traction, the circumferential fold is pulled anterior to the ora serrata (Fig. 4.77C). A trough of varying width and depth is present between the circumferential retinal fold and the pars plana ciliaris. A moderate degree of traction produces a shallow and wide trough (Fig. 4.77A). Severe membrane traction produces a deep and narrow trough (Fig. 4.77C).

A vitrectomy including the vitreous base is performed in order to relieve circumferential traction. Scleral depression and lensectomy are performed routinely to provide optimum visualization of the region of the vitreous base. When a wide retinal trough is present, the membrane bridging it and the condensed vitreous base within it are removed with a vitrector (Figs. 4.77A and 4.78A). Right angled scissors (Fig. 4.79) are used to cut an anterior membrane bridging a narrow trough (Figs. 4.77C and 4.78B).

Traction by the anterior membrane causes the peripheral retina to become stretched, thinned, and atrophic. This atrophic retina is prone to developing retinal breaks during attempts to peel preretinal membranes. With scleral depression and a widely dilated pupil, it is possible to illuminate the peripheral retina with the light from the operating microscope so that a bimanual technique can be used to peel and cut the membrane with less traction to the retina. Additional illumination may be obtained using picks, forceps, or spatulas to which a fiber optic bundle is attached. The preretinal membrane is grasped with forceps held in the surgeon's nondominant hand and then separated from the retina with a spatula held in the dominant hand (Fig. 4.80). Holding the membrane in this manner reduces excessive tractional movements during attempts to peel it and decreases the incidence of iatrogenic retinal break.

Anterior Proliferative Vitreoretinopathy

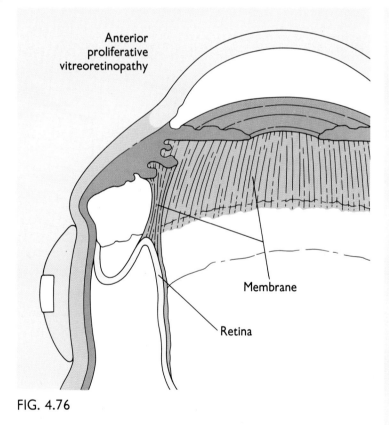

FIG. 4.76

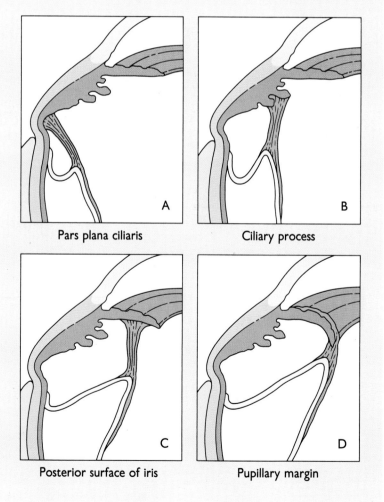

Pars plana ciliaris

Ciliary process

Posterior surface of iris

Pupillary margin

FIG. 4.77

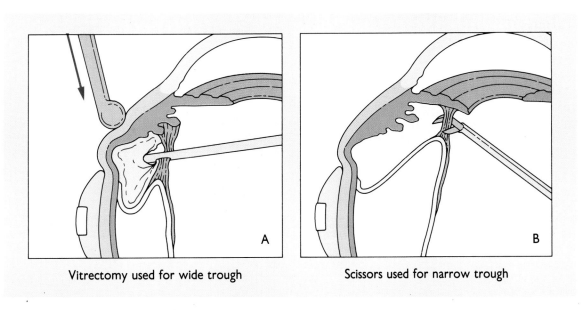

Vitrectomy used for wide trough   A

Scissors used for narrow trough   B

FIG. 4.78

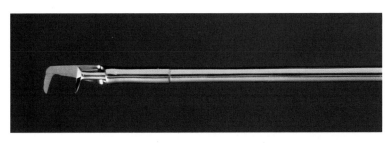

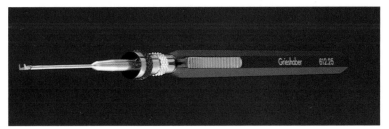

FIG. 4.79

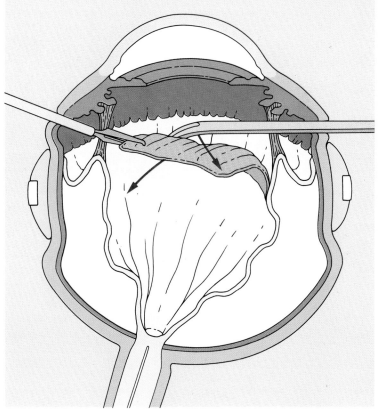

FIG. 4.80

Relaxing Retinotomy

A relaxing retinotomy is performed in eyes in which severe preretinal organization makes it impossible to peel peripheral membranes or cut the anterior membrane (Fig. 4.81A). The retinotomy is made slightly posterior and parallel to the vitreous base and extending over the circumference of the unrelieved traction. An air–fluid exchange is performed to tamponade the posterior edge of the retinotomy where endolaser is applied.

Retinectomy

Penetrating injury involving the region of the ciliary body periretinal and intraretinal organization may result in peripheral retina that is opaque, thickened, immobile, and organized into a mass of radial retinal folds. If efforts to peel preretinal and subretinal membranes and a relaxing reti-notomy are unsuccessful, the organized retina is removed by retinectomy (Fig. 4.81B). In order to avoid excising an excessive amount of retinal tissue, the slowest possible cutting speed of the vitrectomy probe and low suction pressure are used. Retinectomy is continued posteriorly until smooth, relatively mobile retina of normal thickness is reached. An air–fluid exchange is performed in conjunction with internal drainage of subretinal fluid in order to tamponade the posterior retinal flap of the retinectomy against the pigment epithelium. The posterior edge of the retinectomy is mechanically fixed in position with intraocular tantalum retinal screws inserted every 30° using an intraocular screwdriver. Endolaser is applied 360° around the fundus and the air is replaced with a mixture of 20% C_3F_8 gas and air or with fluorosilicone oil.

Anterior Proliferative Vitreoretinopathy: Relaxing Retinotomy and Retinectomy

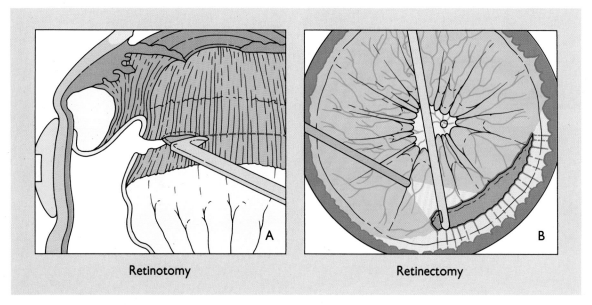

Retinotomy   Retinectomy

A   B

FIG. 4.81

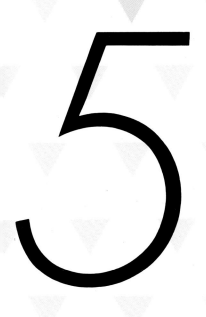

TECHNIQUES IN
STRABISMUS SURGERY

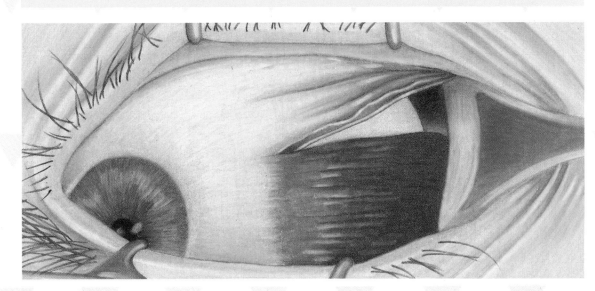

Robert W. Lingua, MD

Preoperatively, one may consider a variety of factors that can assist the surgeon in performing the optimal procedure for the strabismus patient.

The potential of the anticipated surgery to compromise further the blood supply to the anterior segment is to be evaluated in light of previously operated muscles, prior cryotherapy in the vicinity of the long posterior ciliary arteries, the presence or absence of encircling elements, chronic intraocular inflammation, and previous trauma.

Selection of the type and location of the conjunctival incision is based on the number and location of muscles on which to be operated, the anticipated presence or absence of scarring, and the status of the conjunctiva and Tenon's capsule in light of the patient's age and health. Tenon's capsule is typically sparse in the elderly, and the conjunctiva is often friable. In this case, one may select a conjunctival incision that will not require stretching and therefore avoid irregular conjunctival tears. I prefer the cul-de-sac approach in eyes that have not been previously operated on, and especially in the young, where the tissues are more elastic. In patients undergoing reoperation, those with extremely thin conjunctiva, and those intended to undergo an adjustable suture procedure, I employ an incision over the insertion of the tendon (after Swan). When conjunctival recession is planned or in cases involving exploration for the tendon, the exploration begins from the cornea with a limbus-based peritomy. In resections, especially of the medial recti, where one anticipates redundant conjunctiva, I prefer the Swan approach, entering the conjunctiva at the base of the semilunar fold, or employ the limbus-based incision with recession or resection of the conjunctiva in order to minimize chemosis at the nasal limbus postoperatively. Prolonged chemosis may lead to dellen formation and ulceration, especially in the elderly or in the medically compromised patient. When horizontal and oblique or vertical rectus muscles are to be operated on simultaneously, fornix incisions between the muscles will often provide adequate exposure for the entirety of the case, e.g., in A-pattern esotropia with superior oblique overaction or V-pattern exotropia with inferior oblique overaction. Similar planning is necessary when horizontal or vertical transpositions of the recti are to be performed.

Especially in cases of reoperation, at the conclusion of the conjunctival incision, fastidious hemostasis of all conjunctival vessels will minimize the occurrence of hemorrhage in Tenon's capsule, which can obscure tissue planes. A constant awareness of your position relative to the vorticose veins and periocular fat will minimize trauma to these structures. Hemorrhage from a torn vorticose vein will cease with the direct pressure of a cotton tip applicator over its transverse scleral canal, and cautery of its distal aspect in the periocular fascia. Violation of the fat pad can be managed by primary closure with plain gut sutures, and is advised, especially in the presence of any bleeding. Realizing that the horizontal and vertical recti insert between 4 and 8 mm from the limbus, introduction of the muscle hook more posteriorly than the anticipated location of the tendon is to be avoided, since it may draw the posterior Tenon's capsule forward, along with the fat pad, and complicate the dissection. Additional caution is exercised in engaging the lateral rectus, where introduction of the hook along its inferior border more than 8 mm posterior to its insertion is

likely to engage the inferior oblique muscle. Likewise, in surgery of the superior rectus, the superior oblique should be visualized prior to cutting the intermuscular fascia and thus assure its integrity.

As in patients with high myopia, those with a long exposure to alcohol have a rubberlike texture to the sclera, which in the former case may also be very thin. In such cases, the "microtip" spatula needles will pass more easily through the sclera with less tissue drag, but may present a greater risk of perforation. When perforation occurs in the elderly, liquified vitreous may spontaneously drain through the site. In any case of suspected perforation, the pupil is dilated and the area visualized with indirect ophthalmoscopy. When penetration of the retina has occurred, a single small application of cryotherapy over the perforation site is indicated, as well as retinal consultation in the postoperative course.

In general, absorbable suture material can be used when the tendon is secured to the globe at the point of intended attachment. In other situations, e.g., where one might anticipate difficulty in the localization of the tendon if reoperation is necessary (superior oblique tenectomy or large adjustable recessions of the medial or superior rectus), or suspension in the vicinity of a silicone element, or in posterior fixation cases, a nonabsorbable suture may be preferred. When a tendonous insertion is particularly vascularized, as in thyroid eye disease, or as is routinely noted in the vertical recti, light applications of cautery prior to the passage of the spatula needle will minimize hemorrhage in the distal tendon. A hematoma at the insertion can obscure the anatomy and lead to an insecure passage and/or lock of the tendon. Improprer locking of the suture to the Tenon's capsule rather than tendon may lead to muscle slippage. Closure of the conjunctiva can be accomplished with plain gut suture. Passing the needles close to the edge of the conjunctival incision will minimize the risk of inclusion cyst formation.

Recessions alone tend to widen the palpebral fissures, while recess/resect procedures tend to narrow them. The possible consequences of the intended procedure on eyelid position should be discussed with the patient preoperatively and may often be employed to one's advantage when an asymmetry exists preoperatively.

Retrobulbar anesthesia is satisfactory for most adult strabismus surgery. However, caution must be exercised in those with thyroid eye disease, where the necessary volume of anesthetic for anesthesia and akinesia may compromise blood supply to the eye. The longer-acting anesthetics (e.g., bupivacaine) are avoided when one is planning to adjust sutures the following morning. If one intends to perform a passive "spring-back balance" test under general anesthesia, then the use of a long-acting paralytic agent such as Pavulon may be discussed with the anesthetist. If, however, one chooses to elicit a contraction of the extraocular muscle during the procedure, as in certain paralytic, adjustable suture, transposition, or slipped muscle cases, then inhalation anesthesia alone will allow the introduction of succinylcholine as necessary during the case. The skeletal muscle paralysis from succinylcholine will resolve within three minutes of injection, but the increased tension effect in the extraocular muscle typically peaks by 60 seconds after injection and then gradually declines over a period of 10 to

20 minutes. Therefore, when succinylcholine has been used to facilitate general anesthesia, preoperative forced ductions will be influenced by this induced muscular tension.

RECESSION OF A RECTUS MUSCLE

The assistant grasps the eye at the conjunctiva–Tenon's junction with a 0.3-mm forceps and rotates the eye into elevation and abduction (Fig. 5.1). The surgeon then elevates the conjunctiva at the base of the fornix, and incises the conjunctiva the desired distance from the limbus (Fig. 5.2). At this point, all visible conjunctival vessels are lightly cauterized to ensure good visibility through the localization of the tendon. The assistant and the surgeon grasp the fascia within the conjunctival incision with gentle pressure against the sclera, and elevate it from the globe (Fig. 5.3). The scissors are then used to incise Tenon's capsule at this point, exposing bare sclera (Fig. 5.4). Visualization is maintained with the posterior forceps.

Recession of a Rectus Muscle

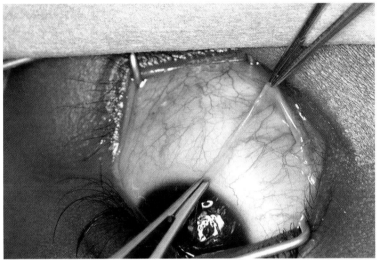

FIG. 5.1

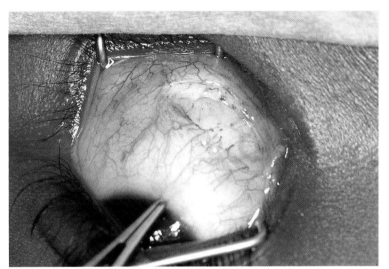

FIG. 5.2

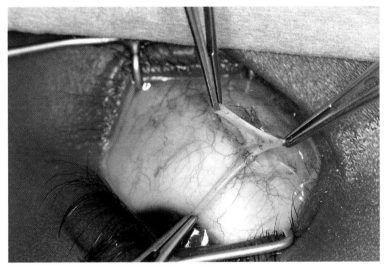

FIG. 5.3

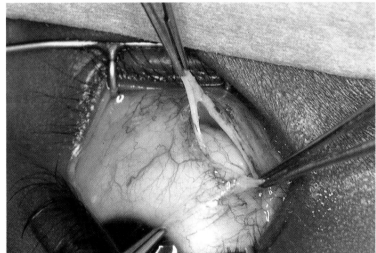

FIG. 5.4

The large muscle hook can then be passed behind the medial rectus muscle without any further posterior movement of the hook than the site of the incision itself (Fig. 5.5). When the medial rectus is on the hook, one should confirm that the entire tendon has been engaged. The posterior arm of the 0.3-mm forceps can be used as a probe to locate the superior pole of the muscle (Fig. 5.6). Securing it with the forceps, the muscle hook is withdrawn to the inferior aspect of the tendon (Fig. 5.7), being sure to release the hook from entrapment in the insertion. Then, it is passed beyond the superior pole held by the forceps (Fig. 5.8). In this way, one can be certain of having completely secured the full length of the tendon. A large Jameson muscle hook, or the Greene hook, will assist in the following dissection.

The small tenotomy hook is introduced between the insertion of the tendon and Tenon's capsule anterior to it (Fig. 5.9) and used to dissect bluntly the fascia from the surface of the tendon, moving posteriorly along its long axis (Fig. 5.10). Overcoming some resistance to blunt dissection at this point is important in order to visualize adequately the tendon during the remainder of the case. When the conjunctiva and Tenon's capsule have been satisfactorily distracted over the tip of the large muscle hook (Fig. 5.11), the scissors are used to incise the superior aspect of Tenon's fascia (Fig. 5.12). Visualization of bare sclera superiorly is accomplished by the introduction of the closed scissor blades into the fascial incision and rotation of them over the tip of the hook (Figs. 5.13 and 5.14). Two small tenotomy hooks are then passed posteriorly along the tendon, against

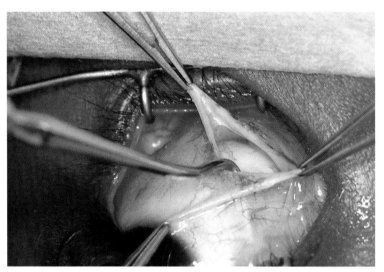

FIG. 5.5

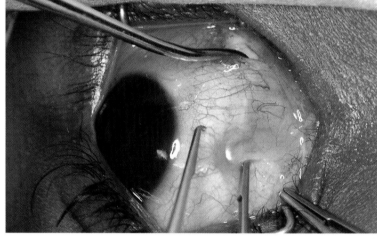

FIG. 5.6

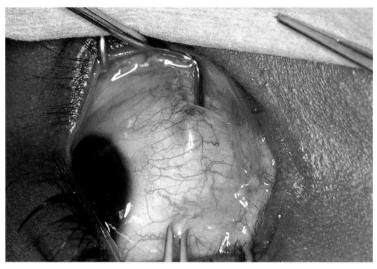

FIG. 5.7

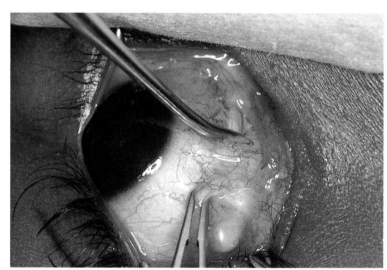

FIG. 5.8

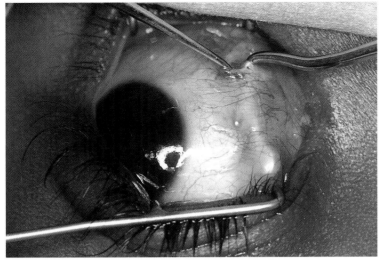

FIG. 5.9

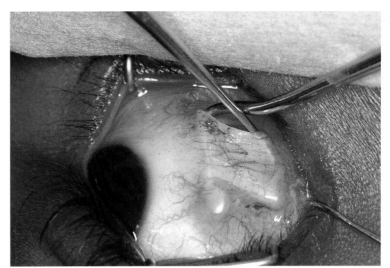

FIG. 5.10

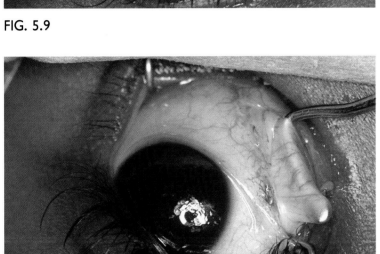

FIG. 5.11

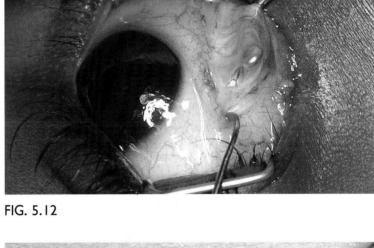

FIG. 5.12

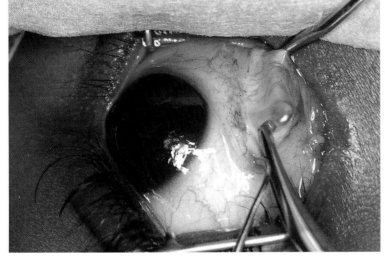

FIG. 5.13

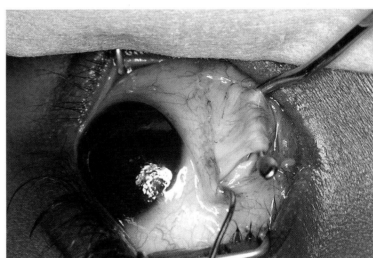

FIG. 5.14

bare sclera, and elevated to expose the intermuscular fascia (Figs. 5.15 and 5.16) for dissection. The 0.5-mm Castroviejo locking forceps are then applied to the distal aspect of the tendon superiorly (Fig. 5.17) and inferiorly. These forceps serve as globe handles throughout the case, obviating the need for traction sutures at the limbus. Also, the superior forceps maintains full exposure of the insertion, keeping the distracted conjunctiva and fascia securely above the superior pole when the inferonasal fornix incision is used.

Gentle traction by the assistant, away from the operated muscle, allows the surgeon to control the hook beneath the tendon and accomplish suture passage at the insertion (Fig.

5.18). The surgeon may then control the forceps during the scleral passes to position optimally and control the globe. The needle is passed from the middle to the superior edge of the tendon, where it is positioned for regrasping. A second "through-and-through" lock to the edge of the tendon (Figs. 5.19 to 5.21) is performed. The Westcott scissors suffices for removing the tendon (Fig. 5.22). Visualization of the tendon may be preserved by passing a dry cotton pledget between the tendon and the globe (Fig. 5.23). The anterior pole of the caliper is positioned at the crotch of the original insertion (Fig. 5.24). The ideal scleral pass imparts

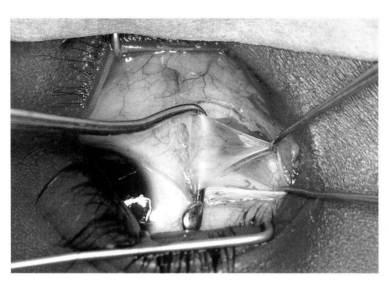

FIG. 5.15

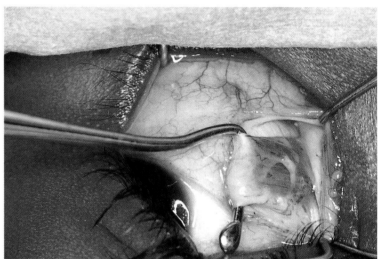

FIG. 5.16

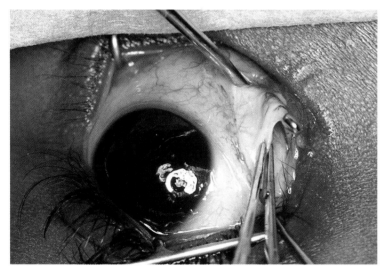

FIG. 5.17

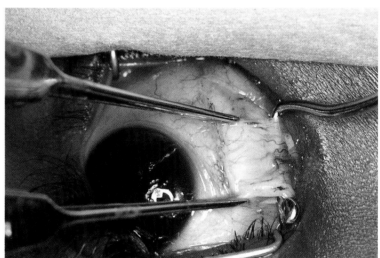

FIG. 5.18

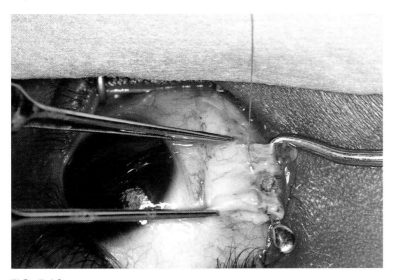

FIG. 5.19

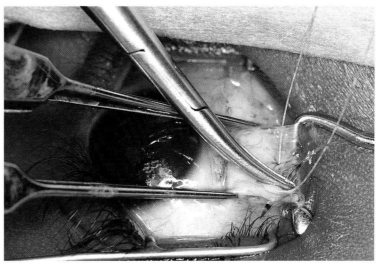

FIG. 5.20

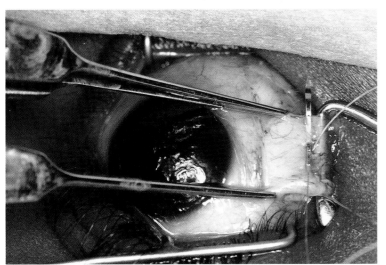

FIG. 5.21

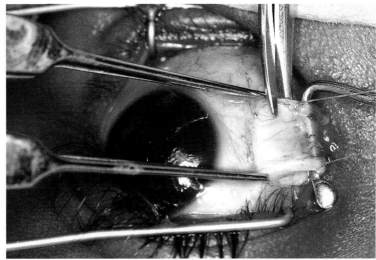

FIG. 5.22

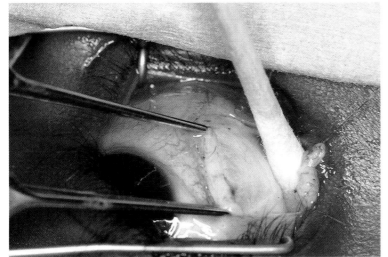

FIG. 5.23

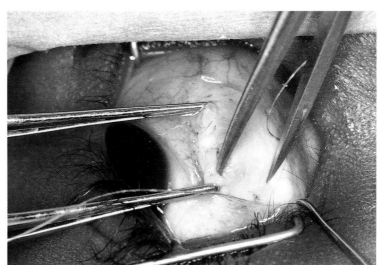

FIG. 5.24

an opaque translucency to the needle (Fig. 5.25).

Because the spatula needle is a "side-cutting" needle, it is important to avoid the tract of the previously passed suture and not inadvertently cut it. Likewise, it is important to have the exits of the sutures not so far apart as to create a buckling effect when the knot is tied (Fig. 5.26). The sutures are then drawn in the direction they were passed (Fig. 5.27) to avoid pulling the sutures through their scleral paths. The recessed muscle is demonstrated where one has attempted to preserve the original orientation of the tendon to the globe at its normal width (Fig. 5.28). After securing the tendon to the globe, the tenotomy hook is then introduced above the superior pole of the old insertion and the fascia is rotated inferiorly (Figs. 5.29 and 5.30) over the operative site. The incision is then closed with a single 6-0 plain suture in a "bury-the-knot" fashion, to minimize a foreign body sensation (Fig. 5.31). In the young, the conjunctiva is routinely closed, since the complication of Tenon's capsule prolapse can require additional anesthesia for management.

RESECTION OF A RECTUS MUSCLE

Elevating the semilunar fold (Fig. 5.32), its junction with the bulbar conjunctiva can be visualized and incised (Fig. 5.33). The conjunctival vessels are cauterized and Tenon's fascia entered. The large muscle hook is passed beneath the

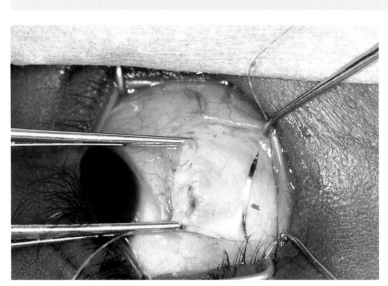

FIG. 5.25

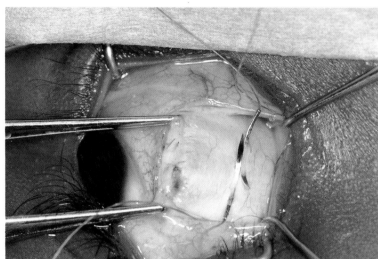

FIG. 5.26

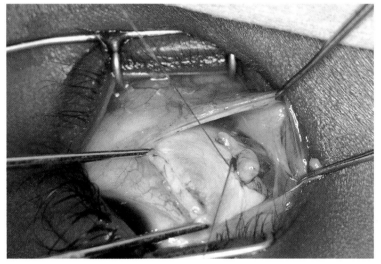

FIG. 5.27

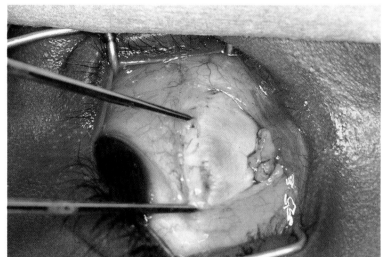

FIG. 5.28

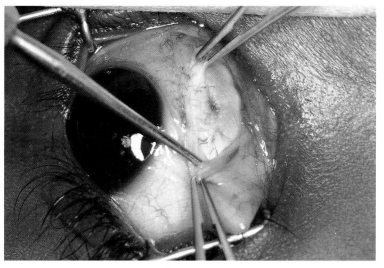

FIG. 5.29

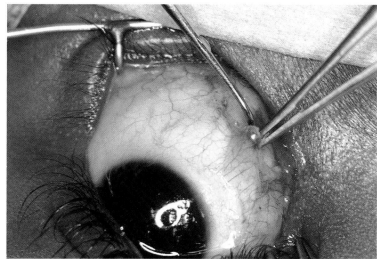

FIG. 5.30

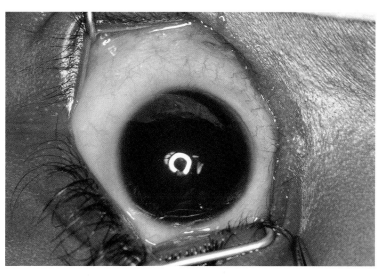

FIG. 5.31

Resection of a Rectus Muscle

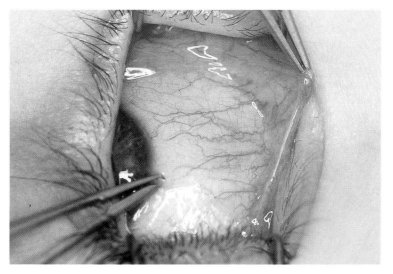

FIG. 5.32

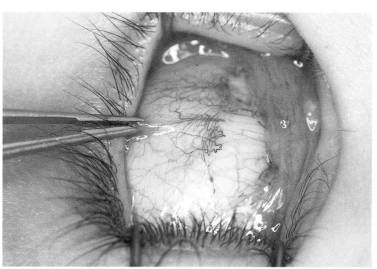

FIG. 5.33

tendon, going no further posteriorly than the insertion itself (Figs. 5.34 and 5.35). The Tenon's capsule beneath the olive tip of the large muscle hook is incised (Fig. 5.36) in order to visualize bare sclera at both poles of the tendon. Two small tenotomy hooks are passed along the long axis of the tendon in order to expose the perimuscular fascia for incision (Fig. 5.37). A second large muscle hook is passed beneath the tendon and traction is applied between the two, keeping the insertion and both hook tips parallel. The anterior arm of the caliper is placed on the midportion of the anterior hook, and the posterior portion delineates the site for needle passage (Fig. 5.38). A marking pen or the cautery may be used if remeasuring during suture passage is not desired.

The same technique of suture passage is employed as was used for recession. The needle is passed tangentially to the tendon and globe and woven through the tendon from its midportion to the superior pole and then locked upon itself.

The needle at the opposite end of the suture is then passed from the midportion to the inferior pole and once again locked, securing the tendon at the point of desired resection (Fig. 5.39). A "mosquito" hemostat is placed across the tendon just ahead of the suture (Fig. 5.40). The tendon is then cut ahead of the clamp (Fig. 5.41), and the resection of tendon then completed at the original insertion (Fig. 5.42). The hemostat can remain on the tendon until all scleral passes have been performed, permitting a clean operating field.

Passage of the needles through the original insertion takes advantage of the differential scleral width at this location. Since the scleral thickness is at its minimum just posterior to the insertion, there is a differential step of 0.5 to 0.7 mm from just behind to just in front of the insertion. Orienting each needle tangentially to the globe just posterior to the insertion will allow a forward movement of the needle through the step of sclera, accomplishing a secure

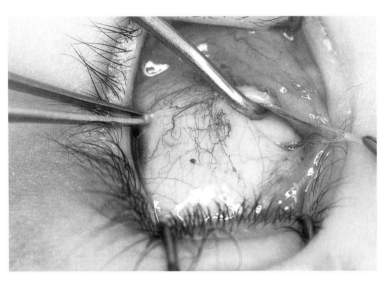

FIG. 5.34

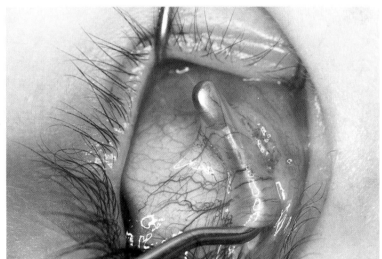

FIG. 5.35

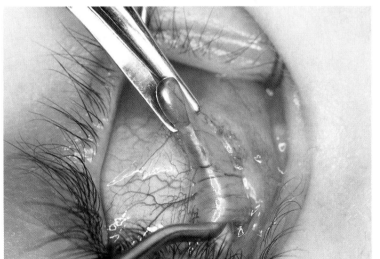

FIG. 5.36

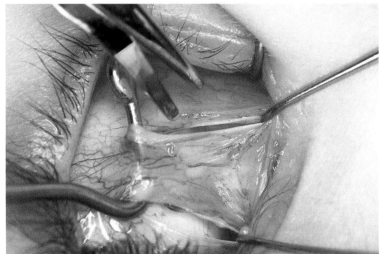

FIG. 5.37

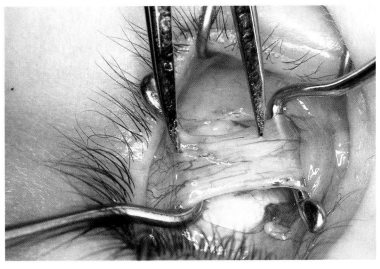

FIG. 5.38

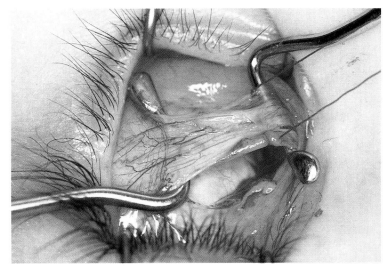

FIG. 5.39

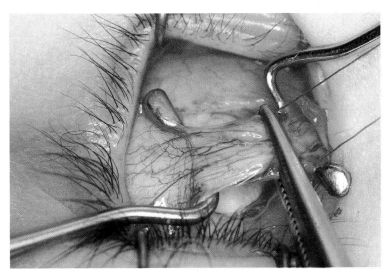

FIG. 5.40

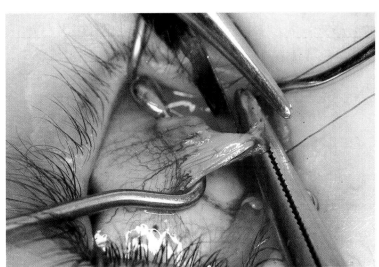

FIG. 5.41

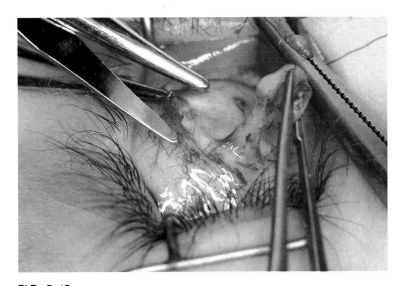

FIG. 5.42

attachment, without ever having to direct the tip of the needle toward the globe (Fig. 5.43). The passage of the needles through the insertion can be in a diagonal fashion in order to maintain the normal width of the tendon at the posterior insertion, and yet have their exit points approximate one another to facilitate tying (Fig. 5.44). Once one is satisfied with the location and depth of the scleral pass, the first suture throw is placed before the muscle is pulled forward. The hemostat is removed from the distal tendon and the muscle drawn forward and knotted (Figs. 5.45 and 5.46). The assistant may slightly adduct the globe at this time to minimize the suture tension required to complete the knot. The conjunctiva can be closed with two interrupted 6-0 plain sutures in a bury-the-knot fashion (Fig. 5.47). The conjunctiva from the limbus to the insertion is left undisturbed.

Resections of the lateral recti and superior recti should include visualization and preservation of the neighboring oblique muscles prior to performing the procedure. The frenulum between the superior rectus and superior oblique should be visualized and incised, and the common fascial attachments between the lateral rectus and inferior oblique

likewise removed to avoid undesired effects on oblique muscle functions.

LEAVING THE RECESSED OR RESECTED MUSCLE FOR ADJUSTMENT

In this case of dysthyroid ophthalmopathy, the inferior rectus has been exposed through a modified Swan incision and placed on a large muscle hook (Fig. 5.48). After placing the locking forceps at the nasal and temporal aspects of the insertion and securing the 6-0 Vicryl suture to the distal aspect of the tendon, the muscle is removed from the globe (Fig. 5.49). In order to facilitate engagement of the sclera during the subsequent needle pass, 1 to 2 mm of tendon is left at the insertion (Fig. 5.50). As in the resection procedure, the tip of the spatula needle is oriented tangentially to the globe at the posterior aspect of the insertion. While the assistant maintains the eye in an elevated position with the use of the locking forceps, the surgeon may gently elevate the residual tendon (Fig. 5.51). The needle is advanced forward through the "shelf" of sclera ahead of the insertion

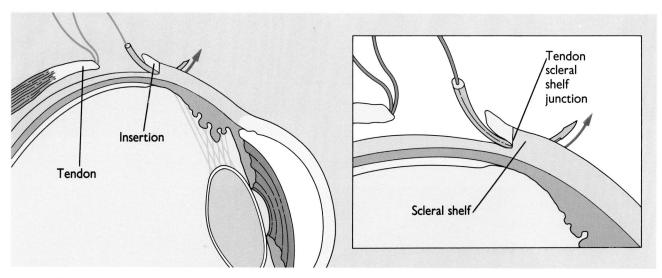

FIG. 5.43

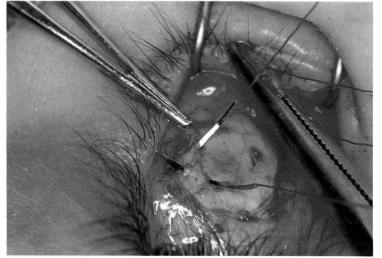

FIG. 5.44

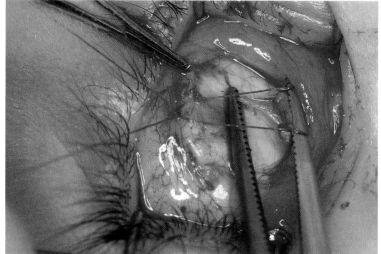

FIG. 5.45

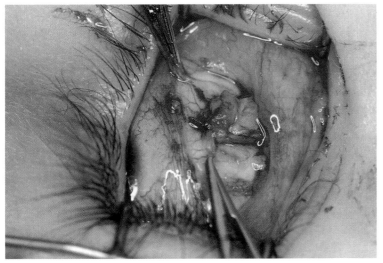

FIG. 5.46

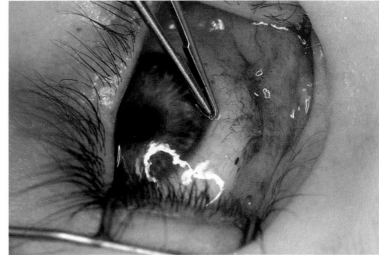

FIG. 5.47

Leaving the Recessed or Resected Muscle for Adjustment

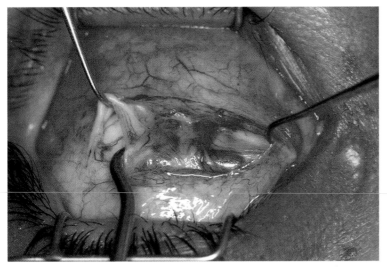

FIG. 5.48

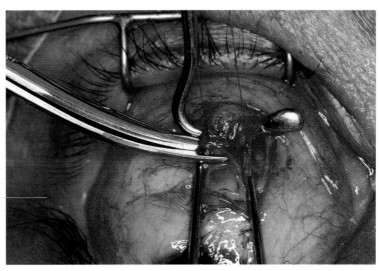

FIG. 5.49

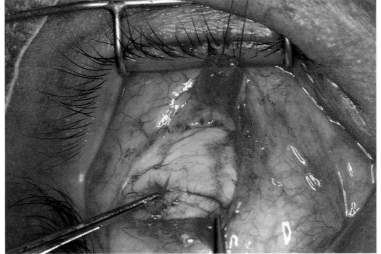

FIG. 5.50

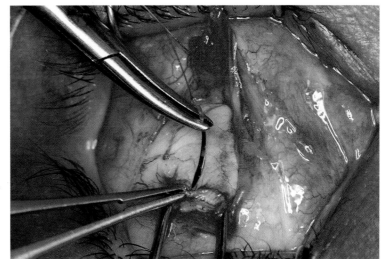

FIG. 5.51

(Fig. 5.52). A gentle elevation effort, prior to releasing the needle, should reveal a satisfactory engagement of the sclera. If a pass is too superficial, involving only the tendon, the needle will easily pull through. Two such passes are performed in parallel, approximately 3 mm apart.

Once both passes have been accomplished, the first double throw of a surgeon's knot is performed (Fig. 5.53). The tendon is then suspended from the insertion by the suspected amount of appropriate recession (Fig. 5.54), or drawn forward to the insertion in the case of resection. The second throw of the suture should accomplish a single bow knot (Figs. 5.55 and 5.56). The bow and both ends of the suture are left 4 to 5 inches long. In vertical muscle cases where exposure of the tendon can be difficult postoperatively, an additional globe handle can be placed consisting of a 5-0 Prolene suture knotted as a loop (Fig. 5.57). The conjunctiva may be closed (Fig. 5.58), and both the loop *and* two ends of the suture are taped to the lateral (or nasal) canthal area to avoid any disturbance of the knot until the time of adjustment (Fig. 5.59). An antibiotic–steroid ointment is placed between the lids, the eye is securely patched, and the area of the sutures protected until the following morning.

If, on the following morning, the patient has had a satis-

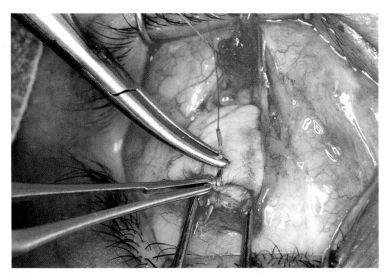

FIG. 5.52

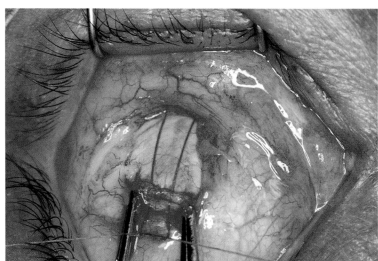

FIG. 5.53

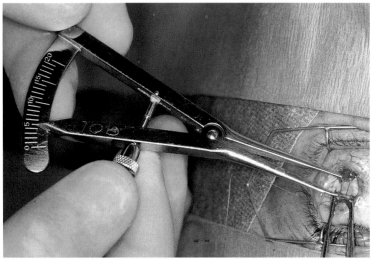

FIG. 5.54

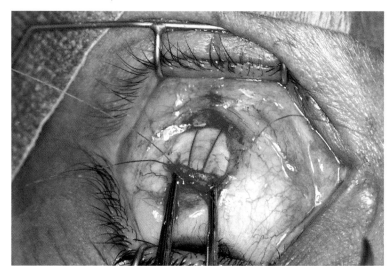

FIG. 5.55

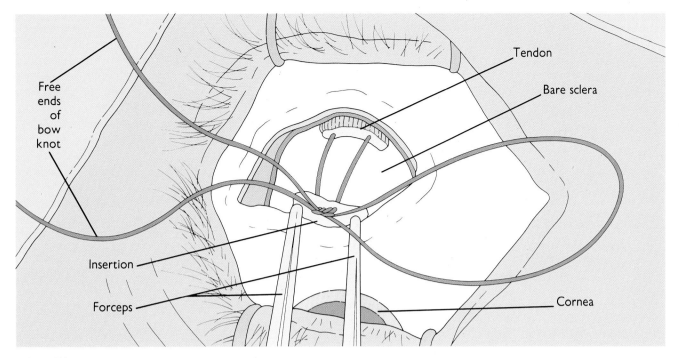

FIG. 5.56

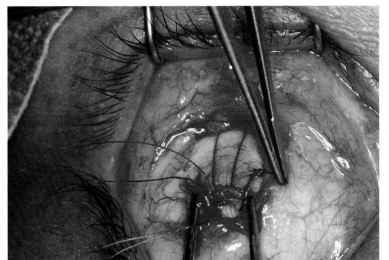

FIG. 5.57

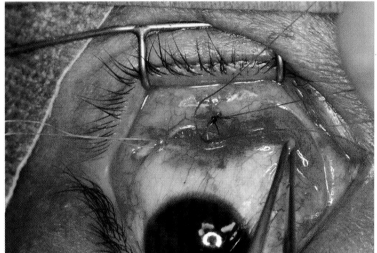

FIG. 5.58

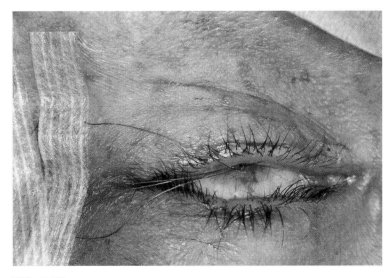

FIG. 5.59

factory amount of surgery performed, then one may expand the loop of the knot, pulling the free end through, and thereby complete the fist square knot without disturbing the position of the muscle (Fig. 5.60). If, however, the position of the muscle needs to be adjusted, the free end of the suture may be pulled to reduce the size of the loop until the second throw has been pulled through (Fig. 5.61). In the latter case, a single double throw exists that can be loosened or drawn forward to adjust the position of the tendon before the square knot is completed.

POSTERIOR FIXATION SUTURE

The medial rectus muscle has been exposed through a conjunctival incision over the distal tendon (Fig. 5.62). The fascia is dissected posteriorly for at least 1 cm from the insertion (Fig. 5.63). After the application of the locking forceps at the insertion, a double-armed 6-0 Vicryl suture is woven and locked at the distal tendon (Fig. 5.64). The tendon is removed from the globe and the Desmarres retractor placed beneath the medial rectus to accomplish exposure of the globe 10–12 mm posterior to the original insertion (Fig. 5.65). If resistance is encountered, a larger conjunctival incision is performed.

A double-armed 5-0 Mersilene suture is passed through the superficial sclera at the desired point of posterior fixation, leaving equal amounts of suture to either side of the scleral canal (Figs. 5.66 and 5.67). The Desmarres retractor is removed, and, visualizing the global aspect of the medial rectus, the inferior half of the Mersilene suture is then introduced into the junction of the middle with the inferior

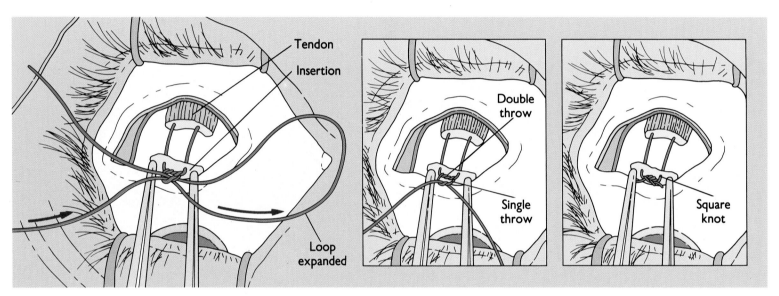

FIG. 5.60

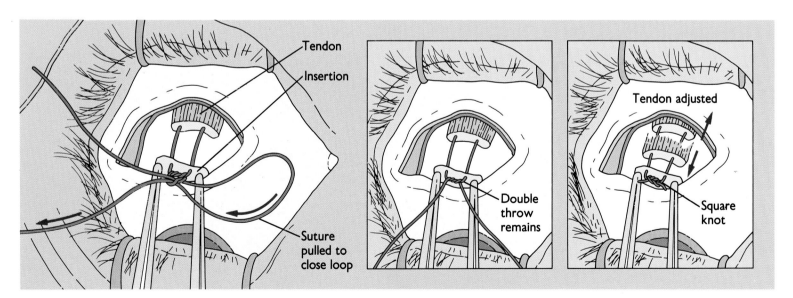

FIG. 5.61

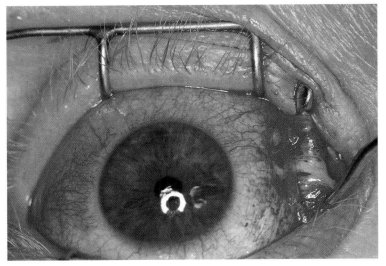

FIG. 5.62

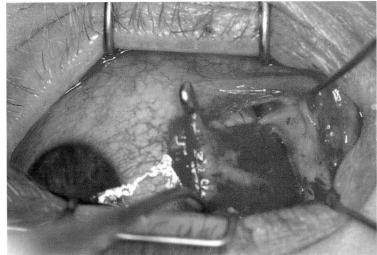

FIG. 5.63

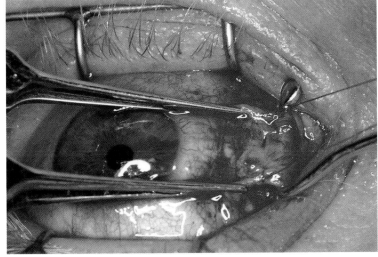

FIG. 5.64

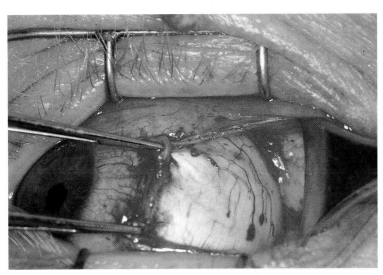

FIG. 5.65

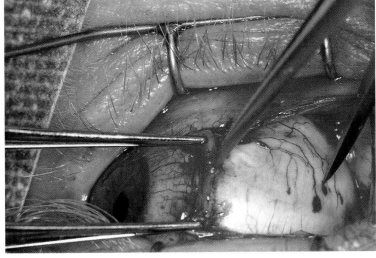

FIG. 5.66

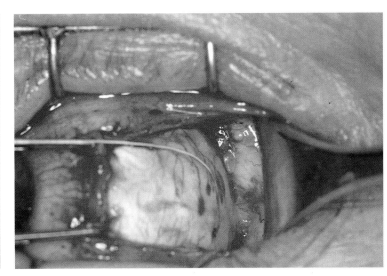

FIG. 5.67

third of the medial rectus tendon (Fig. 5.68). The point of introduction through the medial rectus is determined by the desired amount of accompanying recession that will minimize muscle slack between the anterior and posterior fixation. If the posterior fixation distance is intended to be 12 mm posterior to the original insertion, and the accompanying recession of the anterior insertion 5 mm posterior to the original insertion, then the sutures are passed through the muscle at a point 7 mm from the distal aspect of the tendon.

The tendon is brought against the globe, allowing penetration at the desired distance (Fig. 5.69). The superior half of the suture is similarly passed at the junction of the middle third with the superior third of the medial rectus (Fig. 5.70). The suture is then securely tied on top of the middle

third of the muscle, realizing that any laxity in the knot will defeat the effect of the posterior fixation by allowing slippage of the tendon along the globe at that point (Fig. 5.71). The anterior recession is then completed with passage of the Vicryl sutures (Figs. 5.72 and 5.73) and, after hemostasis, closure of the conjunctival incision can be accomplished with running or interrupted 6-0 plain sutures in a bury-the-knot fashion (Fig. 5.74).

APPROACH TO THE INFERIOR OBLIQUE MUSCLE

With the eye maximally rotated superonasally (Fig. 5.75), Tenon's fascia is elevated between two forceps (Fig. 5.76)

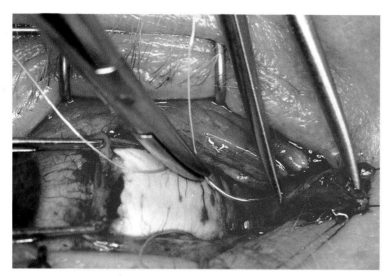

FIG. 5.68

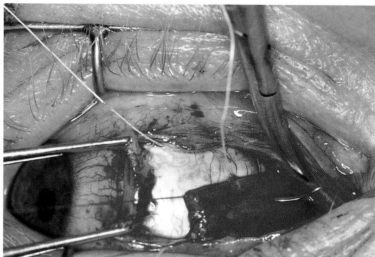

FIG. 5.69

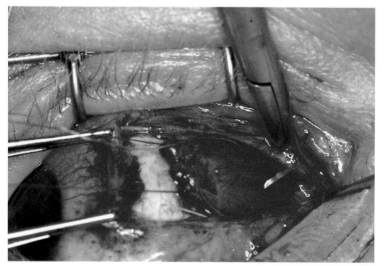

FIG. 5.70

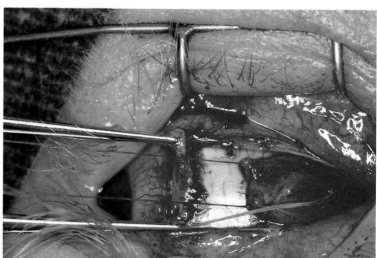

FIG. 5.71

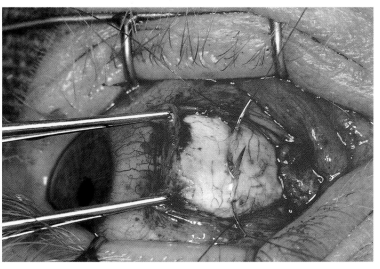

FIG. 5.72

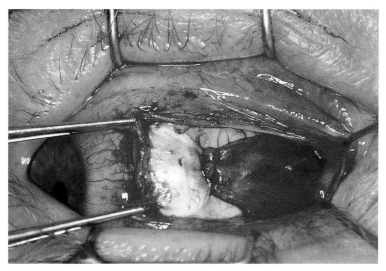

FIG. 5.73

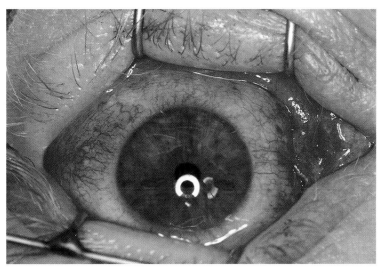

FIG. 5.74

Approach to the Inferior Oblique Muscle

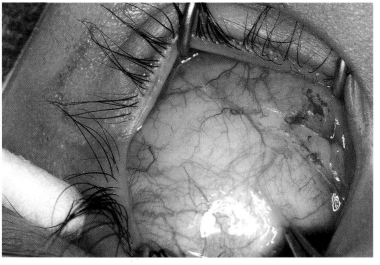

FIG. 5.75

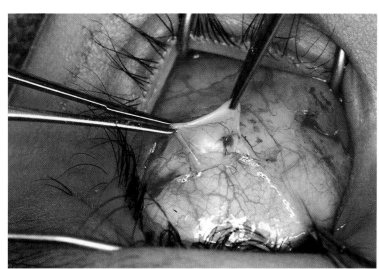

FIG. 5.76

and incised to expose bare sclera (Fig. 5.77). With two large muscle hooks placed beneath the lateral rectus muscle, a single-armed 4-0 black silk suture is passed beneath the tendon (Fig. 5.78). The hooks are removed, and by drawing nasally on the inferior aspect of the suture, the eye will rotate into a superonasal position (Fig. 5.79). The eye is then secured in this position with a clamp to the drapes. Since this may elevate intraocular pressure, one should periodically release the suture, especially with elderly patients. Using a large and a small muscle hook, the inferotemporal fornix is exposed (Fig. 5.80), and the inferior oblique muscle may be seen as a purple discoloration, running in close approximation to the periorbital fat. The small tenotomy hook is introduced against the globe and moved posterior to the inferior oblique. The hook is rotated up to engage the muscle, allowing the point of the hook to

penetrate the fascia between the muscle and the fat (Fig. 5.81). At this point, a myectomy or recession may proceed.

For a myectomy, the large muscle hook supports the inferior oblique muscle and two small tenotomy hooks will expose the intermuscular fascia between it and the lateral rectus (Fig. 5.82). These are then incised and the inferior oblique is removed, flush with the globe (Fig. 5.83). The desired portion of the muscle is then resected, and the stump of the muscle is lightly cauterized (Fig. 5.84) before removal of the clamp, allowing it to retreat beneath the inferior rectus (Fig. 5.85).

In the case of recession, the inferior oblique is placed on a large muscle hook, and distracted inferotemporally. In this way, one may see that no residual muscle remains in the periorbital fat (Fig. 5.86). With nasal traction on the muscle, two small tenotomy hooks elevate the intermuscu-

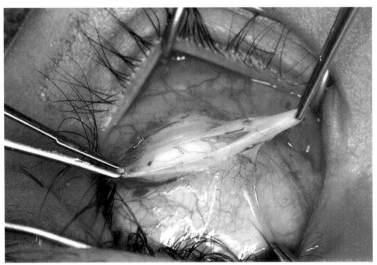

FIG. 5.77

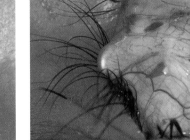

FIG. 5.78

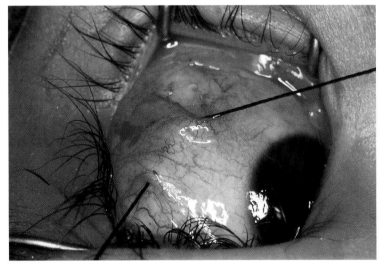

FIG. 5.79

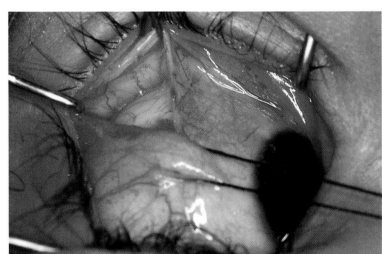

FIG. 5.80

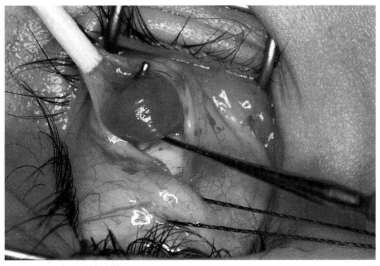

FIG. 5.81

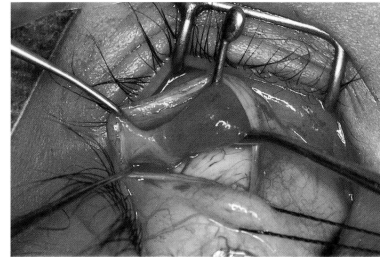

FIG. 5.82

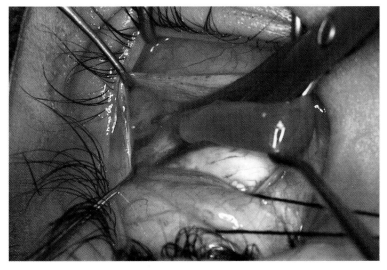

FIG. 5.83

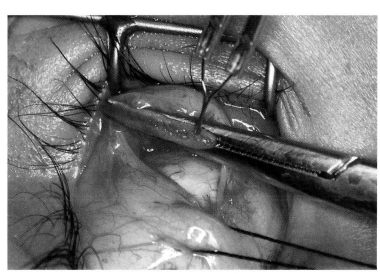

FIG. 5.84

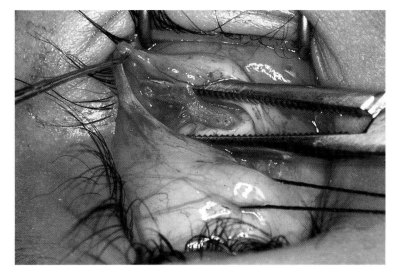

FIG. 5.85

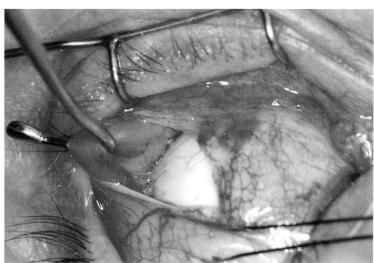

FIG. 5.86

lar connections, which are then incised (Fig. 5.87). The muscle is then removed flush with the globe (Fig. 5.88) and placed on a double-armed 6-0 Vicryl suture (Fig. 5.89). With a large muscle hook beneath the inferior rectus for maximal supraduction, the temporal border of the inferior rectus muscle is exposed and the desired amount of recession performed by two scleral passes (Fig. 5.90). The muscle is thus secured to the globe along its original direction of passage (Fig. 5.91), and the conjunctiva then closed with a gut suture (Fig. 5.92).

APPROACH TO THE SUPERIOR OBLIQUE TENDON

With the eye rotated inferotemporally, a conjunctival incision is made in the superonasal fornix (Fig. 5.93). A large hook is placed beneath the superior rectus muscle and the eye is maximally infraducted (Fig. 5.94). Gently distracting the overlying conjunctiva and Tenon's capsule, the nasal border of the superior rectus is visualized (Fig. 5.95). With the muscle hook maximally distracting the eye inferotem-

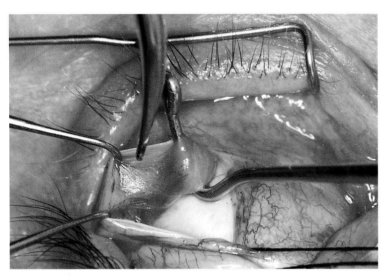

FIG. 5.87

FIG. 5.88

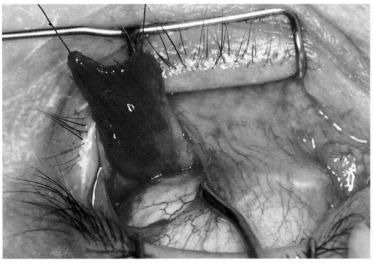

FIG. 5.89

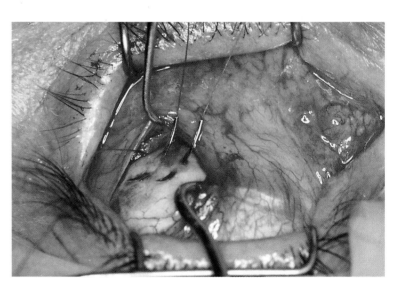

FIG. 5.90

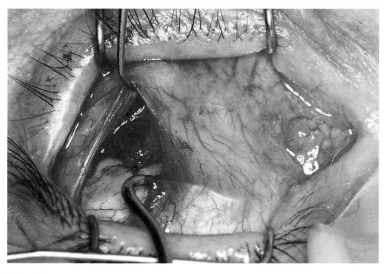

FIG. 5.91

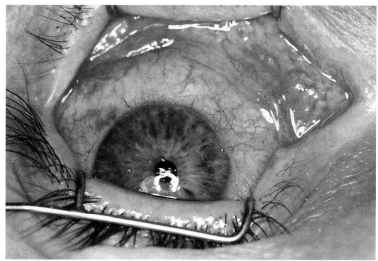

FIG. 5.92

Approach to the Superior Oblique Tendon

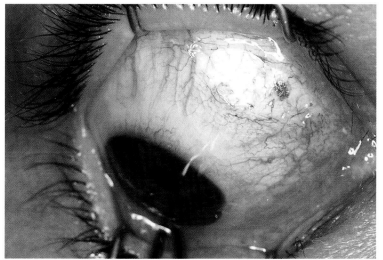

FIG. 5.93

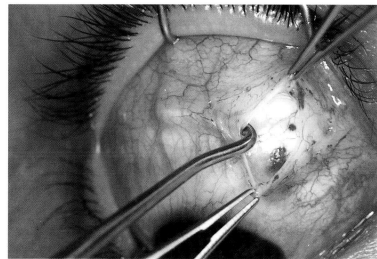

FIG. 5.94

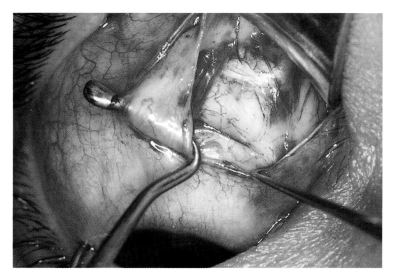

FIG. 5.95

porally, a Desmarres retractor is placed in the incision and used to expose the superonasal quadrant. The oblique tendon is first visualized, and engaged on a tenotomy hook (Figs. 5.96 and 5.97). One can see how the large muscle hook, when passed deeply behind the superior rectus, may engage the posterior fascia and drag the superior oblique tendon into the hook along with the rectus tendon. Furthermore, trauma to the superior oblique tendon can occur if not visualized and preserved prior to a dissection of the intermuscular fascia. The intermuscular fascia ("sheath")

may be dissected from the superior oblique tendon (Fig. 5.98) and, at this point, one may perform a tuck, tenotomy, or tenectomy. A tenotomy may proceed by incising the tendon after protecting the nasal border of the superior rectus with the Desmarres retractor (Figs. 5.99 and 5.100). A tenectomy is performed after grasping the tendon with a hemostat, and sectioned on both sides, removing approximately 4 mm of tendon (Figs. 5.101 and 5.102). The conjunctival incision may then be closed with a running or interrupted 6-0 plain gut suture.

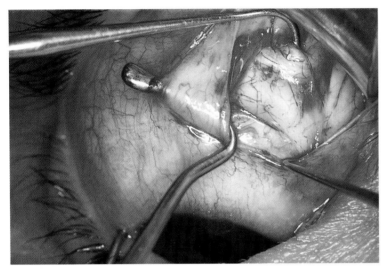

FIG. 5.96

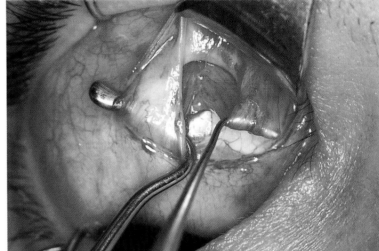

FIG. 5.97

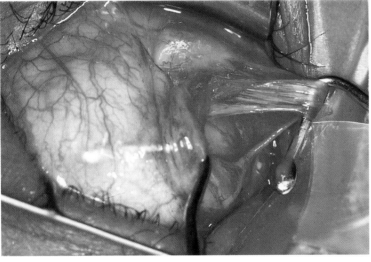

FIG. 5.98

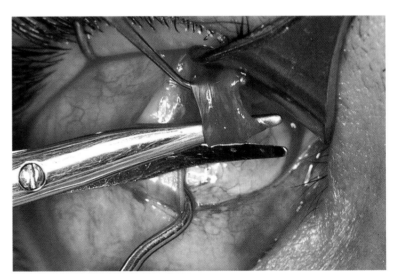

FIG. 5.99

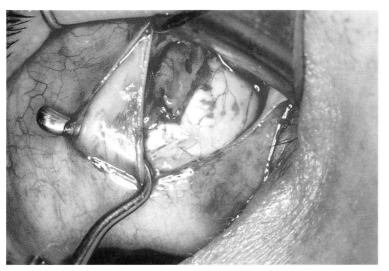

FIG. 5.100

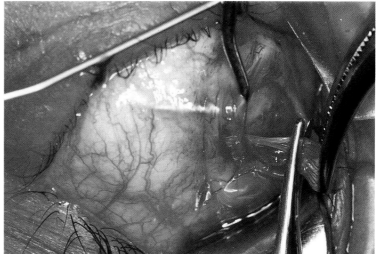

FIG. 5.101

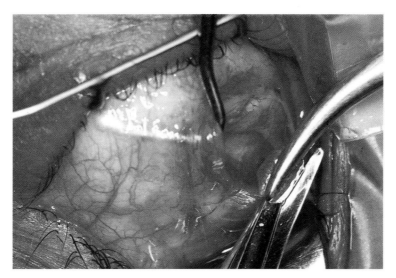

FIG. 5.102

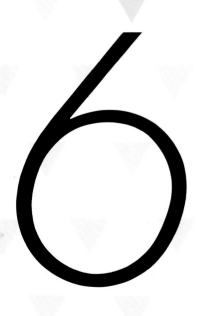

SURGERY OF ACQUIRED LID MALPOSITIONS

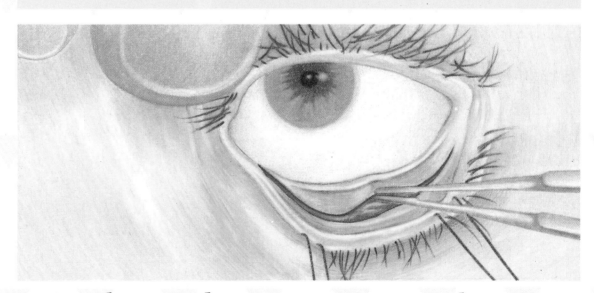

R i c h a r d   R .   T e n z e l ,   M D

This chapter, on the correction of acquired lid malpositions, outlines my preferred technique for each deformity while acknowledging that there are other operations that may correct these abnormalities. I trust that these techniques will aid you in the care of your patient.

Anesthesia is a 50–50 mixture of 2% Xylocaine and 0.75 Marcaine, both with epinephrine. One part of this mixture is combined with nine parts balanced salt solution and given as a preliminary injection. After a two-minute wait, a full-strength anesthetic mixture is injected. The total volume of anesthetic should be kept at a minimum so as not to distort the anatomy of the lids.

Hemostasis is accomplished with the wetfield cautery, using a tip that does not completely close.

SURGERY OF THE UPPER LID RETRACTOR

APONEUROSIS RESECTION FOR ACQUIRED PTOSIS

The anatomy of the upper lid is depicted in Fig. 6.1. The amount of aponeurosis resection is titrated during the procedure; only a local anesthetic is used. In the upright position, the patient is asked to open the eyes and to look at applicator sticks. The height of the lid margin is noted. The lid margin height is rechecked with the patient in the supine position to see if there is a change. If not, all lid levels are checked in the supine position. The lid crease is marked on the lid (Fig. 6.2). In a unilateral case, the crease is matched to the fellow eye. In bilateral surgery, the lid is divided into thirds. The central measurement in women is 10 mm from the base of the lashes; the lateral is 9 mm, and the nasal 8 mm. In men, or women with small eyes, the heights are 1 mm less.

An incision is made with a razor knife through the skin (Fig. 6.3). Picking up both sides of the wound, the underlying subcutaneous tissue can be placed on tension (Fig. 6.4) and cut with scissors, revealing the orbicularis muscle. A strip of orbicularis muscle is either removed (Fig. 6.5) or incised. Dissection is carried out superiorly beneath the orbicularis muscle until the orbital septum is exposed. With pressure on the lids, the fat bulge beneath the septum is buttonholed (Fig. 6.6) and opened across the lid (Fig. 6.7), revealing the levator aponeurosis beneath the septum. After the orbital septum has been opened, the patient is again asked to look at applicator sticks and the difference from the preoperative lid height is noted. If there is a lowering of the lid margin (rarely), the lid is undercorrected by the amount of lowering. If the lid is higher (very frequently), the lid is overcorrected by the amount of rise.

◁ Aponeurosis Resection for Acquired Ptosis

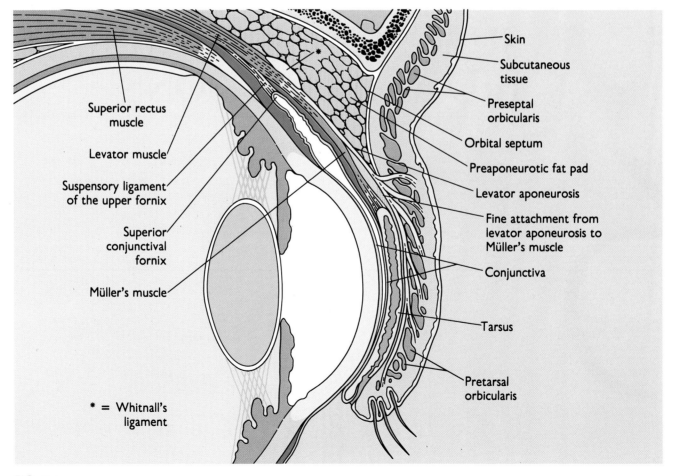

Superior rectus muscle

Levator muscle

Suspensory ligament of the upper fornix

Superior conjunctival fornix

Müller's muscle

* = Whitnall's ligament

Skin

Subcutaneous tissue

Preseptal orbicularis

Orbital septum

Preaponeurotic fat pad

Levator aponeurosis

Fine attachment from levator aponeurosis to Müller's muscle

Conjunctiva

Tarsus

Pretarsal orbicularis

FIG. 6.1

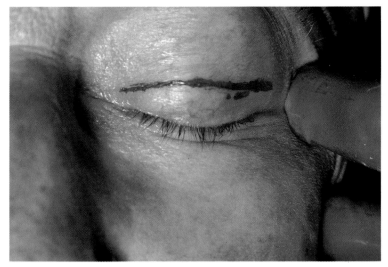

FIG. 6.2

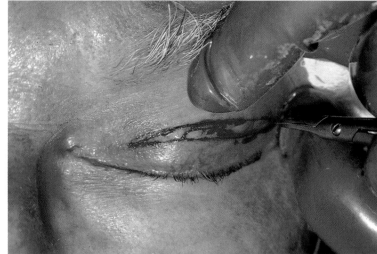

FIG. 6.3

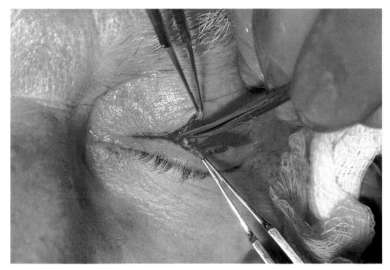

FIG. 6.4

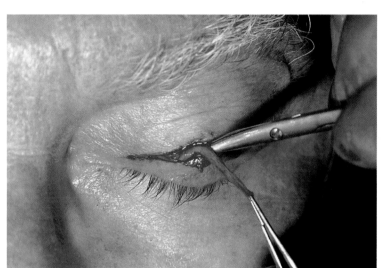

FIG. 6.5

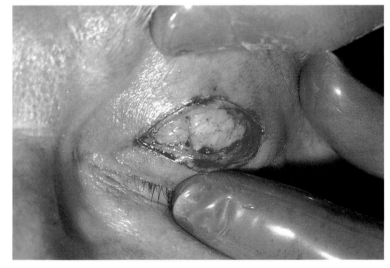

FIG. 6.6

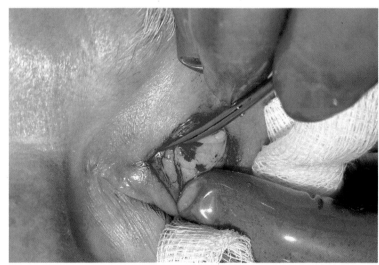

FIG. 6.7

The levator aponeurosis is opened across the midface of the tarsus and dissected from the tarsus (Fig. 6.8). When the dissection reaches the upper edge of the tarsus, the very fine attachments to Müller's muscle found there are separated with sharp and blunt dissection (Fig. 6.9), freeing the levator aponeurosis from the underlying Müller's muscle (Fig. 6.10). A double-armed 6-0 Mersilene suture is placed (partial thickness) in the tarsus at the original central measurement (Fig. 6.11). While the needle is in the tarsus, the lid is everted, each time verifying partial-thickness penetration. Both arms of the suture are brought through the levator aponeurosis and temporally tied (see Fig. 6.14A). The lid *height* is checked by having the patient look at the applicator sticks and the amount of levator resection is adjusted until the lid height is as desired (see Fig. 6.14B).

The medial and lateral sutures are placed in the tarsus, also at the original measurements, and through the aponeurosis. The lid *curvature* is adjusted with these sutures. The sutures are tied, the redundant aponeurosis is excised, and a running 6-0 Mersilene suture is used to attach the edge of the aponeurosis to the aponeurosis, continuing to the lid margin (Figs. 6.12 and 6.14C). One arm of each of the sutures attaching the levator aponeurosis to the tarsus goes through the muscle and subcutaneous tissue at the upper edge of the inferior skin flap, exits just beneath the skin, goes back through, and is tied beneath the orbicularis muscle, recreating the lid crease (Fig. 6.14D). The skin is closed with a subcuticular suture of 6-0 Prolene tied over rubber bands (Figs. 6.13 and 6.14E).

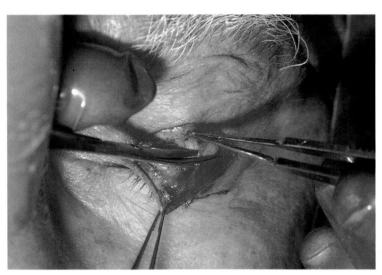

FIG. 6.8

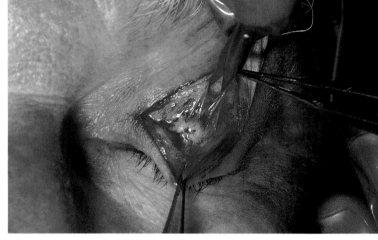

FIG. 6.9

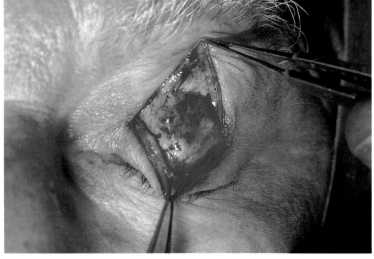

FIG. 6.10

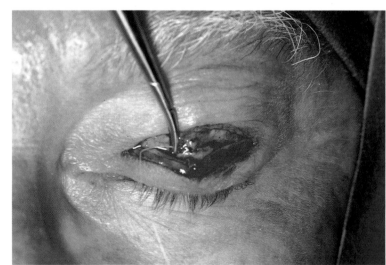

FIG. 6.11

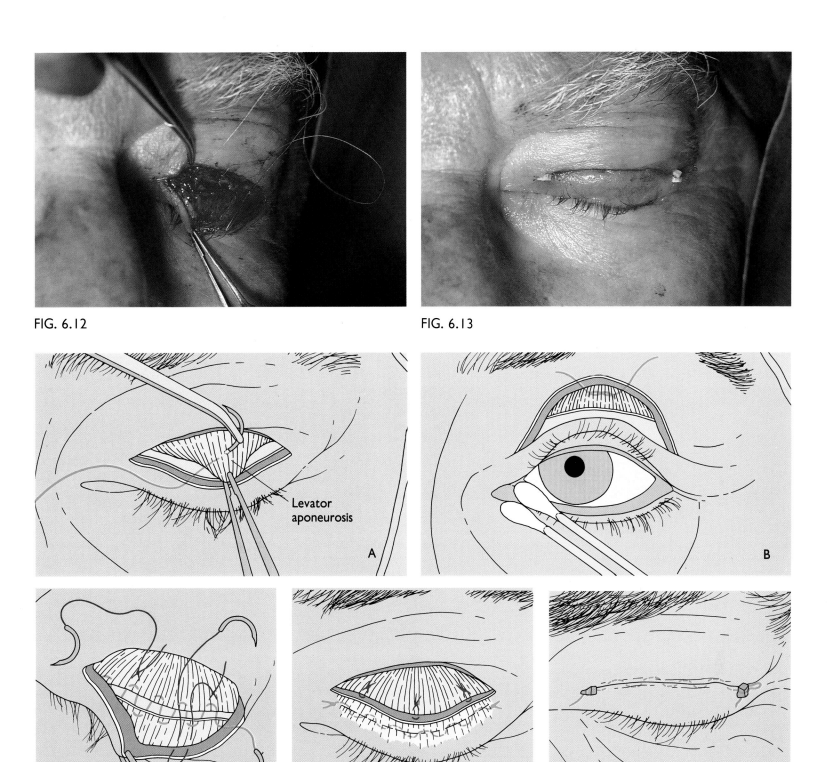

FIG. 6.12

FIG. 6.13

Levator aponeurosis

A

B

C

D

E

FIG. 6.14

Figure 6.15 shows the preoperative appearance with ptosis of the right upper lid post-cataract extraction. Figure 6.16 shows the preoperative upgaze and Fig. 6.17 shows the preoperative downgaze. Figure 6.18 shows the postoperative appearance after aponeurosis repair of the right upper lid. Figure 6.19 shows the postoperative upgaze and Fig. 6.20 shows the postoperative downgaze.

LEVATOR APONEUROSIS— MÜLLER'S MUSCLE RECESSION

This is now the procedure of choice for correction of lid retraction. As described in Figs. 6.2 to 6.8, the orbital septum is opened across the lid. Any anterior adhesions to the levator aponeurosis are released and the levator aponeurosis is cut and dissected from the tarsus. When Müller's muscle is reached, a Desmarres retractor is placed behind the upper edge of the tarsus (Fig. 6.21), putting the conjunctiva on a stretch so that Müller's muscle and the levator aponeurosis can be recessed en bloc (Fig. 6.22). The recession is initially confined to the lateral two-thirds of the lid. During the surgery, the patient is asked to open the lids repeatedly to check their levels. If it is found that more nasal dissection is necessary, it is performed a small segment at a time to prevent nasal overcorrection.

When the desired endpoint is reached, 1 mm higher than the final desired result, a double-arm 6-0 Mersilene suture is placed (partial thickness) at the upper edge of the tarsus and brought through the lid retractors so they will not recede further into the orbit postoperatively (Fig. 6.23).

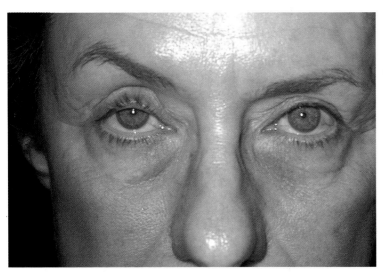

FIG. 6.15

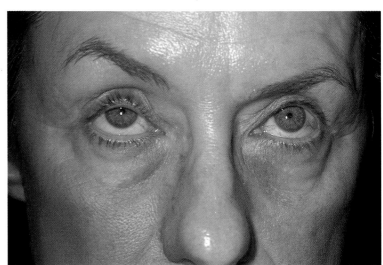

FIG. 6.16

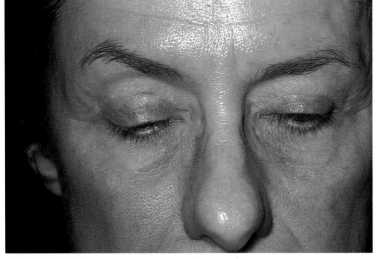

FIG. 6.17

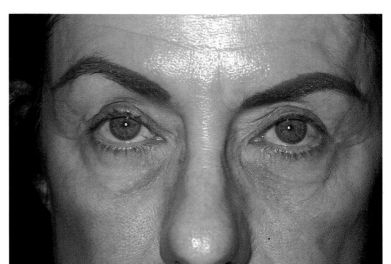

FIG. 6.18

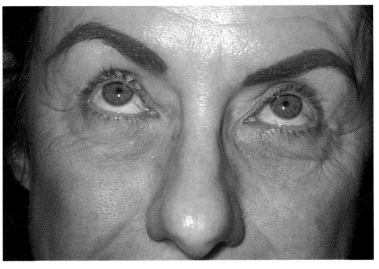

FIG. 6.19

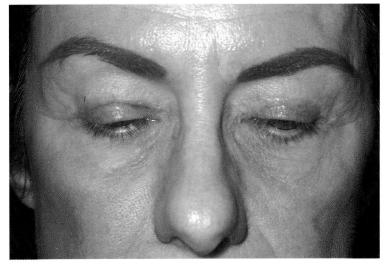

FIG. 6.20

Levator Aponeurosis — Müller's Muscle Recession

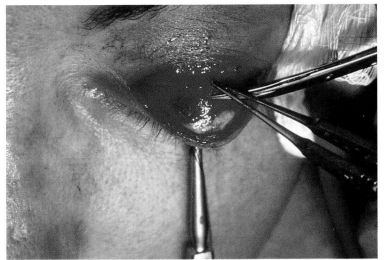

FIG. 6.21

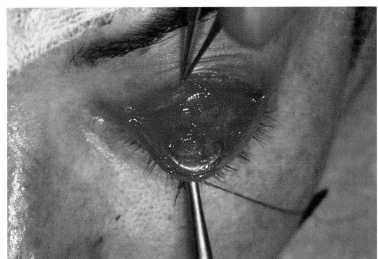

FIG. 6.22

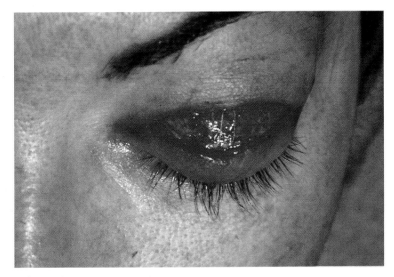

FIG. 6.23

The lid crease is formed with three interrupted horizontal mattress sutures with 6-0 Mersilene. Each suture takes a partial-thickness tarsal bite, goes through the muscle at the upper edge of the inferior skin flap, comes out just beneath the skin, goes back through, and is tied under the muscle. These sutures will keep the lid crease in its proper position. The skin is closed with a continuous suture of 6-0 Prolene.

Figure 6.24 shows the preoperative appearance of a patient with thyroid eye disease, while Fig. 6.25 shows the postoperative appearance after recession of the upper lid retractors bilaterally. In Fig. 6.26, the patient has overcorrection of ptosis of the right upper lid, and is shown before recession of the lid retractors of the right upper lid. Figure 6.27 shows the postoperative appearance.

SURGERY OF THE LOWER LID RETRACTORS
RECESSION OF LOWER LID RETRACTORS

The anatomy of the lower lid is depicted in Fig. 6.28. Two 4-0 silk traction sutures are placed in the lower lid. An incision is made in the conjunctiva at the lower edge of the tarsus (Fig. 6.29) and the conjunctiva is separated from the lower lid retractors beyond the reflection of the inferior fornix, cutting the fascial connections to the inferior fornix (Fig. 6.30). Dissection then proceeds through the lower lid retractors and the orbital septum at the lower edge of the tarsus (Fig. 6.31) and continues down the anterior face of the orbital septum (Fig. 6.32). This allows the lower lid

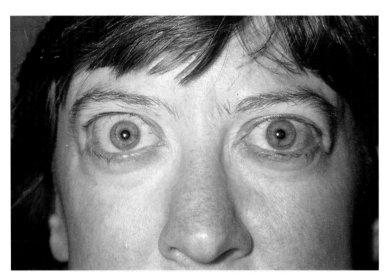

FIG. 6.24

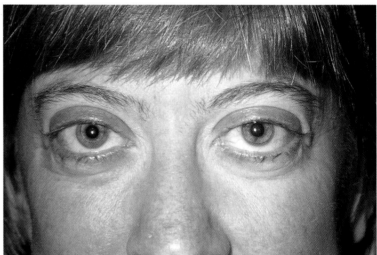

FIG. 6.25

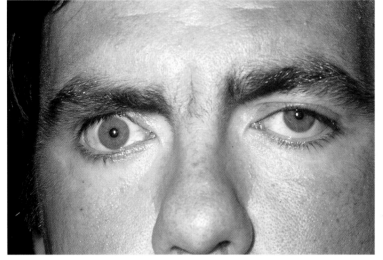

FIG. 6.26

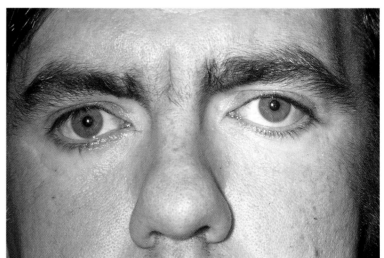

FIG. 6.27

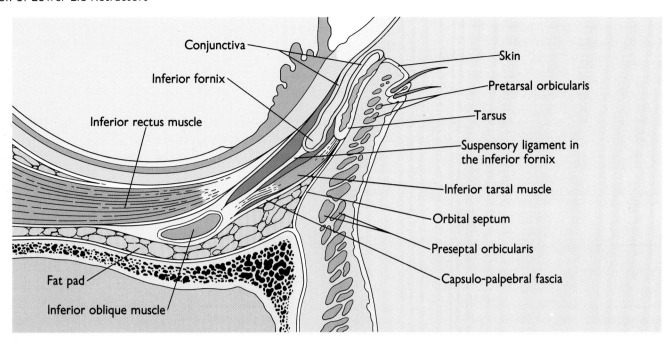

FIG. 6.28

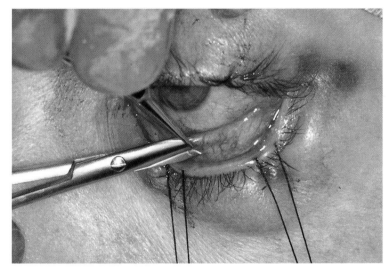

FIG. 6.29

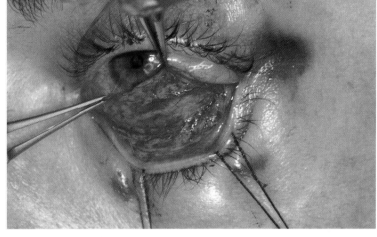

FIG. 6.30

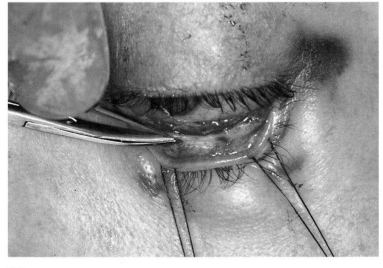

FIG. 6.31

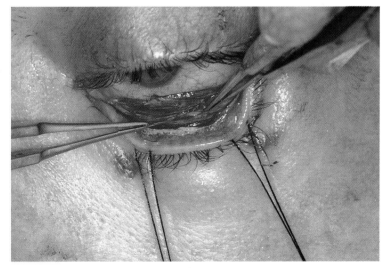

FIG. 6.32

retractors to recede into the orbit en bloc. If necessary, the orbital septum is cut and fat excised (Fig. 6.33).

A strip of sclera 2.5 times the amount of desired recession is placed into the defect and sutured to the upper edge of the lower lid retractors with a continuous suture of 6-0 Vicryl (Fig. 6.34). A 6-0 Prolene suture enters the skin 4 mm below the lid margin, takes a partial-thickness bite of the tarsus (Fig. 6.35), goes through the upper edge of the scleral graft (Fig. 6.36), takes a horizontal subconjunctival bite of the conjunctiva (Fig. 6.37), goes back through the graft (Fig. 6.38), takes a horizontal partial-thickness bite of the tarsus (Fig. 6.39), goes back through the graft, takes another subconjunctival bite of the conjunctiva, and continues across the lid, thereby connecting the upper edge of the graft to the tarsus and bringing the conjunctiva over the scleral graft (Fig. 6.40). When the end of the lid is reached, the suture is brought out through the skin and tied. The suture is left in place for five days. The traction sutures are taped to the brow with the lower lid in an overcorrected position for three to five days (Fig. 6.41).

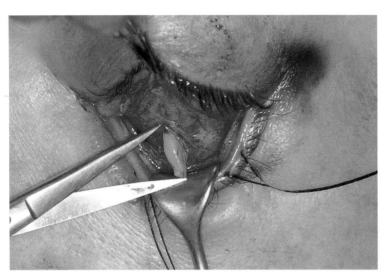

FIG. 6.33

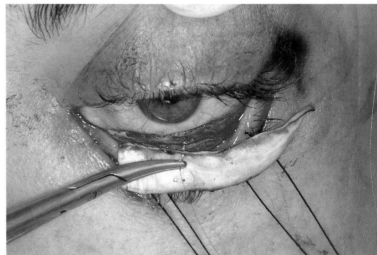

FIG. 6.34

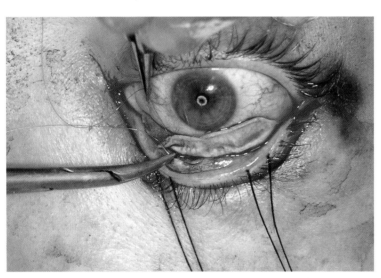

FIG. 6.35

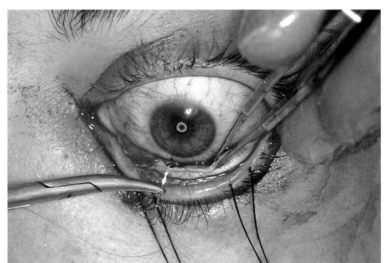

FIG. 6.36

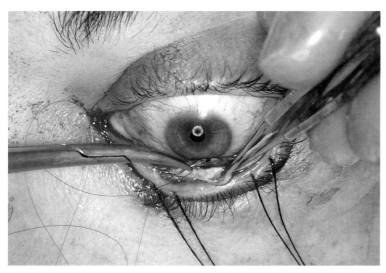

FIG. 6.37

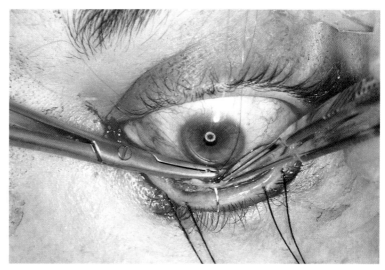

FIG. 6.38

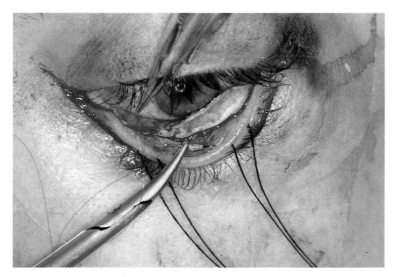

FIG. 6.39

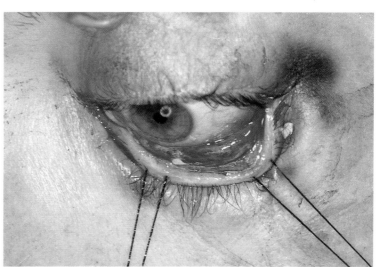

FIG. 6.40

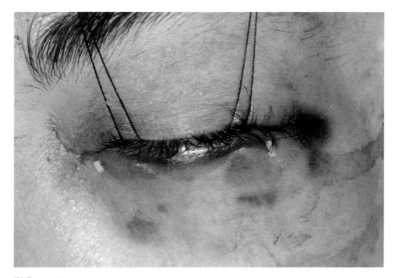

FIG. 6.41

Figure 6.42 shows the preoperative appearance of the patient with retraction of the right lower lid secondary to thyroid eye disease, while Fig. 6.43 shows the postoperative appearance after lower lid recession and scleral graft insertion.

REPAIR OF INVOLUTIONAL LOWER LID ENTROPION

An incision is made inferior temporally, at a 30° angle, starting at the lateral canthus (Fig. 6.44). A flap is formed by blunt dissection beneath the muscle with scissors. One blade of the scissors is placed in the pocket, another beneath the lashes, and the flap is opened by cutting the tissue immediately beneath the lashes (Fig. 6.45). There are three fat pockets in the lower lid: nasal, central, and lateral.

The fat pockets are opened by putting pressure on the globe and buttonholing a pocket. The orbital septum is opened across the lower lid and the fat is made to prolapse with pressure on the lids. The fat is clamped with a hemostat (Fig. 6.46), cut, and cauterized. The fat pedicle is grasped with forceps before releasing the hemostat to make certain there is no bleeding before the fat is allowed to drop back into the orbit (Fig. 6.47).

A 2-mm lateral canthotomy is performed (Fig. 6.48). A full-thickness cut of the lower lid is made at the canthotomy (Fig. 6.49), the lid is overlapped (Fig. 6.50), and the redundant lid excised (Fig. 6.51). Three 7-0 Vicryl sutures are placed from the lateral cut edge of the tarsus to the medial cut edge of the lateral tendon. This tendon is immediately anterior to the conjunctiva (Fig. 6.52). The orbicularis mus-

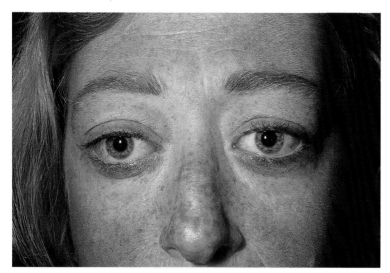

FIG. 6.42

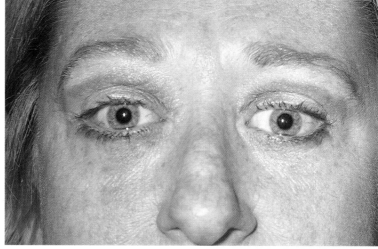

FIG. 6.43

Repair of Involutional Lower Lid Entropion

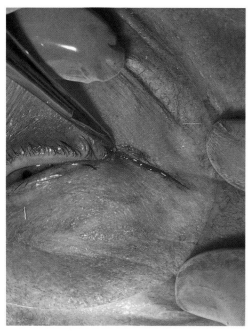

FIG. 6.44

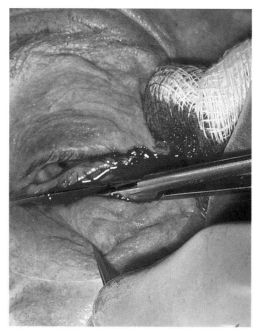

FIG. 6.45

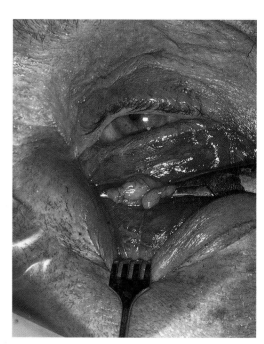

FIG. 6.46

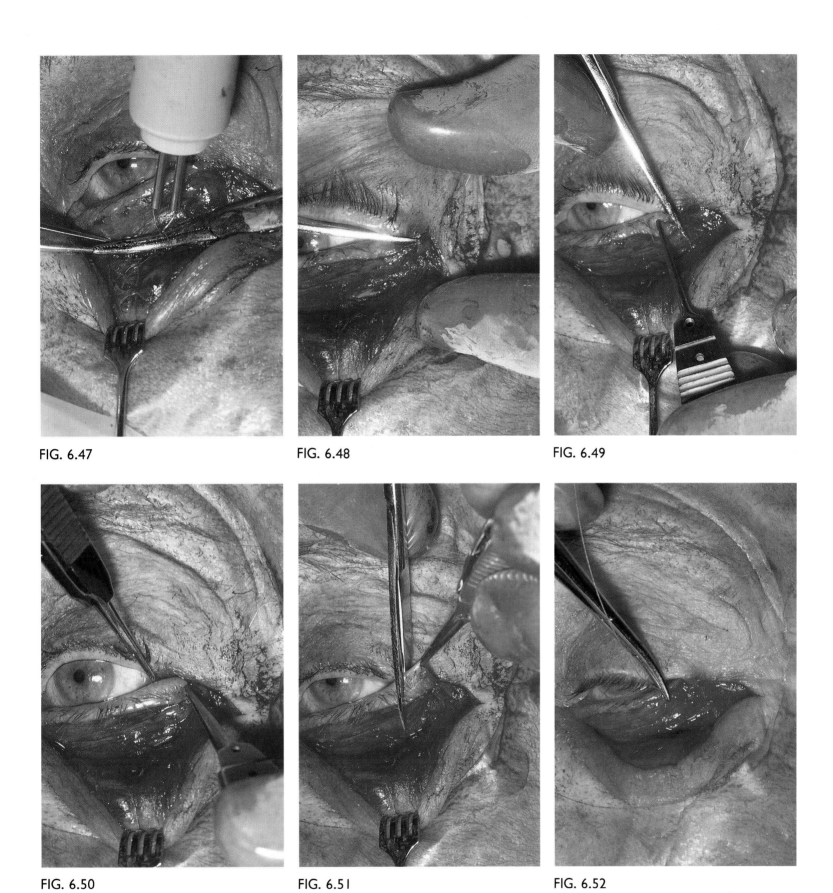

FIG. 6.47

FIG. 6.48

FIG. 6.49

FIG. 6.50

FIG. 6.51

FIG. 6.52

cle is closed with buried sutures of 7-0 Vicryl (Fig. 6.53). Figure 6.54 illustrates poor fixation of the lower lid retractor to the inferior tarsus.

At least three interrupted, 7-0 Vicryl sutures are placed from the lower lid retractors to the inferior edge of the pretarsal orbicularis muscle (Fig. 6.55). One suture is in the center of the lid, one is lateral to the punctum, and one is medial to the lateral canthus. After the sutures are tied, the lid margin should not be able to be forcefully rotated into an entropion position (Fig. 6.56).

The amount of redundant skin is ascertained by using posterior-inferior pressure on the globe through the upper lid (Fig. 6.57) or having the patient look up at the time of the procedure. These techniques flatten out the depression in the lower lid to prevent excess skin excision. The skin is draped over the wound (Fig. 6.58) and the excess skin removed (Fig. 6.59). All bleeding is stopped prior to closure. The wound is closed with a continuous suture of 6-0 Prolene with very small bites widely scattered across the lower lid and continuing as a vertical mattress suture on the temporal portion of the wound. The deep bites are looped with pull-out sutures to facilitate removal of the mattress sutures (Fig. 6.60).

Figure 6.61 shows the preoperative appearance of a left lower lid entropion, while Fig. 6.62 shows the postoperative appearance.

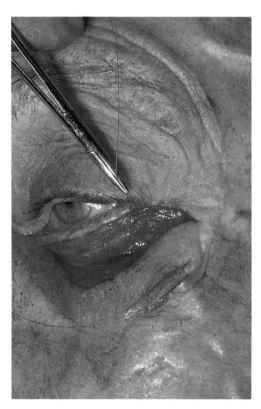

FIG. 6.53

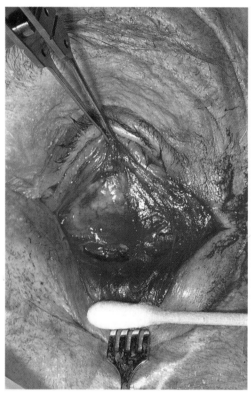

FIG. 6.54

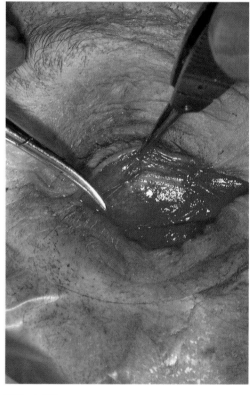

FIG. 6.55

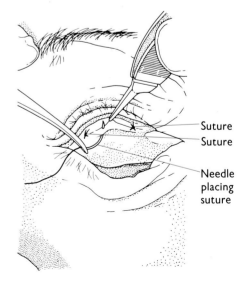

Suture
Suture
Needle placing suture

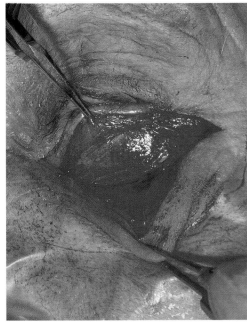

FIG. 6.56

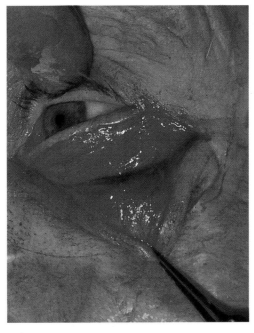

FIG. 6.57

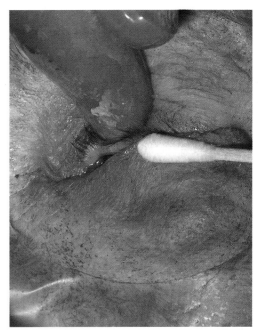

FIG. 6.58

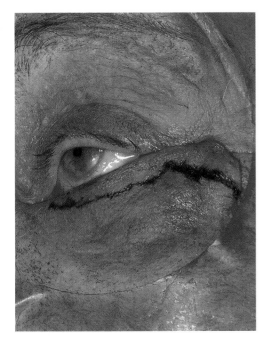

FIG. 6.59

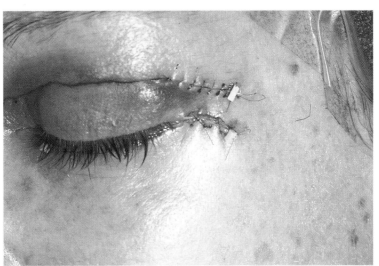

FIG. 6.60

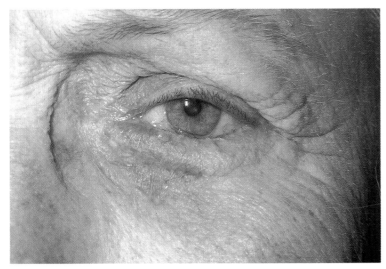

FIG. 6.61

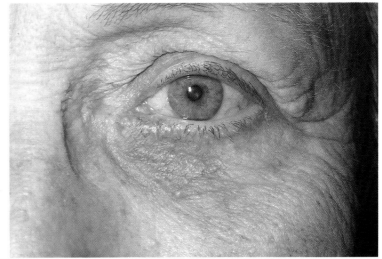

FIG. 6.62

REPAIR OF INVOLUTIONAL ECTROPION: LATERAL CANTHAL SLING PROCEDURE

To perform this procedure, there must be horizontal lid laxity. The greater the laxity, the easier the operation. A lateral canthotomy is made to the orbital rim (Fig. 6.63), where the inferior arm of the canthal tendon is cut (Fig. 6.64). The lower lid is draped across the upper lid and a point is marked on the lower lid where it crosses the beginning of the canthotomy of the upper lid (Fig. 6.65). To this point, the lid margin is removed (Fig. 6.66), the lashes are excised, the skin is separated from the muscle (Fig. 6.67), and the conjunctiva is removed (Fig. 6.68) from the posterior surface of the tarsus. A suture can be placed at the end of the tendon for easier handling of the tissue (Fig. 6.69).

If there is a severe marginal ectropion, an addition is now made to the procedure by a 6-to-7-mm excision of conjunctiva and lower lid retractors. The conjunctiva is picked up 3.5 mm below the tarsus with two forceps. Two hemostats are placed across the base of these tissues, giving a 7-mm excision (Fig. 6.70). A 6-0 Prolene suture enters the skin medially and comes out beneath the hemostat, goes beneath the hemostat at a 45° angle to exit the other side, and continues across the lid (Fig. 6.71). When the lateral end of the wound is reached, the suture is brought out on the skin. The hemostats are removed and the excess conjunctiva and lower lid retractors are excised. The suture is tied over a rubber band on the skin (Fig. 6.72).

Repair of Involutional Ectropion: Lateral Canthal Sling

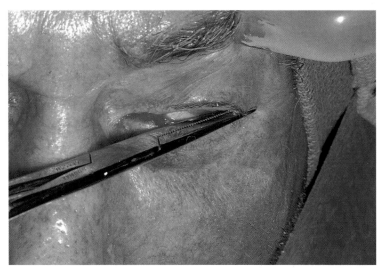

FIG. 6.63

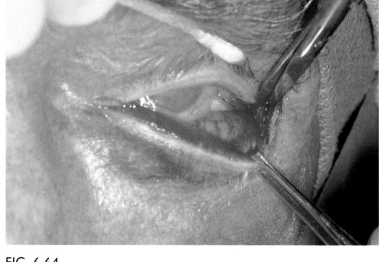

FIG. 6.64

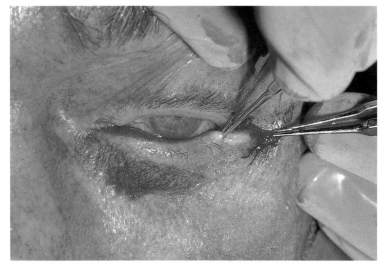

FIG. 6.65

FIG. 6.66

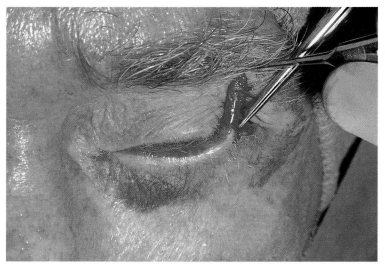

FIG. 6.67

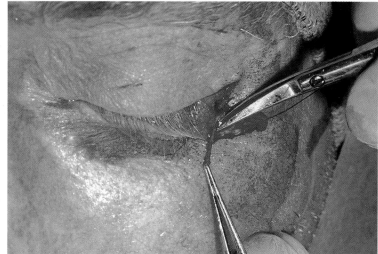

FIG. 6.68

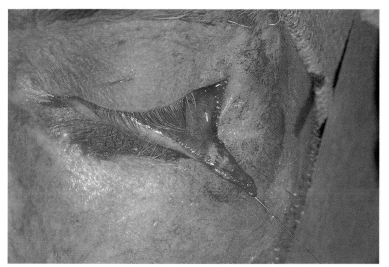

FIG. 6.69

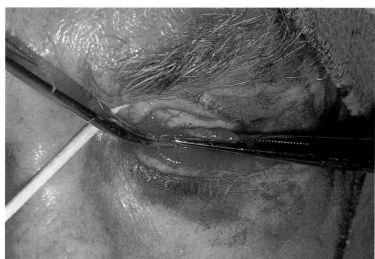

FIG. 6.70

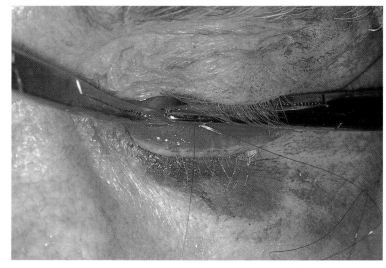

FIG. 6.71

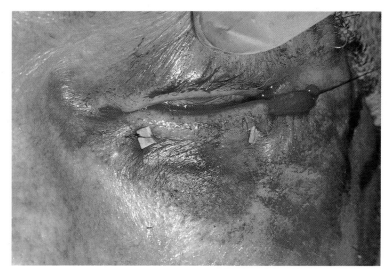

FIG. 6.72

Continuing with the lateral canthal sling, the periosteum is exposed at the lateral orbital rim (Fig. 6.73) by blunt dissection and a buttonhole is made in the upper arm of the canthal tendon (Fig. 6.74). The tarsal strap is brought through this buttonhole (Fig. 6.75) and sutured to the periosteum with a whipstitch of 5-0 nylon on a double-armed half-circle spatula needle (Fig. 6.76). The level should correspond to the level of the lateral canthus on the fellow eye. A second suture is placed superior temporally to the first suture through the periosteum and tarsal strap for better support. The lateral canthus is closed with a full-thickness vertical mattress suture tied over a cotton pledget (Fig. 6.77). The suture stays in place for 8 to 10 days. The remaining wound is closed with deep sutures of 6-0 Vicryl and a continuous suture of 6-0 Prolene on the skin or else near-far-far-near sutures of 6-0 Prolene. These sutures, as well as the sutures beneath the lashes, are removed in five days.

Figure 6.78 shows the preoperative appearance of a patient with involutional ectropion of the right lower lid worse than the left lower lid, while Fig. 6.79 shows the postoperative appearance after repair of the right lower lid with a lateral canthal sling. Figure 6.80 shows the preoperative severe marginal ectropion, while Fig. 6.81 shows the postoperative appearance after a lateral canthal sling and resection of the lower lid retractors bilaterally.

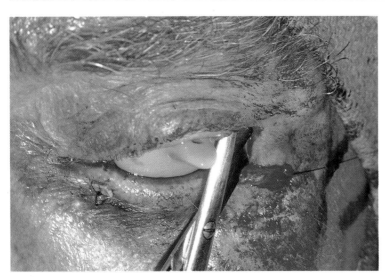

FIG. 6.73

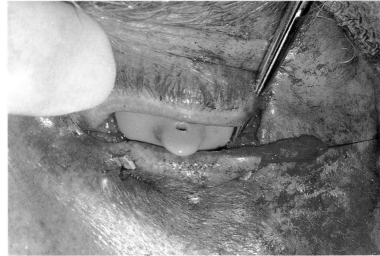

FIG. 6.74

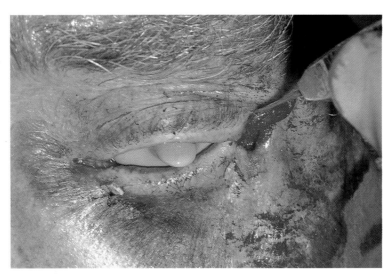

FIG. 6.75

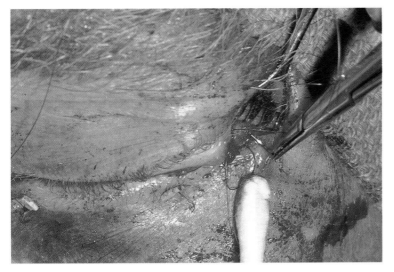

FIG. 6.76

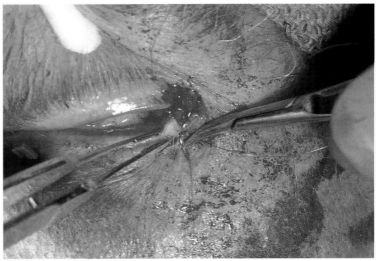

FIG. 6.77

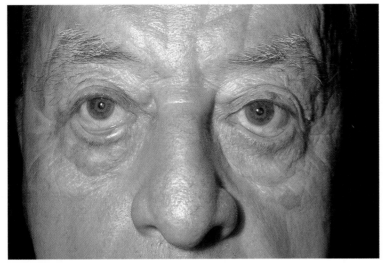

FIG. 6.78

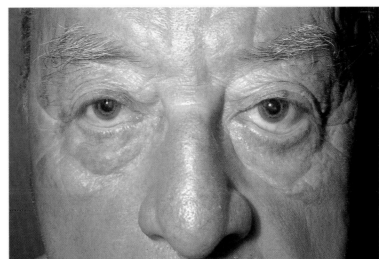

FIG. 6.79

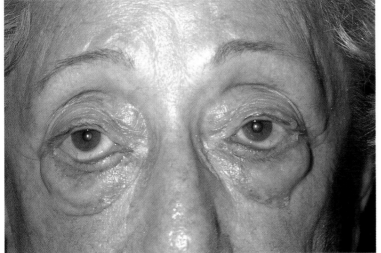

FIG. 6.80

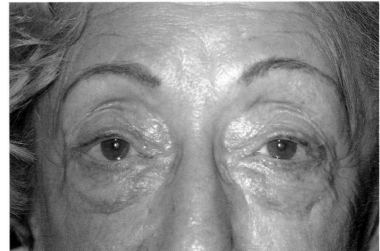

FIG. 6.81

SURGERY OF CONJUNCTIVAL SHRINKAGE DISEASE

CICATRICIAL ENTROPION OF THE LOWER LID

Classically, cicatricial entropion of the lower lid starts in the center of the lid. Slit lamp examination reveals the meibomian gland orifices in this area to be on the posterior lid margin, or even on the posterior palpebral conjunctival surface, rather than almost in the center of the lid margin.

A lid plate behind the lid protects the globe. Two 4-0 silk sutures are placed through the lid 4 mm from the lid margin, one 3 mm medial and the other 3 mm lateral to the entropion (Fig. 6.82). An incision is made through the skin and muscle of the lid between the sutures, staying parallel to the lid margin (Fig. 6.83). The lid is everted over the lid plate. A second incision is made through the conjunctiva and tarsus between the sutures, again staying parallel to the lid margin (Fig. 6.84). The two incisions are joined with scissors, giving a through-and-through transverse blepharotomy (Fig. 6.85). The 4-0 silk sutures are removed and used as horizontal mattress sutures. They enter the skin, just inferior to the lashes, staying anterior to the tarsus (Fig. 6.86), exit the wound, proceed into the small remaining portion of the tarsus of the lower wound, or, if the tarsus is not present, into the lower lid retractors (Fig. 6.87), exit on the conjunctiva, go back into the conjunctiva again, either picking up tarsus or lower lid retractors, exit the lower wound, enter the upper wound, staying anterior to the tarsus, and exit the skin beneath the lashes (Fig. 6.88). Multiple sutures are placed across the lid (Fig. 6.89). When these sutures are tied, the lid should be in a mild ectropion position (Fig. 6.90). The skin can be left open or closed with small interrupted sutures of 7-0 silk. The 4-0 silk sutures are removed in 10 to 12 days.

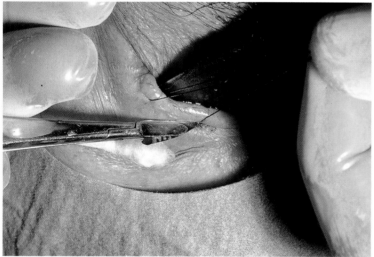
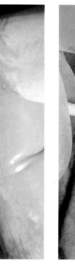

FIG. 6.82

FIG. 6.83

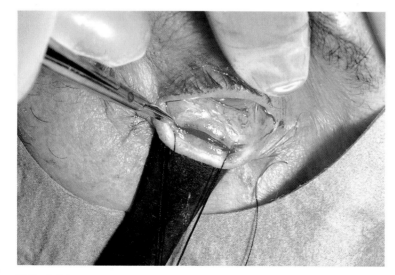

FIG. 6.84

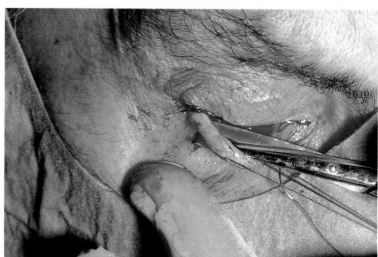

FIG. 6.85

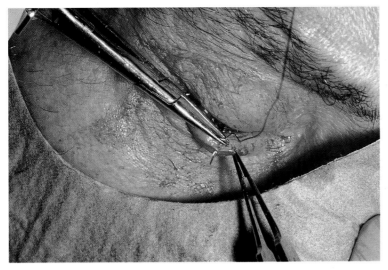

FIG. 6.86

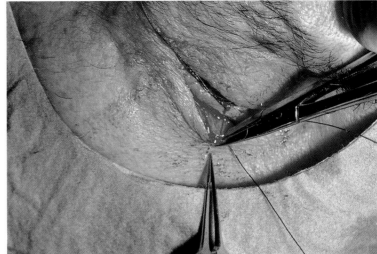

FIG. 6.87

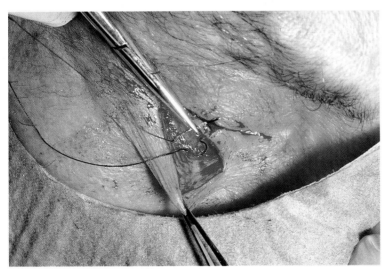

FIG. 6.88

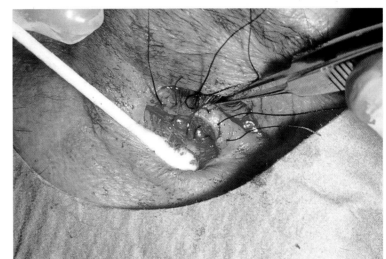

FIG. 6.89

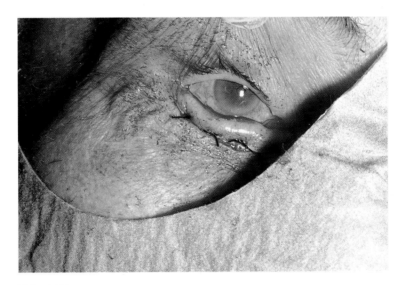

FIG. 6.90

Figure 6.91 shows the preoperative appearance of a cicatricial entropion of the right lower lid, while Fig. 6.92 shows the postoperative appearance.

UPPER LID ENTROPION WITH GRAFT

The upper lid is everted and an incision is made 6 mm from the lid margin through the conjunctiva, tarsus, and levator aponeurosis (Fig. 6.93). The tarsus is separated from the levator aponeurosis to the lash buds (Fig. 6.94). A 6-to-8-mm block of tissue, either sclera, tarsus, or upper palate, is placed in the defect. A horizontal mattress suture enters the skin just above the lashes, comes out the wound with a partial-thickness tarsal bite (Fig. 6.95), takes a horizontal partial-thickness bite in the graft (Fig. 6.96), takes another partial-thickness tarsal bite, and exits on the skin (Fig. 6.97). These horizontal mattress sutures are placed completely across the lid, causing eversion of the lashes (Fig. 6.98). A second row of sutures enters the skin approximately 6 mm higher than the first row (Fig. 6.99), takes a partial-thickness bite in the tarsus (Fig. 6.100), enters the graft in a hor-

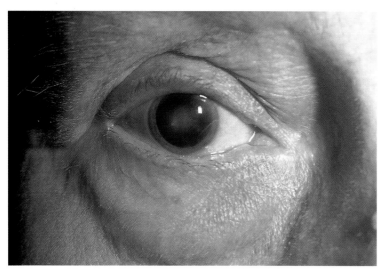

FIG. 6.91

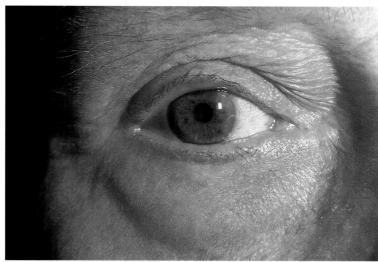

FIG. 6.92

Upper Lid Entropion with Graft

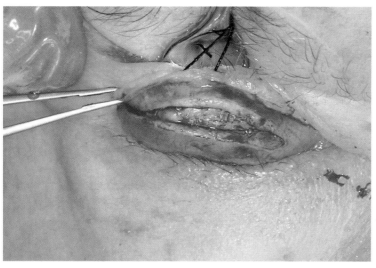

FIG. 6.93

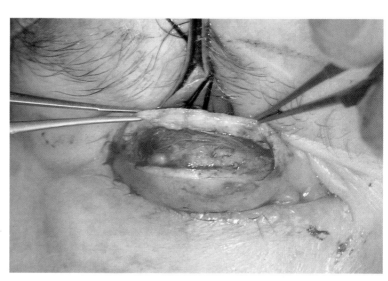

FIG. 6.94

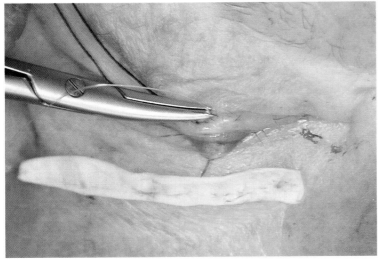

FIG. 6.95

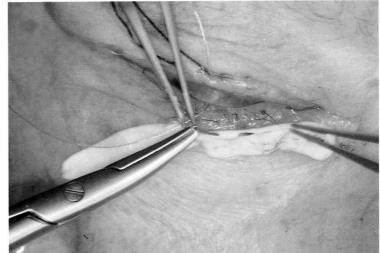

FIG. 6.96

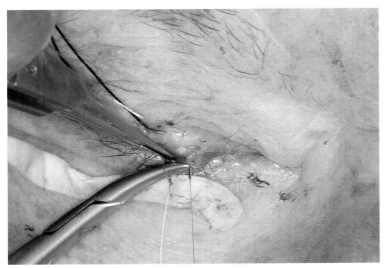

FIG. 6.97

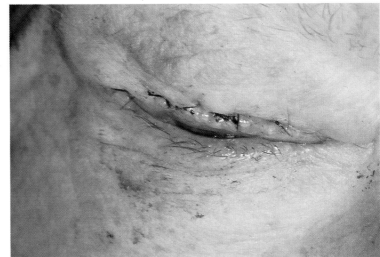

FIG. 6.98

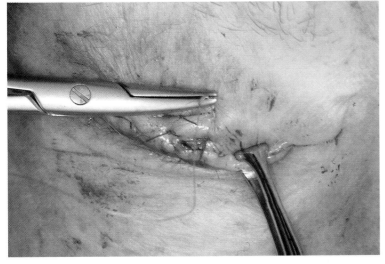

FIG. 6.99

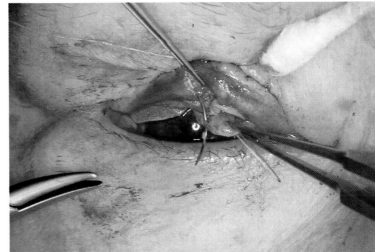

FIG. 6.100

izontal fashion (Fig. 6.101), comes back through the tarsus (Fig. 6.102), and exits on the skin (Fig. 6.103). These sutures are removed in 10 days. It is easier to do this type of suturing with a spatula needle and a 6-0 silk or 6-0 Mersilene suture.

Figure 6.104 shows the preoperative appearance of entropion of the right upper lid, while Fig. 6.105 shows the postoperative appearance.

CICATRICIAL ECTROPION OF THE LOWER LID

An incision is made 2 mm beneath the lashes (Fig. 6.106), two 4-0 silk traction sutures are placed between the incision and the lashes, and skin dissection is carried out until the lid can be brought up into the overcorrected position (Fig. 6.107). The tarsal–tendon resection is performed as described in Figs. 6.48 to 6.53, or a transmarginal horizontal shortening can be used. In this technique, a full-thickness lid margin incision is performed 5 mm from the lateral canthus (Fig. 6.108). The lid is overlapped (Fig. 6.109) to

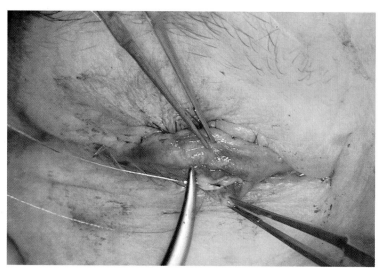

FIG. 6.101

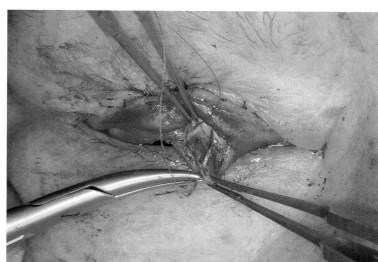

FIG. 6.102

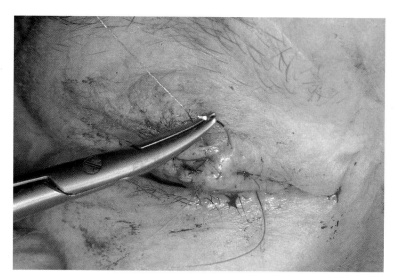

FIG. 6.103

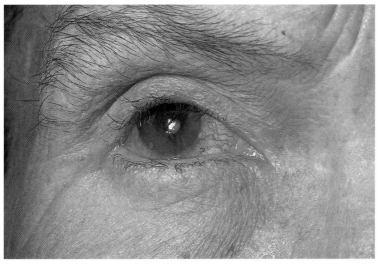

FIG. 6.104

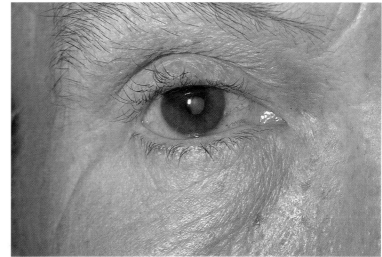

FIG. 6.105

Cicatricial Ectropion of the Lower Lid

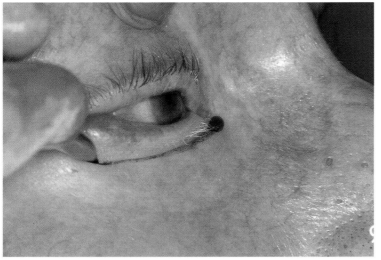

FIG. 6.106

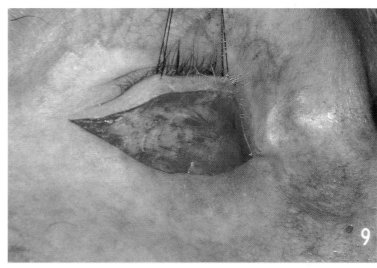

FIG. 6.107

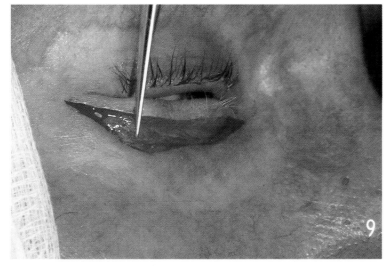

FIG. 6.108

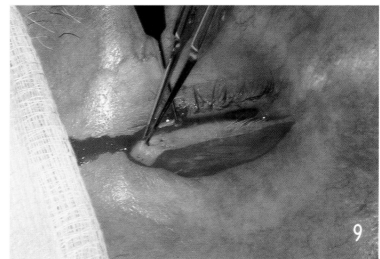

FIG. 6.109

judge the amount of laxity and a second incision is made through the lid margin (Fig. 6.110) parallel to the first incision. A triangulation is taken out at the base for closure. A 6-0 silk suture enters the posterior lid margin 3 mm from the cut edge, exits anterior to the tarsus 3 mm from the lid margin, enters the other side of the wound in the anterior tarsus 3 mm from the lid margin, and exits the posterior lid margin 3 mm from the cut edge (Fig. 6.111). The suture is tied, put on a stretch, and attached to the drapes.

The tarsal and muscle layers are closed with interrupted sutures of 7-0 Vicryl (Fig. 6.112). A second 6-0 silk lid margin suture is placed just posterior to the lashes. Another 6-0 silk suture is placed just beneath the lashes and the two lid margin sutures are tied beneath this suture to prevent corneal abrasion (Fig. 6.113). This two-suture lid margin closure can also be used to repair a lid margin laceration or small tumor excision. The two traction sutures are used to bring the lid back into the overcorrected position and a skin graft is placed in the defect (Fig. 6.114) and sutured with two continuous 6-0 Prolene sutures (Fig. 6.115). One arm of each of the 4-0 silk sutures is placed below the graft (Fig. 6.116). A Telfa bolus is inserted beneath these sutures and these sutures are tied over the bolus (Fig. 6.117). The bolus is removed after 48 hours and the graft sutures in five to seven days.

Figure 6.118 shows the preoperative cicatricial ectropion of the right lower lid postblepharoplasty, while Fig. 6.119 shows the postoperative appearance.

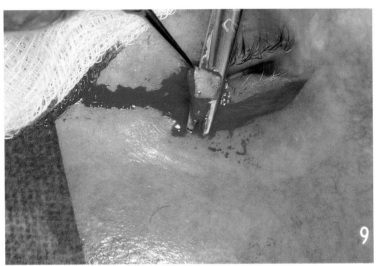

FIG. 6.110

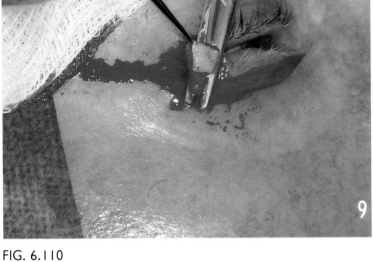

FIG. 6.111

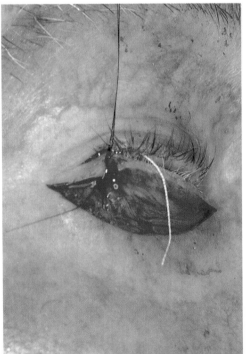

FIG. 6.112

FIG. 6.113

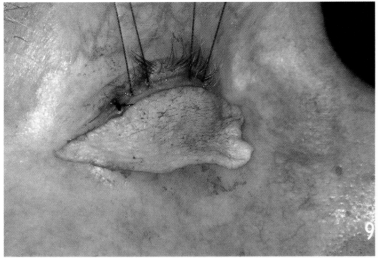

FIG. 6.114

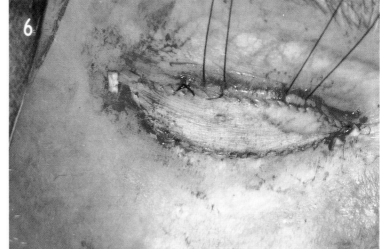

FIG. 6.115

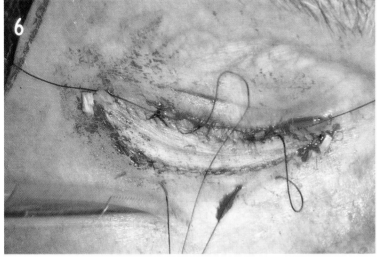

FIG. 6.116

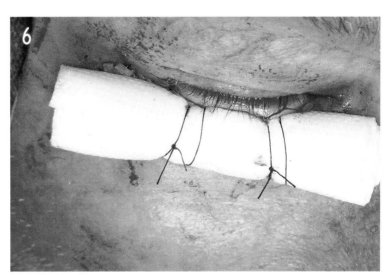

FIG. 6.117

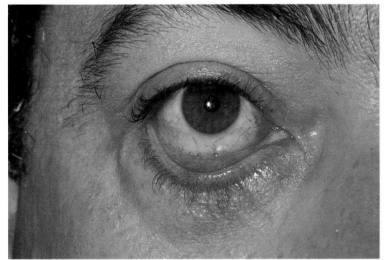

FIG. 6.118

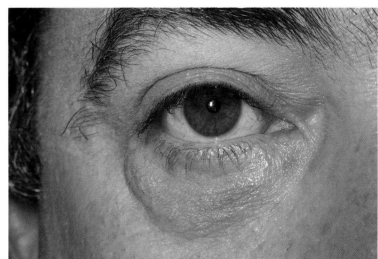

FIG. 6.119

7

REFRACTIVE SURGERY

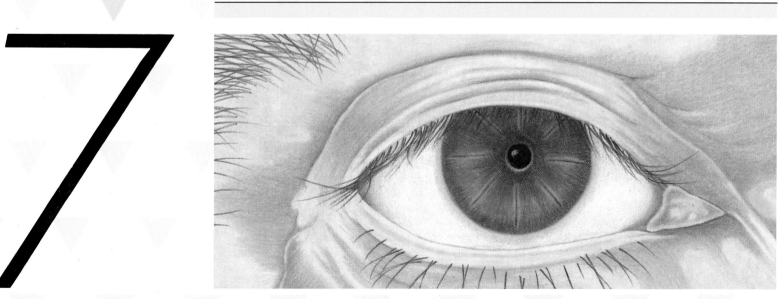

Lee T. Nordan, MD

W. Andrew Maxwell, MD, PhD

Refractive surgery is being performed on a larger scale than ever before. Allowing an ametrope to see without glasses will forever be an honorable, if controversial, endeavor. Someday, refractive error may routinely be considered a disease and surgical treatment the cure.

We present here the general concepts of refractive surgery, as well as our own methodology of performing these techniques. Certainly there are other valid techniques for achieving the same results but we provide here what we feel is a consistent, comprehensive approach. Investigators associated with major principles or procedures are noted in parentheses.

In refractive surgery, success does not require perfection, but let us continue to aspire and strive for even better results.

ANATOMY AND CONCEPTS

The basic corneal structure is shown in Fig. 7.1 and average corneal dimensions are presented in Fig. 7.2. Generally, the superonasal quadrants of the cornea are thicker than the inferotemporal quadrants. The visual axis of the eye corresponds clinically to the patient's "macula–miotic pupil" line and passes through the cornea at a point that is usually nasal to the geometric center of the cornea.

Refractive error is classified as myopia (nearsightedness), hyperopia (farsightedness), or regular astigmatism. Myopia exists when the refractive power of the cornea–lens complex exceeds that necessary to focus a distant object on the macula; hyperopia exists when the refractive power of the cornea–lens complex is less than that necessary to focus a distant object on the macula (Fig. 7.3). Regular corneal

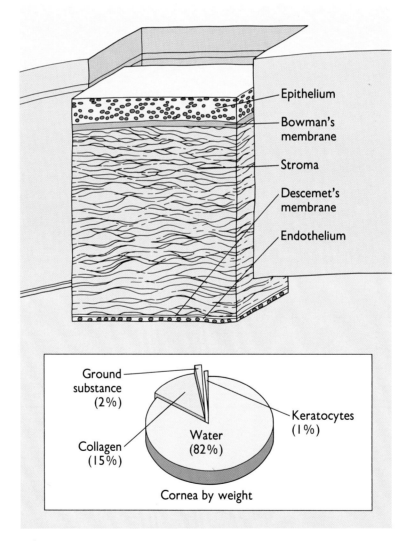

FIG. 7.1

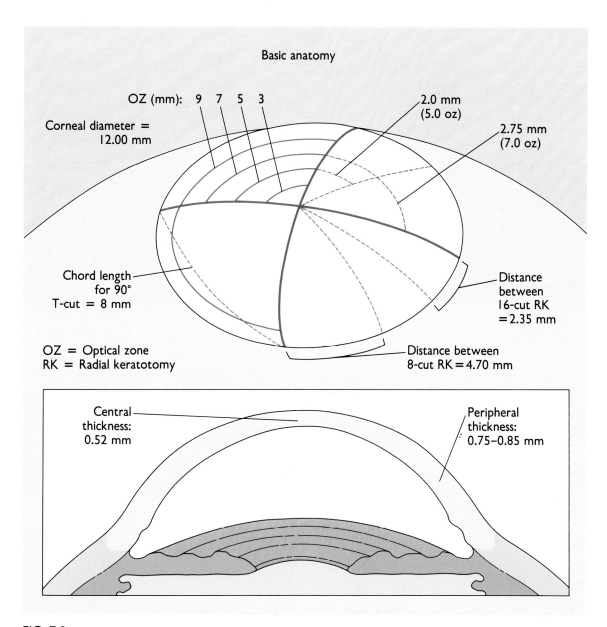

Basic anatomy

OZ (mm): 9 7 5 3

Corneal diameter = 12.00 mm

2.0 mm (5.0 oz)

2.75 mm (7.0 oz)

Chord length for 90° T-cut = 8 mm

Distance between 16-cut RK = 2.35 mm

OZ = Optical zone
RK = Radial keratotomy

Distance between 8-cut RK = 4.70 mm

Central thickness: 0.52 mm

Peripheral thickness: 0.75–0.85 mm

FIG. 7.2

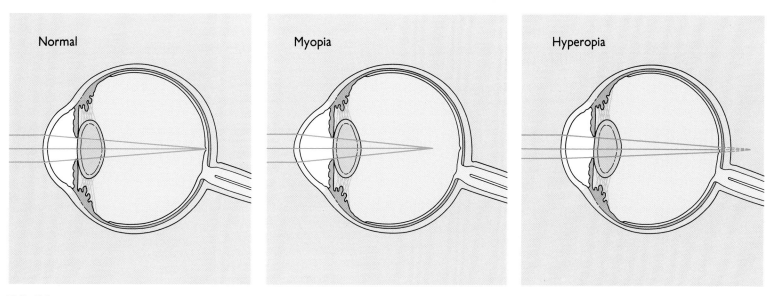

Normal

Myopia

Hyperopia

FIG. 7.3

astigmatism exists when the major and minor meridians of power of the cornea are unequal in refractive power (Fig. 7.4). Irregular astigmatism is a corneal condition in which the epithelial surface is optically distorted. This distortion may be caused by an underlying stromal defect such as scarring or by epithelial pathology such as punctate keratopathy (Fig. 7.5).

Keratorefractive surgery results in central corneal flatten-ing or steepening. Central corneal flattening reduces corneal refractive power, while central corneal steepening results in an increase. The mechanisms by which this flattening or steepening are accomplished, along with the respective procedures, are given in Fig. 7.6. An important phenomenon is the *coupling effect* (Ruiz) (Fig. 7.7). This occurs when the steeper meridian of the cornea is flattened by astigmatic keratotomy, resulting in an associated steep-

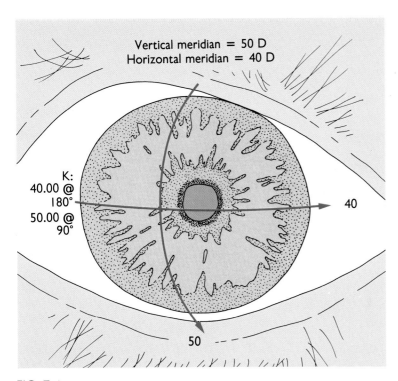

FIG. 7.4

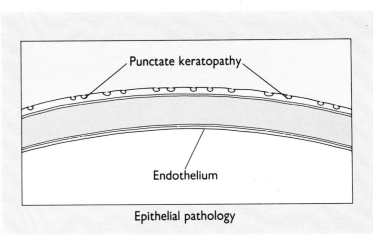

Epithelial pathology

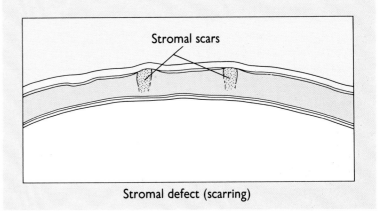

Stromal defect (scarring)

FIG. 7.5

REFRACTIVE SURGERY PROCEDURES

CENTRAL CORNEAL FLATTENING		CENTRAL CORNEAL STEEPENING	
MECHANISM	PROCEDURE USED TO OBTAIN EFFECT	MECHANISM	PROCEDURE USED TO OBTAIN EFFECT
Paracentral weakening of cornea	Radial keratotomy	Central weakening of cornea	Circular or hexagonal keratotomy
Removal of central stroma	Myopic keratomileusis	Removal of peripheral stroma	Hyperopic keratomileusis
	Myopic epikeratophakia		Hyperopic epikeratophakia
	Laser ablation		Laser ablation
		Increase in central thickness	Homoplastic or alloplastic keratophakia
Placement of intracorneal lens	Alloplastic intrastromal implant	Placement of intracorneal lens	Alloplastic intrastromal implant
		Central "ectasia" of cornea	Deep lamellar keratectomy

FIG. 7.6

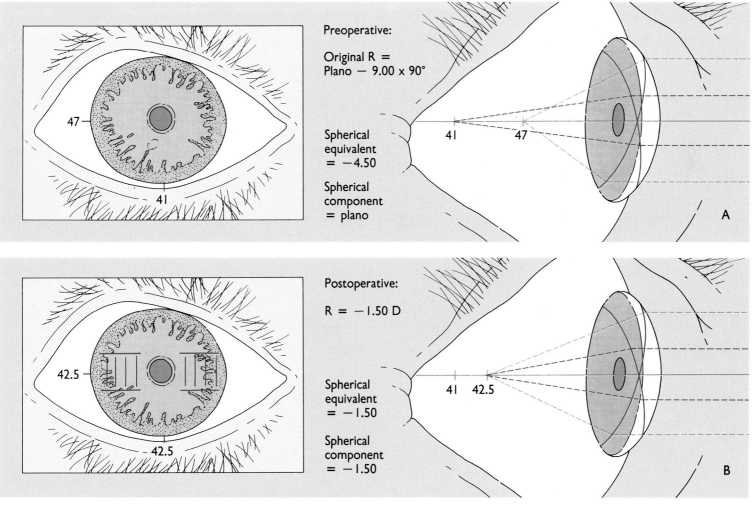

Preoperative:

Original R =
Plano — 9.00 x 90°

Spherical
equivalent
= −4.50

Spherical
component
= plano

A

Postoperative:

R = −1.50 D

Spherical
equivalent
= −1.50

Spherical
component
= −1.50

B

FIG. 7.7

ening of the flatter meridian. The ratio of flattening to steepening varies mainly with the transverse length of the astigmatic keratotomy.

Corneal transplantation procedures are classified in two groups: penetrating keratoplasty (PKP) or lamellar keratoplasty (LKP) (Fig. 7.8). PKP replaces the entire thickness of the patient's cornea and is characterized by the lack of a corneal interface, the possibility of an endothelial graft rejection, and the risks of an intraocular procedure. LKP creates a stromal interface between the donor and recipient but does not involve a clinically significant rejection since aqueous is not in contact with donor endothelium. LKP entails penetration rather than perforation of the cornea (as in PKP), so the patient is not subjected to the risks of an intraocular procedure.

SURGICAL CONSIDERATIONS

Keratorefractive surgery is considered statistically successful when uncorrected visual acuity comes within two Snellen lines of the preoperative best corrected spectacle visual acuity (or presurgical goal) *and* there is no greater than a one-half Snellen line decrease in the postoperative best-corrected spectacle visual acuity. Also, disabling glare or distortion must be absent. Subjective success may occur when a satisfied patient is a statistical failure. A patient's needs, desires, and expectations play a key role in determining clinical success or failure.

When obtaining informed consent, the surgeon must point out that a certain benefit/risk ratio exists for all surgery. No guarantees can be made. The surgeon must be aware of inappropriate patient expectations or psychological difficulties. In addition, previously undiagnosed keratoconus, maculopathy, or amblyopia must be documented in order 'to assess adequately proper refractive surgery capabilities.

RADIAL KERATOTOMY

Radial keratotomy (RK) (Sato, Fyodorov) is by far the most common keratorefractive surgery performed at this time. The elements of RK surgical technique are used in astigmatic keratotomy as well as in hexagonal incisions for hyperopic correction. Therefore, the following description of RK is presented in detail since these considerations are important in a large percentage of patients.

PREOPERATIVE PREPARATION

Calculations
The preoperative calculations to be performed are given in the nomogram in Fig. 7.9. The working sphere is equal to the refractive error $+/-$ factors relating to the patient's age, intraocular pressure, gender, and central corneal thickness. The effect of RK depends greatly on these characteristics. Experience has shown that the least effect from RK is obtained in young females with thin corneas and low intraocular pressure.

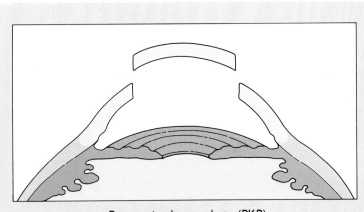
Penetrating keratoplasty (PKP)

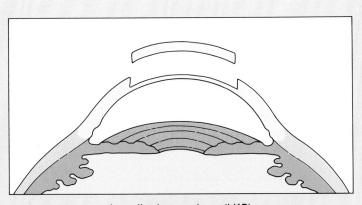
Lamellar keratoplasty (LKP)

FIG. 7.8

RADIAL KERATOTOMY NOMOGRAM, NORDAN/MAXWELL METHODOLOGY

Assumptions: 90% achieved depth; centrifugal incision; noncycloplegic refraction
Factors considered: refractive error; age; gender; IOP; corneal thickness (The sum of these factors = working sphere)
Factors not considered: corneal diameter; keratometry

REFRACTIVE ERROR

REFRACTIVE ERROR (WORKING SPHERE)	NUMBER OF INCISIONS	OPTICAL ZONE		
—0.50	3	5.00		
—0.75	3	4.50		
—1.00	6	4.50		
—1.25	6	4.25		
—1.50	6	4.00		
—2.00	8	4.00		
—2.50	8	3.75		
—3.00	8	3.50		
—3.50	8	3.25		
—4.00	8	3.00		
—4.50	8	3.00	5.00	
—5.00	8	3.00	5.00	7.00
—5.50	8	3.00	5.00	7.00
—6.00	16	3.00	5.00	
—6.50	16	3.00	5.00	7.00
—7.00	16	3.00	5.00	7.00
—7.50	16	3.00	5.00	7.00

AGE

MYOPIA	18–23	24–27	28–31	32–34	35–37	38–41	42–45	46–48	49–53	54–57	58 AND ABOVE
0 to —2.00	—0.75	—0.50	0	+0.25	+0.50	+0.75	+1.00	+1.25	+1.50	+1.50	+1.75
—2.25 to —4.75	—1.00	—0.50	0	+0.25	+0.50	+0.75	+1.00	+1.25	+1.50	+1.50	+1.75
—5.00 + more	—1.50	—0.75	—0.25	0	+0.50	+0.50	+1.00	+1.25	+1.50	+1.50	+1.75

CORNEAL THICKNESS

If central corneal thickness is less than 0.49 mm, add —0.50 D to refractive error
if original refractive error is —2.00 D or greater. If central thickness is greater
than 0.57 mm, add +0.50 to refractive error.

INTRAOCULAR PRESSURE

Add —0.25D for every 2 mm Hg less than 15 mm Hg. If IOP is greater than
22 mm Hg, control IOP as appropriate and consider undercorrection.

GENDER

Females, age 24-34, add —0.50 D to refractive error.

FIG. 7.9

Mechanism

Paracentral weakening of the cornea allows for peripheral steepening with subsequent central flattening (Fig. 7.10). The postoperative "functional" optical zone is smaller than before surgery. Reduced visual acuity may result when the pupil dilates. However, the aspheric corneal curvature of the paracentral cornea often decreases presbyopic symptoms (Fig. 7.11).

Blade Considerations

A modern diamond blade is currently the sharpest and most desirable instrument used for RK. Figure 7.12 summarizes the characteristics of the back-cutting (Fig. 7.13), front-cutting (Fig. 7.14), and double-cutting (Fig. 7.15) blades.

▽ Radial Keratotomy: Mechanism

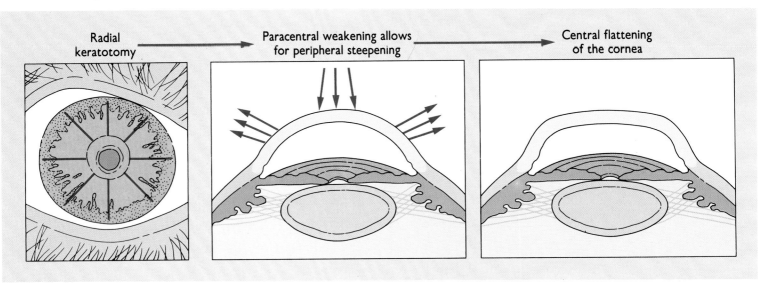

FIG. 7.10

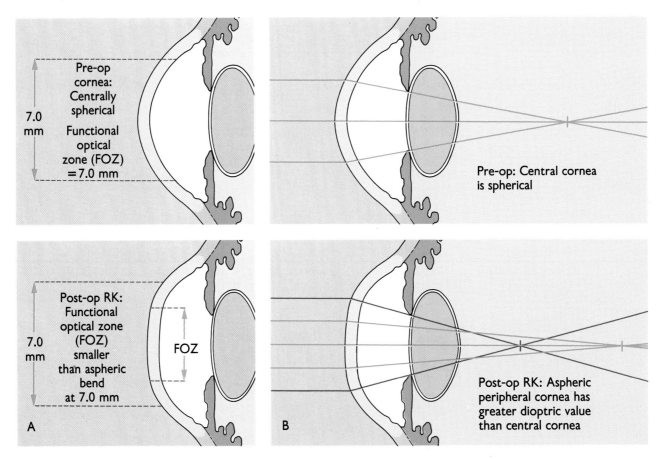

FIG. 7.11

TYPES OF BLADES USED IN KERATOREFRACTIVE PROCEDURES

BLADE TYPE	CUTTING CHARACTERISTICS	ADVANTAGES	DISADVANTAGES
Back-cutting	Tends to surface during incision Used for centrifugal incisions only	Safe Incision will not cross visual axis	Larger optical zone than intended Poor visibility for astigmatic keratotomy
Front-cutting	Tends to remain deep during incision Used for centripetal incisions only	Vertical incision at optical zone Excellent visibility for astigmatic keratotomy	Less safe Incision may cross visual axis unexpectedly
Double-cutting	Excellent penetration	Desired depth achieved easily Excellent for astigmatic keratotomy	Less safe Incision may cross visual axis unexpectedly Tends not to track straight during RK

FIG. 7.12

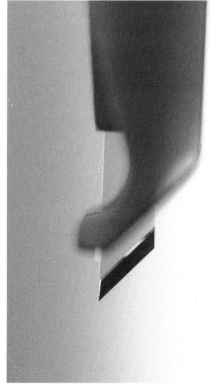

FIG. 7.13

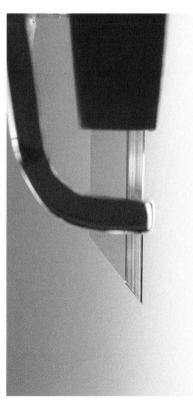

FIG. 7.14

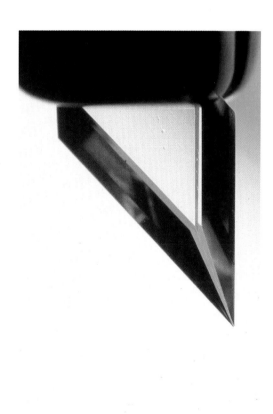

FIG. 7.15

SURGICAL TECHNIQUE

Anesthesia

Topical anesthesia is best achieved with proparacaine. Cocaine disrupts the epithelium and tetracaine stings with each administration. Viscous Xylocaine is a suitable alternative to proparacaine. A pledget of anesthesia is applied to the limbus if desired. Several drops of anesthetic are used 1 to 2 minutes before grasping the conjunctiva. Preoperative sedation p.o. is often useful, as well. No peribulbar or retrobulbar anesthesia is necessary. The rapport between patient and doctor is of the utmost importance. The surgeon should "talk the patient along" without long periods of silence that may cause patient anxiety. Topical anesthetic applied to the nonsurgical eye minimizes blinking.

Pachymetry

Ultrasound pachymetry with a 1,640-mm/sec velocity setting is used. A standardized pattern of measurements is taken using an epithelial marker (Figs. 7.16 and 7.17); the data is recorded. A coaxial microscope is used during the pachymetry and blade depth is changed when a 0.03 mm increase in corneal thickness is encountered (Fig. 7.18).

Preparation

Routine surgical preparation of the involved eye takes place. The surgeon wears sterile gloves but a gown is not necessary. The patient is not draped. The lid speculum is engaged only after the blade has been set in order to minimize desiccation of the cornea. The speculum should be a nonflexible model such as the Lancaster type (Fig. 7.19).

Blade Length and Ocular Fixation

A calibrated gauge block allows for consistent blade length measurements (Fig. 7.20). Initially, a practice globe can be used to correlate pachymetry with blade depth by gradually increasing blade length until perforation.

Various philosophies exist as to the best method of selecting blade depth. It is unresolved whether or not it is better to leave uncut an equal amount of stroma in all meridians or whether the amount of stroma left uncut should be proportional to the original thickness of the cornea in the various meridians. Since we are dealing with uncut tissue equal to 10% of corneal tissue in a range of depth from approximately 0.50 to 0.75 mm, the maximum difference is 10% (0.5) = 0.50 versus 10% (0.75) = 0.75 mm. This maximum disparity of 0.025 mm is most likely insignificant in the clinical action of RK.

Of great significance, however, is the concept that incision depth should be based on either an average or a single paracentral pachymetry reading with an *assumed* increase in the corneal thickness at a given distance from the center of the cornea.

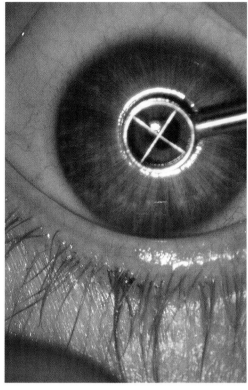

FIG. 7.16

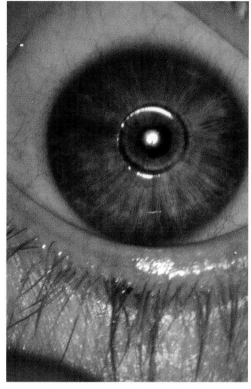

FIG. 7.17

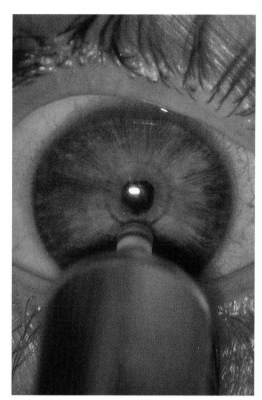

FIG. 7.18

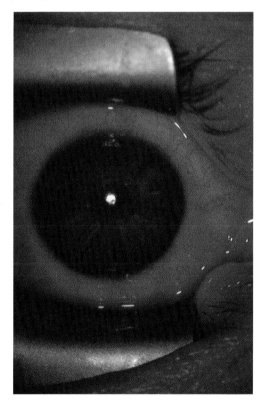

FIG. 7.19

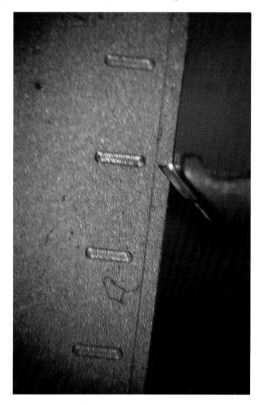

FIG. 7.20

For example, consider a "typical" cornea with corneal thickness as follows (Fig. 7.21A):

Central = 0.52

Temporal = 0.53
Inferior = 0.55
Nasal = 0.58
Superior = 0.61

The average corneal thickness at a 3.50 mm optical zone is

$$\frac{0.53 + 0.55 + 0.58 + 0.61}{4} = 0.568$$

Assume that a 10% blade bias above 100% corneal thickness yields the desired achieved depth of 90%. Therefore, the actual blade length and achieved depth, based on the actual pachymetric measurements at the given optical zone plus a 10% bias, would be as given in Fig. 7.21B. Remember, the blade may be longer than the thickness of the cornea but still achieve a 90% depth cut due to the resistance and inward bowing of the cornea during the incisions.

If the blade length is based on the temporal reading, the uncut tissue induced superiorly would equal $0.61 - 0.48 = 0.13$ mm [0.48 = achieved depth from a 0.59 blade (0.90×0.53)]. There is $0.13/0.61 = 21\%$ of stroma left uncut superiorly compared with 10% temporally.

If the blade length is based on the average of the optical zone measurements $+ 10\%$ bias, then the blade length would equal $0.568 + 10\% (0.568) = 0.62$ mm.

A blade length of 0.62 mm will achieve an incision depth of 0.51 mm:

Temporally, $0.51/0.53 = 96\%$

Superiorly, $0.51/0.61 = 84\%$

This produces an achieved depth of 96% temporally, which is a significantly different result from 84% superiorly. We consider a consistent thickness or percentage of uncut stroma superior to a varying amount of uncut stroma.

A Kremer forceps achieves stable ocular fixation with minimal manipulation (Fig. 7.22). The patient fixates on the microscope light initially but is instructed *not* to follow the apparent movement of the light during incisions.

Incisions

The epithelial marker is again centered on the miotic pupil. Centrifugal incisions are preferred because they are safer.

Proper blade bias allows for the desired achieved depth of 90% of corneal thickness. Entry is made with the blade directed toward the center of the globe to ensure a perpendicular margin for each incision. The surgeon waits until after the initial plunge to allow settling of the blade to its full depth in the cornea. The blade is kept perpendicular to the cornea during the incisions and each incision ends ½ mm before the limbus. Each zone is finished before moving to the next one, and each is started with the shortest blade necessary. Figures 7.23 and 7.24 show the postoperative appearance of the incisions.

Incisions are irrigated only when necessary due to the presence of a foreign body or blood but *never* when a microperforation is present.

POSTOPERATIVE CONSIDERATIONS

Topical intravenous antibiotics (without preservatives) are applied along with a short-acting topical steroid drop. A semipressure patch is used until the epithelium is intact, which usually takes about 12 to 18 hours. Antibiotic and steroid drops are used every six hours for four days and additional patching, artificial tears, or a bandage soft contact lens are used as necessary if the epithelium is not healing well. If transient recurrent erosions occur, they are usually at points of redeepening. At this time, the value of using "epidermal growth factor," or "corneal mortar," to improve corneal healing is not considered clinically significant.

REOPERATION CONSIDERATIONS

Reoperation is considered 2 to 3 months following the procedure. The surgeon determines at that time whether the depths of the original incisions are correct. If they are not, a decision is made either to extend the incisions inward or create new incisions. If good depth was achieved with the first incisions, the effect of a smaller optical zone will be the same as for the original incisions. In an eight-incision case, redeepening yields 0.50 D per redeepened zone; eight additional incisions will yield approximately 20% effect in addition to the original eight incisions. To determine which reoperative procedure to perform, multiply the residual spherical equivalent by 2.5 and add or subtract other factors for age, sex, intraocular pressure, etc., to determine the new working sphere. Choose an optical zone for the eight new incisions based on the new working sphere. If extension of the preexisting incisions is desired, then a front-cutting blade is used.

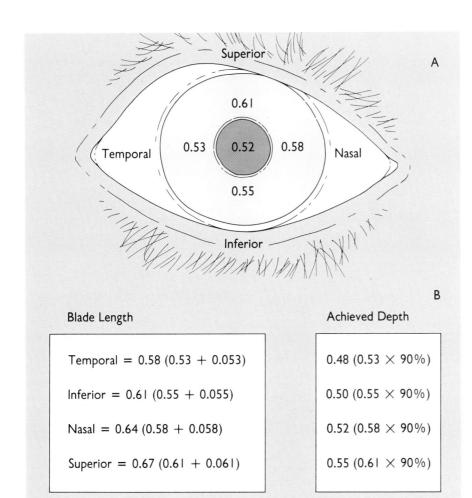

A

B

Blade Length

Temporal = 0.58 (0.53 + 0.053)

Inferior = 0.61 (0.55 + 0.055)

Nasal = 0.64 (0.58 + 0.058)

Superior = 0.67 (0.61 + 0.061)

Achieved Depth

0.48 (0.53 × 90%)

0.50 (0.55 × 90%)

0.52 (0.58 × 90%)

0.55 (0.61 × 90%)

FIG. 7.21

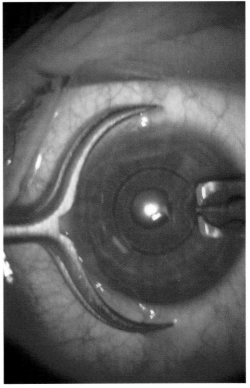

FIG. 7.22

Radial Keratotomy: Incisions

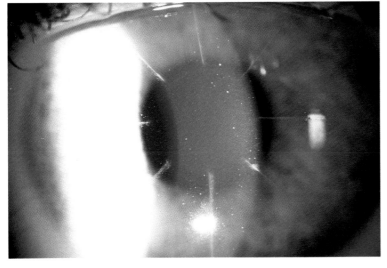

FIG. 7.23

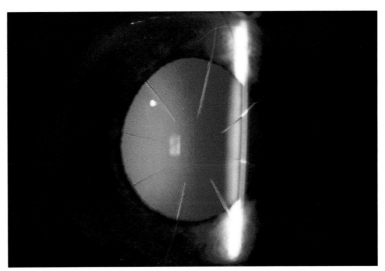

FIG. 7.24

ASTIGMATIC KERATOTOMY

Astigmatic keratotomy (AK) (Fig. 7.25) can be used to correct regular, but not irregular, corneal astigmatism. The coupling effect often determines the length of the transverse component of the AK so that hyperopia and myopia may be minimized while correcting the astigmatism. After AK, the *spherical component* becomes more *myopic* and the *spherical equivalent* becomes more *hyperopic* (see Fig. 7.7).

AK is performed on the steeper keratometric meridian, but the power of the AK is based on the refractive astigmatism. Postoperatively, keratometry usually does *not* correspond exactly to the refractive astigmatic power. The transverse incisions (T-cuts) of a simple AK are performed at the 7.0-mm optical zone (Fig. 7.26). If the same optical zone and achieved depth are used for all single AKs, the effect will be directly proportional to the length of the transverse incisions (not Ruiz procedures), thereby increasing the consistency of performance. Also, a 7.0-mm optical zone ensures no glare from the T-cuts when the pupil dilates. A Ruiz procedure is used to correct astigmatism greater than 4.00 D (Figs. 7.27 and 7.28). Unlike RK, age, intraocular pressure, and gender have no significant effect on AK calculations. However, previous RK, AK, PKP, or cataract surgery cause overcorrection if routine calculations for AK are used. The surgeon is wise to aim for 60% of the astigmatic error in these cases.

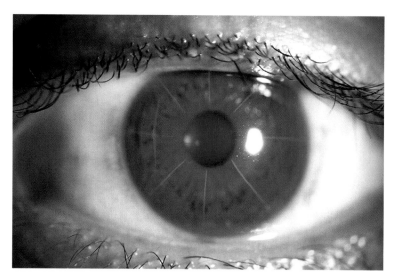

FIG. 7.25

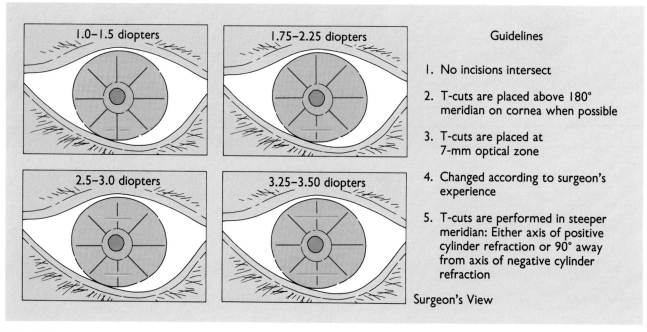

| 1.0–1.5 diopters | 1.75–2.25 diopters | Guidelines |
| 2.5–3.0 diopters | 3.25–3.50 diopters | |

Guidelines

1. No incisions intersect

2. T-cuts are placed above 180° meridian on cornea when possible

3. T-cuts are placed at 7-mm optical zone

4. Changed according to surgeon's experience

5. T-cuts are performed in steeper meridian: Either axis of positive cylinder refraction or 90° away from axis of negative cylinder refraction

Surgeon's View

FIG. 7.26

RUIZ TECHNIQUE—CORRECTION OF ASTIGMATISM

LENGTH OF STEP-LADDER INCISIONS	DIOPTERS OF ASTIGMATISM					
	3	4	5	6	7	8
(Small) 2.5 mm	4.75 (−0.5)	4.25 (−0.7)	3.75 (−0.9)	3.50 (−1.0)	3.50 (−1.2)	3.50 (−1.3)
(Large) 4.5mm	5.00 (−0.8)	4.50 (−1.00)	4.00 (−1.3)	3.75 (−1.5)	3.50 (−1.8)	3.50 (−2.00)

INSTRUCTIONS

1. Refraction is given in negative cylinder format.
2. Column is found for diopters of astigmatism correction desired.
3. Either the middle or lower box of column is chosen, depending upon amount of induced myopia desired (number in parentheses).
4. The number above the parentheses is the proper optical zone.
5. The box to the extreme left of the chosen row is the length of the stepladder incision.
6. Surgeon's own factor for patient age, etc., must be taken into account.
7. If the spherical component is less than or equal to 0, then 1.5-mm stepladder incisions are used. This is combined with radial keratotomy if desired.
8. Technique is adjusted according to surgeon's experience.
9. This chart assumes 85% depth for all incisions.

REMINDER

Ruiz technique performed at steeper meridian equals axis of plus cylinder refraction, or 90° away from negative cylinder refraction.

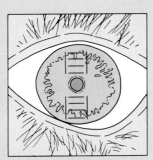

Ruiz at 90°

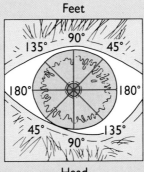

Feet

Head
Surgeon's view

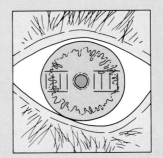

Ruiz at 180°

FIG. 7.27

Several modifications of trapezoidal keratotomy for correction of astigmatism (Ruiz procedure)

FIG. 7.28

Fyodorov originally proposed using parallel radial incisions and an oval optical zone to correct astigmatism. These techniques have been abandoned, largely due to a lack of consistency (Fig. 7.29). An effective AK incorporates a transverse incision that allows for quantifiable central flattening of the involved meridian. In order to minimize scarring, glare, and irregular astigmatism, no crossing of the transverse and radial incisions of the AK is done.

The surgical technique of AK is similar to RK with several important points emphasized. A front-cutting blade allows for better visibility. The desired achieved depth is 85% to 90% of the corneal thickness. The procedure is performed on the steeper meridian of the cornea, which is the same as the positive cylinder axis. It is very advantageous to mark the appropriate meridian on the cornea before globe fixation so that inadvertent torsion does not occur. Postoperative care for AK is similar to RK except that patching is often necessary for a day or two longer than with RK due to gaping of the transverse incisions.

KERATOMILEUSIS

Keratomileusis (KM) was first performed by Barraquer in 1964. Myopia of up to approximately −15.00 D can be corrected by myopic keratomileusis (MKM) and hyperopia of up to about +12.00 D can be corrected by hyperopic keratomileusis (HKM) (Fig. 7.30). Age, intraocular pressure, and gender are not predictive factors in KM. A 6.0-mm optical zone provides the best combination of maximum power capability with minimum glare. The rate of irregular astigmatism following MKM is 6% to 12%; it is lower for HKM. Radial keratotomy and AK may be performed 6 months after KM to improve the original KM result.

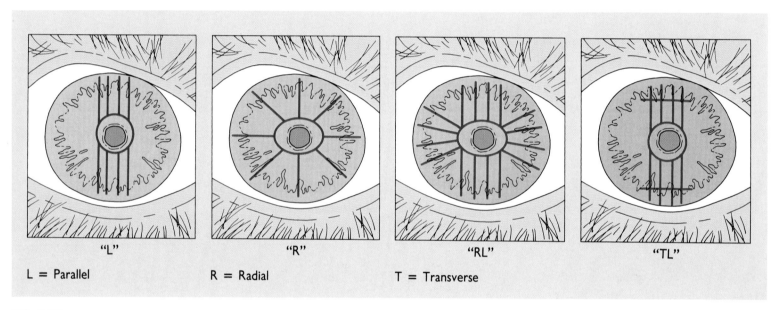

"L"   "R"   "RL"   "TL"

L = Parallel   R = Radial   T = Transverse

FIG. 7.29

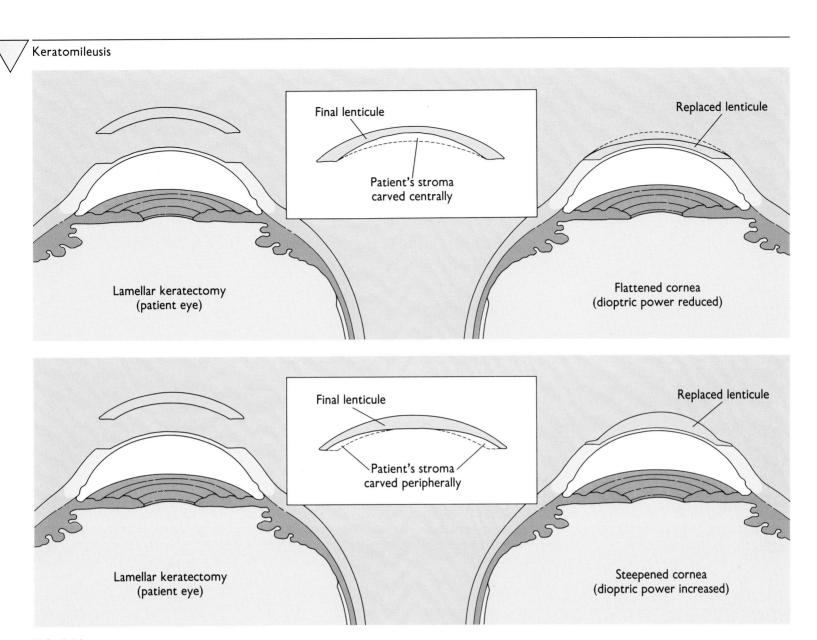

FIG. 7.30

Shaping the patient's corneal disk into a lenticule during KM may be achieved by use of the Steinway Barraquer cryolathe (Figs. 7.31 and 7.32) or the nonfreeze BKS-1000 (Fig. 7.33). The cryolathe freezes the corneal tissue and produces an exact optical zone dimension; The BKS-1000 does not allow for a consistent optical zone. Currently, the Steinway Barraquer cryolathe is the standard of excellence in creating accurate results.

The basic steps of KM are as follows. *Retrobulbar anes-* *thesia*, in a 4-to-5-cc dose, is given to increase exposure. *Keratectomy* is performed next, using the microkeratome and suction ring (Fig. 7.34). After suction is established (Fig. 7.35), the intraocular pressure (Fig. 7.36) and expected diameter of the patient's corneal disk (Fig. 7.37) are confirmed, prior to the actual keratectomy (Figs. 7.38 and 7.39). This is the most difficult aspect of KM. A refractive cut, with or without freezing, is made (Fig. 7.40). Anti-torque sutures are used to reposition the lenticule on the

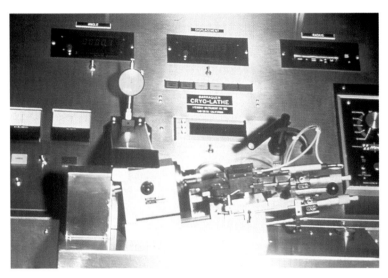

FIG. 7.31

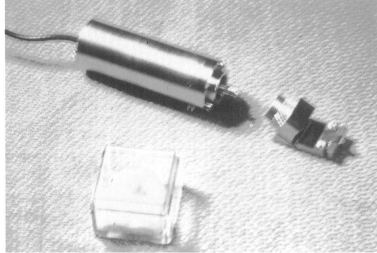

FIG. 7.32

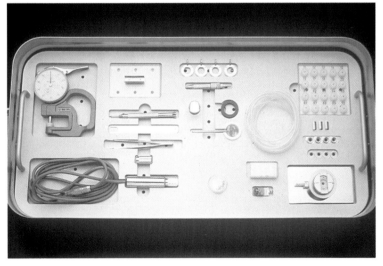

FIG. 7.33

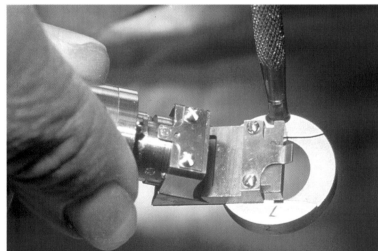

FIG. 7.34

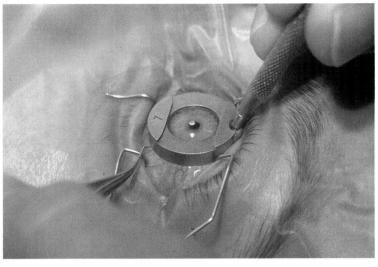

FIG. 7.35

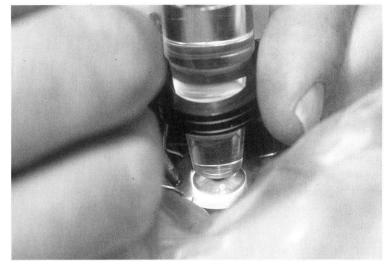

FIG. 7.36

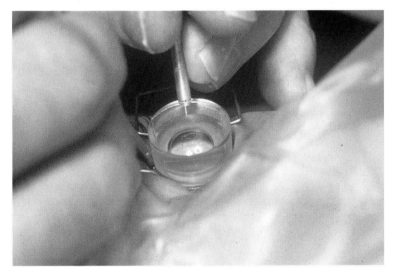

FIG. 7.37

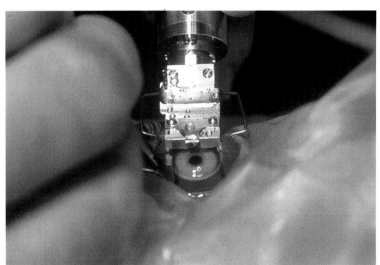

FIG. 7.38

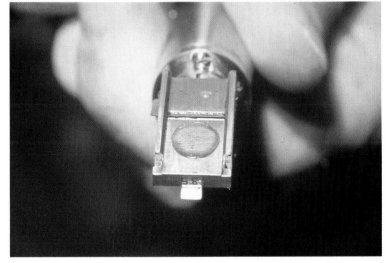

FIG. 7.39

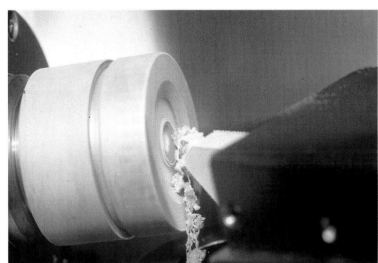

FIG. 7.40

recipient cornea (Figs. 7.41 to 7.45). The postoperative course requires a patch for two to three days and a steroid/antibiotic drop for 2 weeks. Suture removal takes place 2 to 3 weeks postoperatively.

EPIKERATOPHAKIA

Epikeratophakia (EPI) (Kaufman, Werblin) is used to correct myopia and hyperopia (Fig. 7.46). It is a modification of KM using a donor cornea, obviating the need for a keratectomy of the patient's cornea. Myopic epikeratophakia (M-EPI) can correct myopia of up to approximately −18.00 D, but the incidence of irregular astigmatism is significantly higher than that of KM and the quality of vision is often decreased. Hyperopic epikeratophakia (H-EPI) may be used for hyperopia of +3.00 D to +16.00 D and is equivalent to HKM in accuracy and incidence of irregular astigmatism. The quality of vision decreases in H-EPI as the central corneal thickness increases and the optical zone decreases.

Epikeratophakia may also be used to correct keratoconus (Fig. 7.47). Benefits include low surgical risk, improved uncorrected acuity, improved contact lens tolerance, and improved spectacle-corrected acuity. The procedure should be considered for central corneal thickness of approximately 0.3 mm or greater and minimal central scarring. Of course, a PKP may be performed if the EPI proves inadequate for any reason.

Shaping of the lenticule during EPI may be done by either the Kaufman-McDonald (KME) or Nordan (NET)

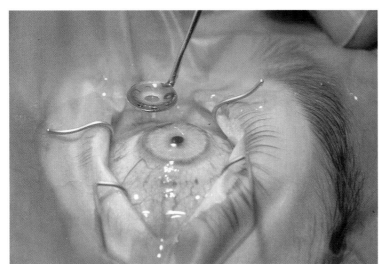

FIG. 7.41

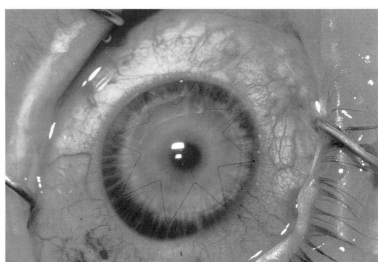

FIG. 7.42

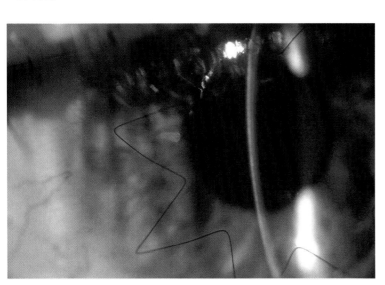

FIG. 7.43

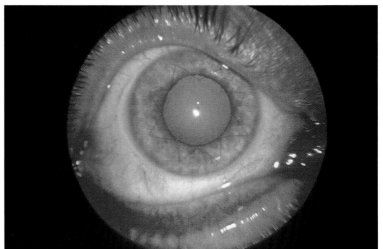

FIG. 7.44

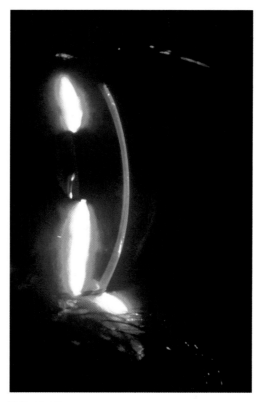

FIG. 7.45

Epikeratophakia

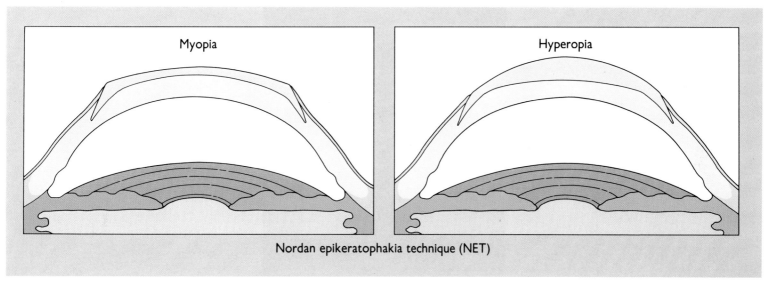

Myopia

Hyperopia

Nordan epikeratophakia technique (NET)

FIG. 7.46

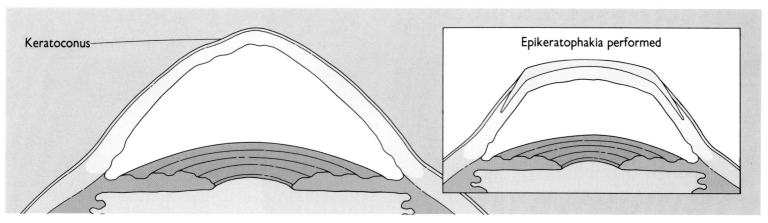

Keratoconus

Epikeratophakia performed

FIG. 7.47

techniques (Figs. 7.48 and 7.49). Lenticule power is based on the refractive error at the corneal plane for M-EPI and H-EPI. In KME, a planar donor is used for keratoconus; NET uses a donor power equal to two-thirds of the preoperative spherical equivalent in an attempt to optimize uncorrected visual acuity. Classic KME uses a keratotomy and keratectomy to allow for EPI fixation to the recipient cornea. NET requires only an oblique keratotomy, without removal of any recipient corneal tissue (Fig. 7.50). Future methods may reduce the need for suturing by other fixation methods such as glue or spot-welding laser techniques.

Surgery begins with administration of general or local anesthesia. The epithelium is removed by mechanical debridement rather than with chemicals in order to promote faster reepithelialization and avoid stromal haze. Centration of the miotic pupil (the visual axis indicator) is extremely important. Keratotomy is performed using the Baron trephine and/or hand dissection (Fig. 7.51). The keratectomy of the KME technique is performed with Vannas scissors (Figs. 7.52 to 7.55). Suturing is done with 10-0 nylon, using either combined sutures—eight interrupted and eight bite antitorque sutures—or 16 interrupted

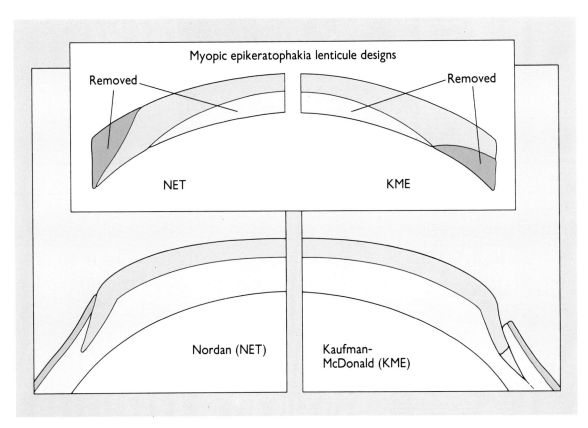

FIG. 7.48

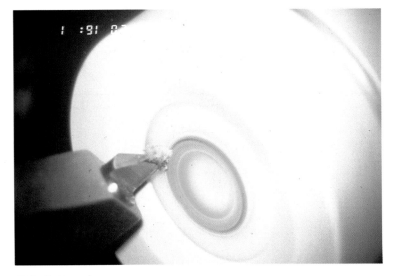

FIG. 7.49

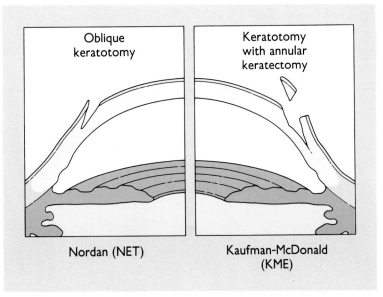

FIG. 7.50

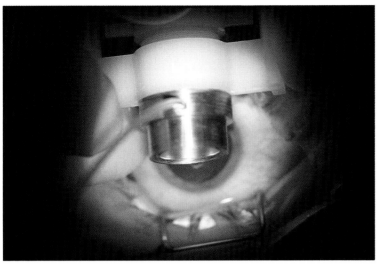

FIG. 7.51

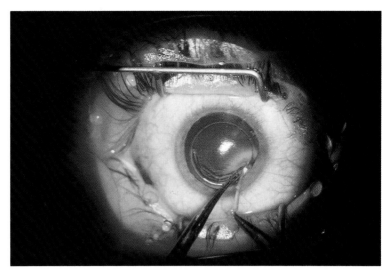

FIG. 7.52

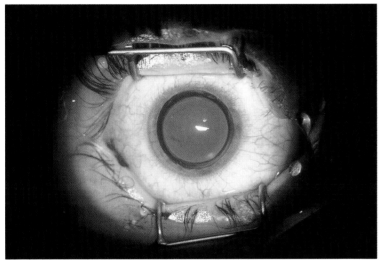

FIG. 7.53

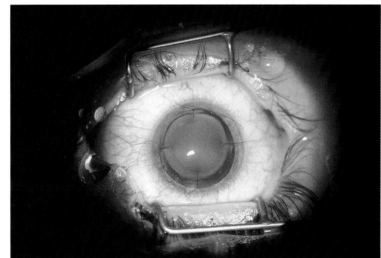

FIG. 7.54

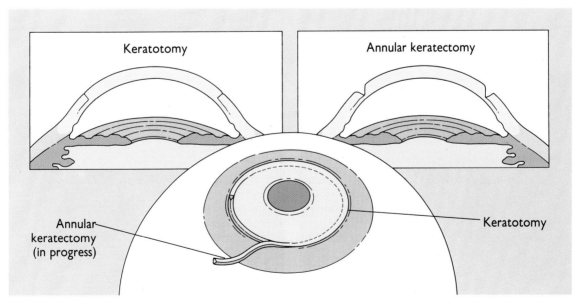

FIG. 7.55

sutures. Postoperative care includes patching, usually for three to four days, until the eye is fully epithelialized. The interrupted sutures are then removed to control astigmatism. A soft bandage contact lens is used only if necessary. Steroid and antibiotic drops are administered for 2 weeks. If nonepithelialization or scarring occurs after 2 weeks, the EPI is removed and the procedure repeated if desired. The running suture should remain in place for 2 to 8 weeks in hyperopes, and 3 to 4 months in myopes and keratoconus patients (Figs. 7.56 to 7.58). Figure 7.59 shows a pathologic example of human EPI.

INTRAOCULAR LENS IMPLANTATION

Intraocular lens (IOL) implantation for the correction of refractive error presents great potential risks and benefits to the patient. Risks of IOL surgery include those associated with intraocular surgery, such as infection, retinal detachment (early and late), and iritis with cystoid macular edema (CME). A phakic anterior chamber IOL may promote cataract formation. Intraocular lens implantation creates an absolute presbyopia that is poorly tolerated by younger patients. However, IOL implantation undoubtedly provides the most accurate correction of high ametropia. The accuracy of IOL power determination decreases as the axial length becomes very long or short. Use of ultrasound axial length-measuring devices that would assure proper visual axis orientation is desirable.

Our philosophy concerning IOL implantation for the correction of refractive error attempts to balance the aforementioned risk/benefit ratio. Clear lens extraction with posterior chamber (PC) IOL in-the-bag implantation is useful in selected cases of older severe ametropes. Routine clear lens extraction with PC IOL implantation in high myopes and prepresbyopes is *not* advocated due to the risk factors discussed. The incidence of complications related to cataract extraction and PC IOL implantation has been estimated at 5% if one considers improper IOL power, CME, retinal detachment, infection, iritis, and corneal decompensation. This incidence of complication is too high to advocate routine IOL–clear lens extraction.

LESS COMMON AND THEORETICAL PROCEDURES

KERATOPHAKIA

Keratophakia (KF) (Barraquer) (Fig. 7.60) requires a keratectomy so that a convex donor lenticule of stroma may be inserted into the recipient cornea to create a steepening of the anterior curvature, thereby correcting severe hyperopia. A corneal pocket dissection is not satisfactory, since in this instance the donor causes a backward bowing of the posterior corneal layers without significantly affecting the anterior curvature of the cornea. The double stromal interface of keratophakia is often deleterious to visual acuity and 6 to 12 months are necessary to achieve the best corrected acuity. Keratophakia is rarely used these days considering the success of IOLs.

Alloplastic Keratophakia

In alloplastic keratophakia (McCarey), a donor material such as hydrogel (a soft contact lens material) (Figs. 7.61 and 7.62) is used in a manner analogous to the stromal donor of keratophakia. The ability to correct myopia by this method is currently unknown and the difficult step of keratectomy is still necessary.

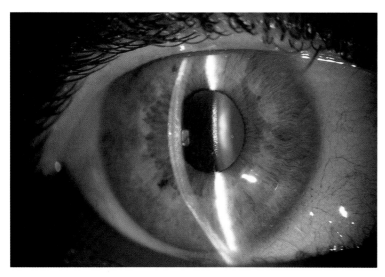

FIG. 7.56

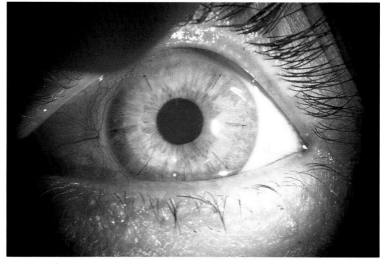

FIG. 7.57

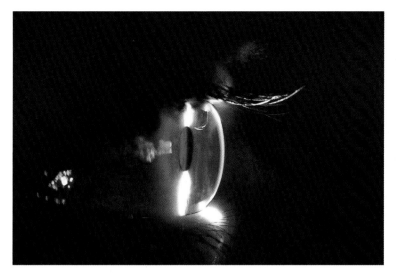

FIG. 7.58

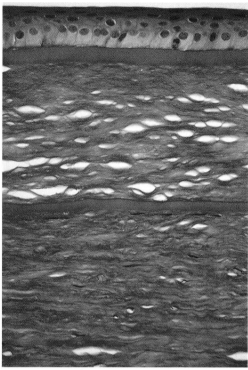

FIG. 7.59

Keratophakia

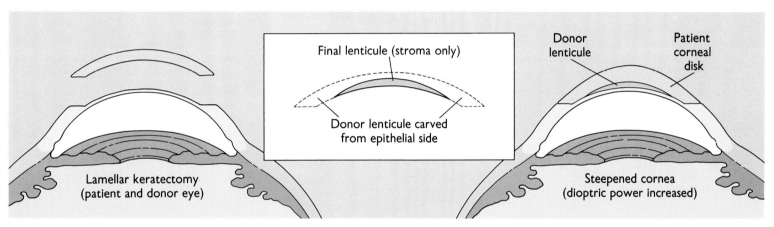

Lamellar keratectomy
(patient and donor eye)

Final lenticule (stroma only)

Donor lenticule carved
from epithelial side

Donor
lenticule

Patient
corneal
disk

Steepened cornea
(dioptric power increased)

FIG. 7.60

Alloplastic Keratophakia

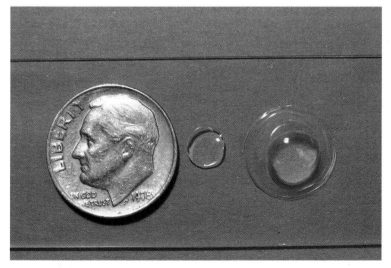

FIG. 7.61

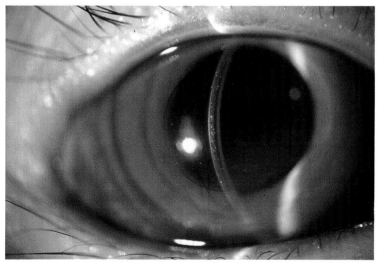

FIG. 7.62

INTRACORNEAL LENS PLACEMENT

Placement of an intracorneal lens (ICL) (Choyce) with a high index of refraction can correct hyperopia and myopia. A corneal pocket dissection may be used rather than a keratectomy. Nutrition of the anterior cornea and lens erosion through the stroma with time are major long-term concerns. The current material of the ICL, polysulphone (Fig. 7.63), has an index of refraction of 1.633, is impenetrable to water and nutrients, and is rather rigid. Current technique calls for deep implantation of the ICL near Descemet's membrane (Figs. 7.64 and 7.65).

WEDGE RESECTION

Wedge resection (Troutman, Barraquer) (Fig. 7.66) is performed on the flatter meridian of the cornea in an attempt to cause steepening. This surgery is not as accurate as AK on the steeper meridian since initial overcorrection must be achieved and stability wanes with suture biodegration or removal.

HEXAGONAL KERATOTOMY

A hexagonal keratotomy (Mendez) may correct +1.00 to +3.00 D of hyperopia (Fig. 7.67). The effect increases as the diameter of the hexagon decreases. The hexagonal incisions must be joined together to get the desired effect, but the potential instability of the isolated central cornea is of concern (Figs. 7.68 and 7.69).

DEEP LAMELLAR KERATECTOMY

Deep lamellar keratectomy (Ruiz) may be performed with a microkeratome to correct low levels of hyperopia. The

▽ Intracorneal Lens Placement

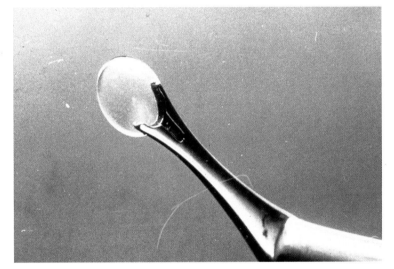

FIG. 7.63

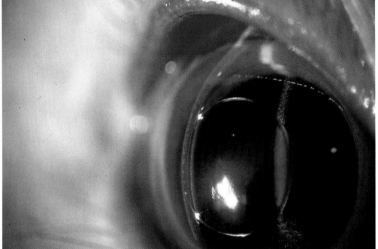

FIG. 7.64

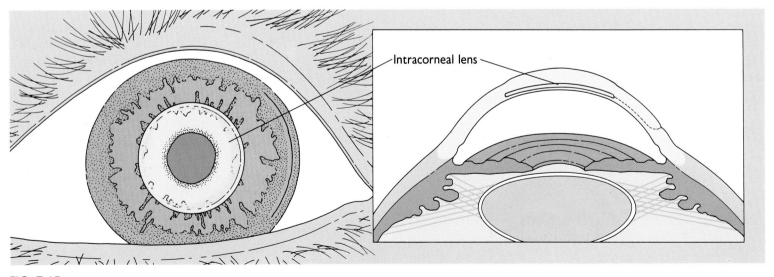

Intracorneal lens

FIG. 7.65

Wedge Resection

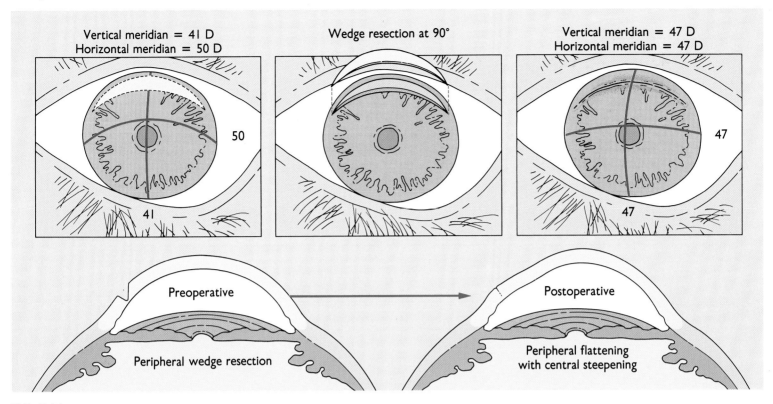

Vertical meridian = 41 D
Horizontal meridian = 50 D

50

41

Wedge resection at 90°

Vertical meridian = 47 D
Horizontal meridian = 47 D

47

47

Preoperative

Peripheral wedge resection

Postoperative

Peripheral flattening with central steepening

FIG. 7.66

Hexagonal Keratotomy

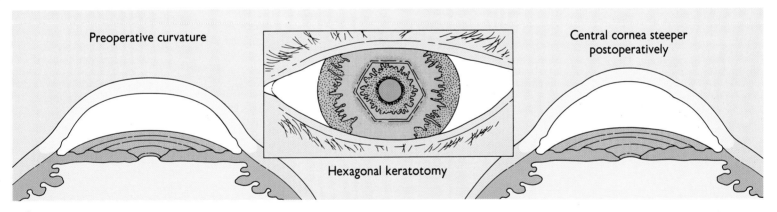

Preoperative curvature

Hexagonal keratotomy

Central cornea steeper postoperatively

FIG. 7.67

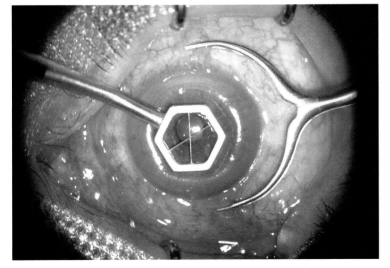

FIG. 7.68

FIG. 7.69

central cornea steepens due to "controlled ectasia," but the precision of this approach is questionable (Fig. 7.70).

LASER CORNEAL REFRACTIVE SURGERY

Theoretically, lasers may be employed to create the radial and transverse incisions of RK, AK, and hexagonal keratotomy, to reshape the anterior surface of the cornea, and to produce intrastromal ablation of tissue. The Excimer (ultraviolet) laser cuts the corneal surface by repeated removal of surface tissue (Fig. 7.71). The Automated Laser System (ALS) uses yellow-orange light (523 nm) and functions by ablating tissue in a 6-to-20-μm area and making these small plasma fields of destruction confluent both vertically and laterally.

Excimer laser research has produced RK, but clinical delivery to a patient is difficult. Anterior corneal reshaping by this laser destroys Bowman's membrane, thus creating potential reepithelialization and subepithelial haze problems (Fig. 7.72). In myopia, enough tissue must be removed to avoid glare from the transition zone between tissue that has and has not been removed.

The visual light of the ALS system can be delivered to the cornea through a clear fixation contact lens (Fig. 7.73) and

Deep Lamellar Keratectomy

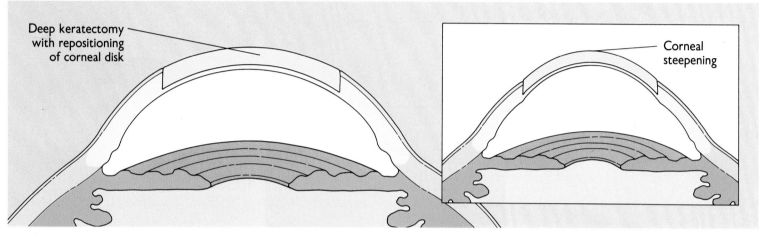

Deep keratectomy with repositioning of corneal disk

Corneal steepening

FIG. 7.70

Laser Corneal Refractive Surgery

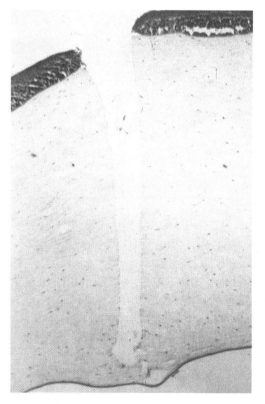

FIG. 7.71

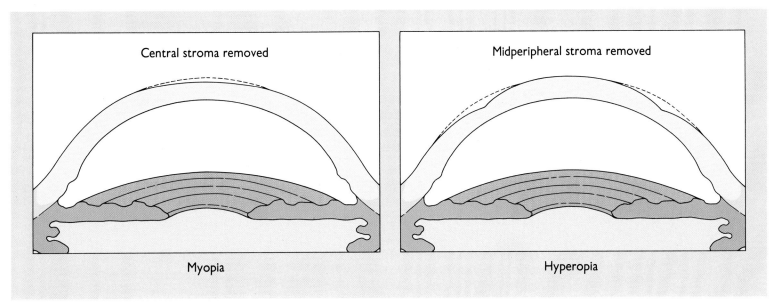

FIG. 7.72

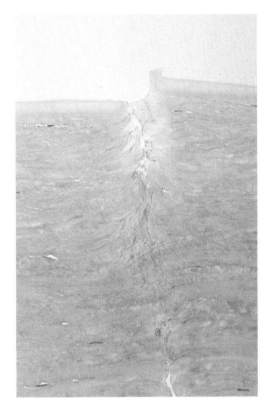

FIG. 7.73

has the potential to keep epithelium intact during RK or AK. This would eliminate pain and infection during the procedure. The precise nature of the ALS technology theoretically would allow for intrastromal ablation of stromal tissue to correct for myopia, hyperopia, and astigmatism (Fig. 7.74), but the clinical aspects of such a procedure have yet to be mastered.

Laser corneal refractive surgery would allow for increased consistency and decreased complications. The laser could be computer driven to improve upon the surgeon's hand (Fig. 7.75).

CONCLUSION

Undoubtedly, high technology will play an ever-expanding role in refractive surgery and allow for improved consistency and reduced complications. Hopefully the day soon will come when all of civilization is capable of excellent unaided visual function; then the dreams of the great refractive surgery pioneers and their patients will have been fulfilled.

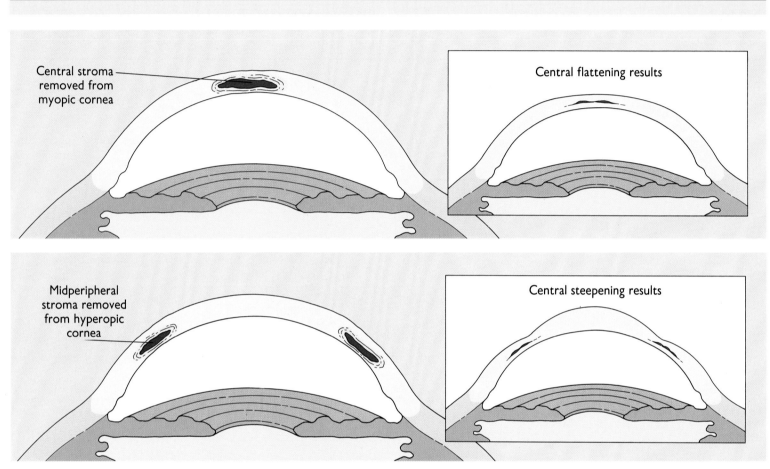

FIG. 7.74

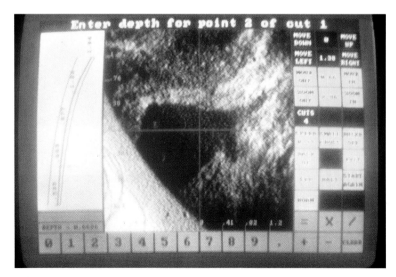

FIG. 7.75

Picture credits for this chapter are as follows: Figs. 7.13 and 7.14 courtesy of CooperVision Cilco; Fig. 7.15 courtesy of Metico, Inc.; Figs. 7.61 and 7.71 courtesy of Allergan Medical Optics; Fig. 7.62 courtesy of Bernard McCarey, PhD, Emory University School of Medicine, Atlanta, Georgia; Fig. 7.65 C courtesy of Surgidev Corp.; Figs. 7.68 and 7.69 courtesy of Antonio Mendez, MD; Fig. 7.73 courtesy of Automated Laser Systems, Inc. (Slide preparation and photomicrography provided by Harry Brown, MD—Ophthalmic Pathology Laboratory, Jules Stein Eye Institute, UCLA).

LASER SURGERY OF CHORIORETINAL DISEASES

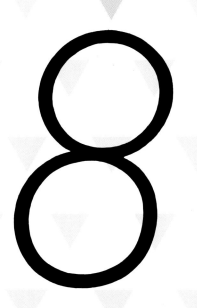

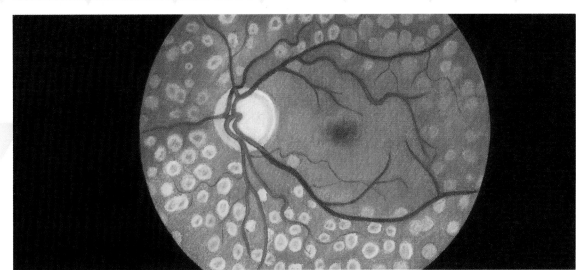

Peter H. Judson, M D

Lawrence A. Yannuzzi, M D

Several chorioretinal diseases are amenable to laser photocoagulation treatment. They may be conveniently divided into two groups: retinal diseases and retinal pigment epithelial–choroidal diseases. Diseases within each group are listed in Fig. 8.1. Clinical and fluorescein angiographic features, along with the indications for laser photocoagulation treatment, will be described for each of these entities. Where appropriate, laser technique guidelines, complications, and postoperative management are included.

RETINAL DISEASES

DIABETES MELLITUS

More retinal laser procedures are performed for patients with diabetic retinopathy than for any other patient group. This disease is the leading cause of blindness in persons 25–74 years of age. There are over 10 million Americans with diabetes, and the prevalence and severity of retinopathy (and consequent need for laser intervention) are strongly related to the duration of the disease and patient age.

For example, younger-onset insulin-dependent diabetics (under age 30) with less than 2 years of disease have only a 2% incidence of retinopathy. They rarely have proliferative diabetic retinopathy (PDR) or clinically significant macular edema. However, diabetics who have had their disease for at least 15 years have a 98% chance of retinopathy. Most significantly, 26% progress to PDR and at least 15% have macular edema. Laser treatment may be considered for this group of diabetics as they begin to show clinical signs of retinopathy as well as for older-onset diabetics who do or do not require insulin.

It should be remembered that older-onset diabetics often develop retinopathy more rapidly than younger-onset diabetics (at least 20% by 2 years). Older insulin-requiring diabetics develop PDR and macular edema with a greater frequency than those who are controlled by diet or hypoglycemic medication.

Laser photocoagulation is most effective when it is considered in these groups of patients to ameliorate macular edema or to prevent the progression of fibrovascular proliferation and associated vision-threatening vitreous hemorrhage and retinal detachment.

Macular Edema

The single greatest cause of visual impairment in diabetics is macular edema. As the severity of the overall retinopathy increases, the proportion of eyes with macular edema also increases: 3% of eyes with mild nonproliferative diabetic retinopathy (NPDR), 38% with moderate-to-severe NPDR (equivalent to preproliferative retinopathy) and 71% with PDR.

There are now several randomized clinical photocoagulation trials for diabetic macular edema that have concluded that laser treatment tends to stabilize vision in most eyes and, less often, to improve it. The largest of these trials, the Early Treatment Diabetic Retinopathy Study (ETDRS) Research Group, showed that at 3 years' follow-up, 50% more untreated than treated eyes with "clinically significant macular edema" had vision loss of 3 or more lines on the ETDRS chart.

Laser treatment may be effective by closing off leaking microaneurysms [reestablishing the inner blood–retinal barrier (BRB)] or by debriding the retinal pigment epithelium (RPE) (reestablishing the outer BRB). Figure 8.2 shows a patient with extensive exudative maculopathy with serous edema surrounded by heavy lipid deposition. Note in Fig. 8.3 the same patient following focal laser treatment. Laser photocoagulation burns were directed at leaking microaneurysms under fluorescein guidance. There has been complete resolution of the serous and lipid exudation.

According to Bresnick, it is important clinically and prognostically to subdivide diabetic macular edema into four categories, some of which overlap: focal macular edema, diffuse macular edema, macular edema associated with significant ischemia, and macular edema following panretinal photocoagulation (PRP).

Focal Macular Edema Venous–capillary microaneurysms are the site of focal inner BRB breakdown. Serum leaks from these partly incompetent vessels and the water content is later incompletely reabsorbed, leaving lipid-rich material (exudates) in the extracellular spaces of the retina (outer plexiform layer). Circinate rings of hard lipid exudates and retinal edema surround clusters of leaking microaneurysms, which can usually be seen clinically and by fluorescein angiography. Intraretinal microvascular

CHORIORETINAL DISEASES AMENABLE
TO LASER PHOTOCOAGULATION TREATMENT

RETINAL DISEASES	RETINAL PIGMENT EPITHELIAL-CHOROIDAL DISEASES

Diabetic retinopathy
  Nonproliferative
  Proliferative
Vein occlusions
  Central
  Branch
Peripheral vascular occlusive disease
  Sickle cell retinopathy
  Eales' disease (idiopathic)
Arteriolar macroaneurysms
Retinal telangiectasia
Angiomatosis retinae
Retinal breaks and detachments
	Age-related macular degeneration
	Retinal pigment epithelial detachments
	Other diseases associated with
	subretinal neovascularization
	  Presumed ocular histoplasmosis syndrome
	  Idiopathic
	  Angioid streaks
	  Pathologic myopia
	  Others
	Central serous chorioretinopathy
	Miscellaneous
	  Tumors
	  Subretinal parasites
	  Inflammations

FIG. 8.1

Diabetes Mellitus: Macular Edema

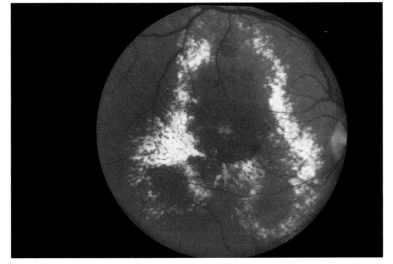

FIG. 8.2

FIG. 8.3

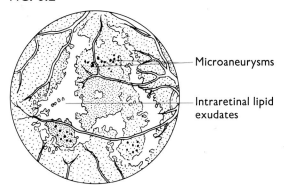

— Microaneurysms

— Intraretinal lipid exudates

abnormalities (IRMA) also may be responsible for focal leakage. In Fig. 8.4, note the circinate ring of lipid exudation surrounding leaking telangiectatic and aneurysmal changes. There is also some patchy hemorrhage. The exudation is confluent at the fovea. The same patient is seen following laser treatment in Fig. 8.5. Very few laser burns were needed in the treatment of this patient. Direct photocoagulation of aneurysms under fluorescein guidance eliminated the edema.

Contact lens biomicroscopy is essential prior to laser treatment to confirm that the patient has macular edema that is amenable to focal laser treatment. Fluorescein angiograms from the arteriovenous and late phases should be compared to determine which areas leak.

Published studies have reported using xenon arc and argon blue-green lasers, but most retinal specialists now advocate the use of argon green lasers for treatment within the xanthophyll-containing macular tissue. Others have suggested the use of yellow light (dye laser) because of its higher percentage of hemoglobin absorption and its transmission by xanthophyll pigment. Most microaneurysms are 25–100 μm in size; thus precisely focused 50–200-μm spot sizes are used. Burns of moderate intensity (to cause a grayish-white retinal color change) lasting 0.05–0.2 s are advocated. Preoperative confirmation of foveal fixation, preferably with a different color aiming beam, is important. The microaneurysm is obliterated in a "target" fashion with as little energy as possible. Dot hemorrhages that do not leak angiographically are not treated. Treatment of lesions further than 3,000 μm from and closer than 500 μm to the center of the foveal avascular zone (FAZ) is optional. Care must be taken not to treat confluently in areas of perifoveal capillary net dropout and in the papillomacular bundle.

The patient should be advised that visual acuity often declines in the immediate postoperative phase. While improvement of vision is the ideal goal, it is more realistic to advise patients that, at best, visual stabilization can be achieved. Patients should also be counseled regarding the realistic possibility of insidious and permanent loss of vision from progressive exudative maculopathy if not treated.

Diffuse Macular Edema In diffuse edema, the inner BRB is diffusely involved, with widespread dilation of the capillary bed and widened intercapillary spaces on fluorescein angiography. Hard exudates are less frequent since the generalized defect in the BRB is insufficient to allow larger lipoprotein molecules to pass into the extravascular space. Diffuse edema may also be the result of decompensating telangiectatic capillaries rather than multifocal aneurysms, which tend to be associated with lipid deposition. Renal failure with fluid retention and hypertension are often associated with this condition, and correction of these systemic abnormalities often ameliorates the edema. Cystoid macular edema (CME) with foveal cyst formation and macular ischemia has a particularly poor visual prognosis.

Since few if any focal microaneurysmal leaks are seen on fluorescein angiography, grid photocoagulation is advocated. Mild to moderate laser burns 100–200 μm in size of 0.05–0.2 s duration are placed throughout the macula in areas of retinal thickening and/or capillary nonperfusion surrounding the perifoveal capillary network. Burns are placed at least one burn width apart. In the patient in Fig. 8.6, note the distribution of laser photocoagulation burns surrounding the central macula but sparing the perifoveal area. There is still perifoveal edema where treatment was not carried out. The same patient is shown in Fig. 8.7 following placement of additional burns in the perifoveal area. There has been complete elimination of the perifoveal edema.

Burns should not be placed closer than 500 μm to the center of the FAZ or the optic nerve. If focal microaneurysms are additively treated, this is termed a "modified grid." Using a modified grid with argon blue-green laser photocoagulation, Olk found, at 1- and 2-year's follow-up, a significant number of patients whose vision improved at least 2 lines compared with untreated patients with and without CME. Similarly, the ETDRS Research Group noted a 50%–70% reduction in the decrease of visual acuity when using a combination of focal and grid photocoagulation.

The mechanism of grid treatment is largely unknown. Debridement of the RPE may remove some abnormal cells and stimulate others to reabsorb retinal fluid via a competent outer BRB or reduce the metabolic needs of the outer retina by destroying a number of photoreceptor cells. This would allow more oxygen to reach the ischemic inner retina. Alternatively, a type of endothelial cell repair process in the retinal vessels may help to restore the inner BRB.

Macular Edema Associated With Ischemia Good-quality fluorescein angiography is necessary to fully evaluate capillary nonperfusion and is important since macular isch-

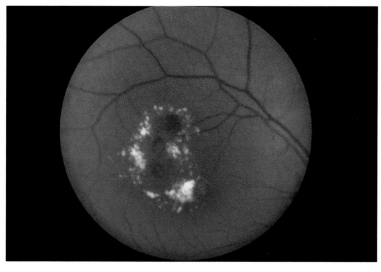

FIG. 8.4

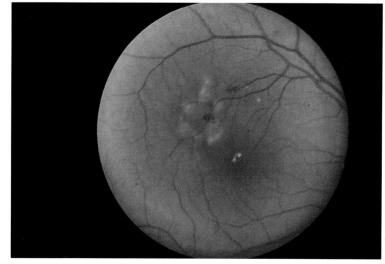

FIG. 8.5

Diabetes Mellitus: Diffuse Macular Edema

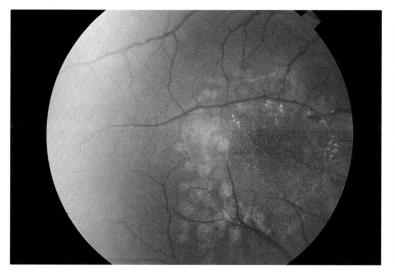

FIG. 8.6

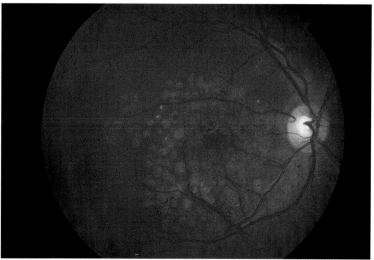

FIG. 8.7

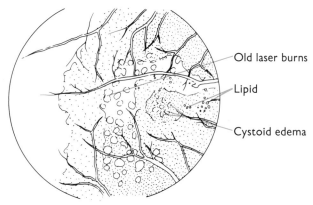

Old laser burns

Lipid

Cystoid edema

emia portends a poor visual prognosis with or without treatment. In Fig. 8.8, note the perifoveal nonperfusion and the temporal macular ischemia. There is also a patch of neovascularization in the superior macula. This condition is underdiagnosed and often overlooked. Enlargement of the FAZ (normally 250–600 μm in diameter) and especially notchlike areas of capillary and arterial closure of the FAZ seen on the fluorescein angiogram may be associated with cotton wool spots (soft exudates) and clinically evident retinal edema. FAZs over 1 mm in diameter are found almost exclusively in eyes with PDR.

Macular Edema Following Panretinal Photocoagulation

Many eyes that receive PRP for PDR develop macular edema for the first time or show a worsening of edema 6–10 weeks after treatment. This edema is usually of the diffuse variety, and may or may not persist. It has been the impression of many clinicians that macular edema is more common following single-treatment PRP. However, it has recently been found that no long-term difference in macular edema exists between eyes that were completely treated in one session compared with eyes given three or more treatments spaced at least 1 week apart.

PRP has been postulated to raise inner retinal oxygen levels by destroying photoreceptors. Autoregulated arteriolar vasoconstriction in the midperipheral retina might decrease blood flow there while increasing it to the macula. Incompetent dilated macular capillaries may then leak. Data from the Diabetic Retinopathy Study (DRS) show that eyes with macular edema prior to PRP are more likely to lose 2 lines of vision than eyes without macular edema by a 2:1 ratio. This is above and beyond the acceptable degree of expected vision loss from the photocoagulation itself. The DRS suggests that patients with macular edema have focal photocoagulation before PRP to minimize the chance of vision loss.

All patients about to undergo PRP should be reminded that the beneficial effects of laser treatment outweigh the negative early effects after 2 years. A treatment plan in which smaller amounts of laser are placed in and around the posterior pole during routine PRP has been suggested to decrease subsequent macular edema and vision loss.

Proliferative Diabetic Retinopathy

The now-classic DRS determined that scatter photocoagulation in eyes with "high-risk" characteristics (neovascularization of the disk (NVD) with vitreous hemorrhage, moderate-to-severe NVD [more than ¼ disk diameter (DD)], or neovascularization of the retina (NVE) with vitreous hemorrhage) produced a 60% overall reduction in the rate of severe visual loss compared with untreated eyes. Figure 8.9 shows disk neovascularization. The same patient following panretinal photocoagulation is seen in Fig. 8.10. Note the laser burns surrounding the posterior pole. There has been complete regression of the neovascularization.

The ETDRS Research Group is attempting to answer the question of whether patients with severe NPDR ought to undergo PRP if, as the DRS Research Group showed, 50% of such eyes progress to PDR in 1–2 years. Eyes with severe NPDR treated with PRP progress to PDR (as measured by onset of NVD) at a rate 30%–40% slower than untreated controls. At this time, it may be prudent to treat one eye with severe NPDR with PRP and to observe the fellow eye.

When a patient is suspected clinically of having PDR or severe NPDR, a fluorescein angiogram and color photographic sweep of the fundus ought to be done. If at least two high-risk characteristics exist, the patient should be considered for PRP. A frank discussion with the patient explaining that the aim of treatment is first to stabilize the retinopathy and protect vision (rather than improve it) is helpful. Patients must be informed that their central vision may decrease after PRP due to macular edema, as well as their peripheral vision and night vision. The DRS Research Group suggested that concomitant macular edema may indicate that focal laser treatment should be done first, but not if this will significantly delay completion of PRP.

It is not necessary for the experienced ophthalmologist to project the angiogram or color photographs unless macular treatment is planned. The treatment should be divided into at least three sessions since heavy doses of laser energy are usually associated with more postoperative pain, macular edema, and a higher rate of complications (e.g., ischemic papillitis, traction retinal detachment, angle closure, choroidal effusions).

The Rodenstock and Mainster panfunduscopic lenses (Figs. 8.11 and 8.12, respectively) are especially helpful in performing the posterior and midperipheral laser applications (Stages 1 and 2), and help to avoid skip areas in treatment. Stage 1 treatment includes placing a ring of burns around the macula to create a "border" to protect against inadvertent macular burns as the remainder of the PRP is performed. The superior optics and magnification of the Mainster lens are ideally suited for this stage.

The inferior retina should be treated initially if there is any history of vitreal hemorrhage, since this region will become obstructed in the event of future bleeding between

Diabetes Mellitus: Macular Edema Associated With Ischemia

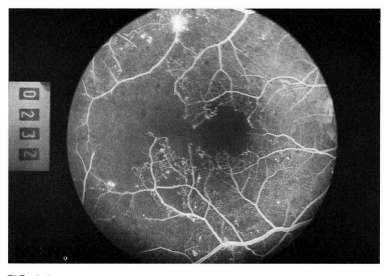

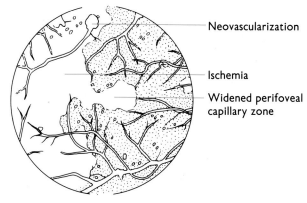

Neovascularization

Ischemia

Widened perifoveal capillary zone

FIG. 8.8

Diabetes Mellitus: Proliferative Diabetic Retinopathy

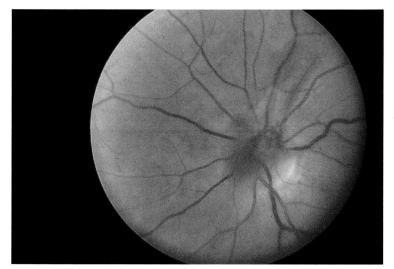

FIG. 8.9

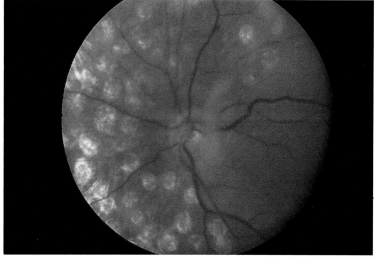

FIG. 8.10

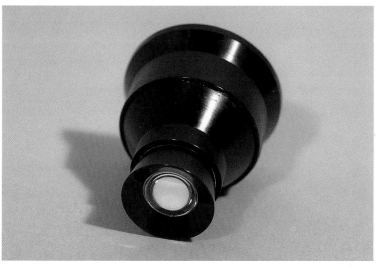

FIG. 8.11

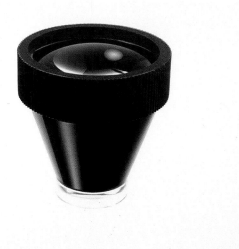

FIG. 8.12

sessions. Figure 8.13 shows the distribution of the laser burns following the first stage of treatment. Figure 8.14 shows the distribution of the burns following the secondary stage of PRP. The peripheral mirrors of the Goldmann lens may be used for the rest of the peripheral applications (Stage 3) (Fig. 8.15).

Usually, the patient's tolerance to pain decreases as the treatment becomes more peripheral, due to a higher concentration of ciliary nerves. In treating peripheral to the equator, it is best to leave the nasal and temporal regions (in the vicinity of the long posterior ciliary nerves) until last due to extreme sensitivity to laser burns. Most patients can be effectively treated without retrobulbar anesthesia, especially if their sessions are short and multiple. Also, some patients benefit from pretreatment analgesics or tranquilizers. Pain can sometimes be reduced by reducing the burn size duration and intensity appropriately. Nonetheless, retrobulbar anesthesia is effective for extremely sensitive or uncooperative patients, especially for treating the peripheral retina and juxtafoveal areas, though it is not without inherent risks. Three to four cubic centimeters of 2% xylocaine, with or without Wyedase, are injected via a sharp or blunt retrobulbar needle into the peribulbar or retrobulbar space, while the globe is constantly observed for movement. The patient is instructed to look straight ahead during the injection rather than up and in, a method commonly taught in the past. Immediately afterward, the patient should be observed for any change in breathing pattern or consciousness and appropriate CPR measures taken if necessary (rare).

Laser burns 200–500 μm in diameter (using the largest spot size that can be focused for most efficient coverage) of moderate intensity and of 0.1–0.5 s duration are placed in a scatter fashion in order to turn the retina and underlying RPE gray-white. Care should be taken to allow at least 3 DD (slightly less if macular ischemia occurs temporally) of temporal macula away from the fovea to remain untreated and to spare 500–1,000 μm around the optic nerve. All burns are placed one burn width apart. Neovascular disk tissue is not treated directly, but flat NVE away from the macula may be treated confluently (ETDRS protocol) with a 500-μm "safety zone." Adequate coverage, rather than the actual number of burns, is important. In some patients treated with large spot sizes, 1,200 burns may be sufficient. In patients with especially aggressive proliferative disease, 4,000 or more burns, applied in multiple sessions, may be needed.

The mechanism whereby PRP effectively causes regression of NVD and NVE is unknown. Figure 8.16 shows disk and peripapillary neovascularization. Figure 8.17 shows the same patient following ablation photocoagulation. Note the transformation of actively proliferating vessels into a fibrous scar. Sometimes there will be some residual perfusion of these regressed vessels. PRP probably destroys some hypoxic retinal tissue and/or photoreceptors to allow other tissues preferentially to obtain a better retinal blood flow and oxygenation and to decrease the production of a vasoproliferative factor.

Follow-up may be scheduled at monthly intervals once PRP has been completed, unless concomitant problems such as rubeotic glaucoma necessitate more frequent visits. It should be emphasized that successful PRP does not always result in total regression of neovascularization, especially NVD. Figure 8.18 shows fibrovascular proliferation along the course of the superior temporal arcade, exhibiting traction on the retina. The same patient following krypton laser ablation is seen in Fig. 8.19. There is marked regression of the neovascularization with minimal contraction of the surface of the retina and secondary fibrous proliferation.

Xenon arc and argon laser treatments were used in the DRS, but krypton red and dye yellow or red wavelengths may be equally effective; theoretical advantages exist in certain patients with different pigmentary patterns, degrees of vitreoretinal traction, or media opacities. The Krypton–Argon Regression of Neovascularization Study (KARNS) was designed to analyze this question.

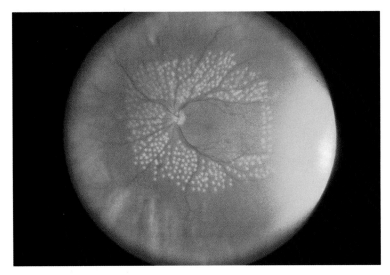

FIG. 8.13

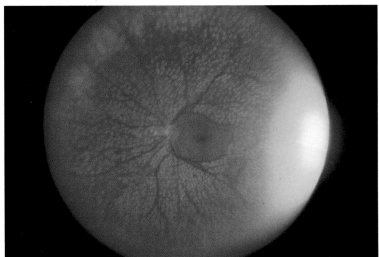

FIG. 8.14

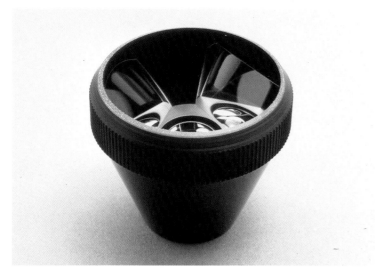

FIG. 8.15

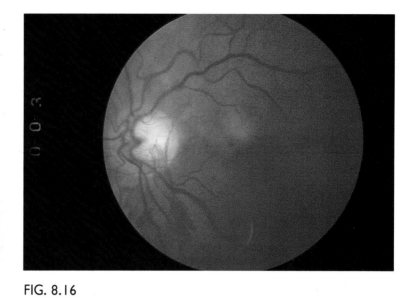

FIG. 8.16

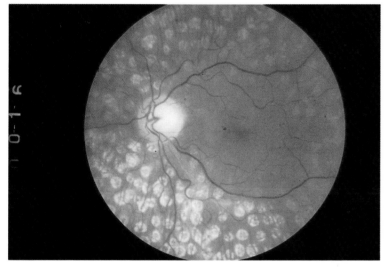

FIG. 8.17

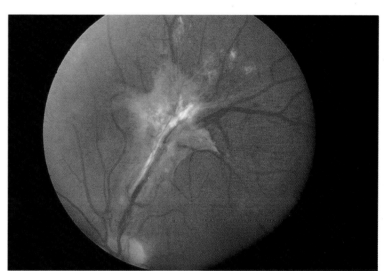

FIG. 8.18

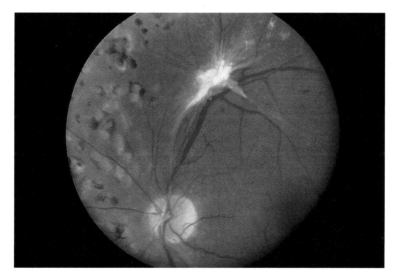

FIG. 8.19

VENOUS OCCLUSIVE DISEASE

Venous occlusive disease can be divided into *central* retinal vein occlusion (CRVO), including hemispheric vein occlusion, and *branch* retinal vein occlusion (BRVO). Associated risk factors for all venous occlusions include hypertension and cardiovascular disease; for CRVO exclusively, risk factors also include hyperviscosity states and glaucoma.

Central Retinal Vein Occlusion

Fifteen percent of all retinal venous occlusions involve the central vein. CRVO occurs when venous outflow is blocked by a thrombus at the level of the lamina cribrosa. It is important to differentiate ischemic from nonischemic cases. Approximately 20% of all patients with CRVO go on to develop neovascular glaucoma. However, close to 60% of ischemic CRVOs are associated with rubeosis, while less than 2% of nonischemic CRVOs develop this complication. Most, but not all, eyes with rubeosis will develop neovascular or hemorrhagic glaucoma. The visual prognosis is extremely poor for the ischemic group, with only 10% of eyes achieving vision better than 20/400.

Ischemia causes a severe chronic breakdown of the inner BRB with consequent diffuse retinal edema and hemorrhage due to vascular endothelial dysfunction. Few viable capillaries capable of proliferation remain in ischemic cases of CRVO; consequently, the risk of neovascularization of the retina (NVE) is low (less than 8%–10%). Vitreal hemorrhage, either from NVE or retinal vascular rupture, is rare. Grid photocoagulation for chronic macular edema from CRVO has been suggested but the value of such treatment is still unproven. The National Institutes of Health has funded a National Collaborative Trial to assess the efficacy and safety of this form of therapy. Studies are currently in progress comparing antiplatelet agents (aspirin, persantine) alone or in combination with lytic agents [tissue plasminogen activator (TPA)] and anticoagulants (heparin, coumadin) for partial and complete CRVOs.

At this time, the main management consideration for CRVO is PRP, which is extremely effective in eliminating the risk of neovascularization of the iris (NVI) or hemorrhagic glaucoma in ischemic CRVO (90% protective in one study). Since most cases of neovascular glaucoma occur within the first 3–5 months following the occlusion, and since advanced neovascular glaucoma does not respond well to treatment, PRP should be considered in all cases of ischemic CRVO and performed as expeditiously as possible. Argon, dye, or krypton laser treatment may be used as in PRP for PDR.

Although speculative, PRP seems to work by destroying ischemic retinal tissue responsible for production or liberation of "angiogenic" factors, by facilitating drainage of vasoproliferative factors into the choroidal circulation, and/or by enhancing choroidal oxygenation of hypoxic retinal tissue.

Branch Retinal Vein Occlusion

Branch retinal vein occlusions (BRVOs) are thought to occur when arteriovenous sclerotic changes within the common adventitial sheath cause venous constriction, turbulence of flow, endothelial cell damage, and thrombotic occlusion. Usually a secondary or tertiary branch of the central retinal vein is involved, and the superotemporal branch vein is implicated in over 65% of the cases. Management centers around laser treatment for macular edema and retinal or disk neovascularization, which are potential visually damaging sequelae of BRVO.

Macular Edema   Chronic macular edema is the most common complication impairing central vision, occurring in nearly 50% of patients with BRVO. The Branch Vein Occlusion Study Group showed that argon grid laser photocoagulation performed 3–18 months after the onset of occlusion is beneficial in the management of eyes with macular edema with a visual acuity of 20/40 or worse. Similar favorable results have been found in other studies.

It may be helpful to distinguish at least two types of macular edema in BRVO. The most common form of edema results from a "back-up pressure" in the involved macular capillaries. This edema appears early in the course of BRVO, and is characterized on fluorescein angiography by a typical cystoid pattern in the macular area drained by the occluded vein. The increased capillary pressure due to the venous stasis results in macular capillary decompensation or leakage. Late in the course of BRVO, other forms of edema may evolve from chronic leakage by venules. These vascular abnormalities combine with microaneurysms and decompensated macular capillaries to produce a markedly thickened retina and the accumulation of hard exudates.

Figure 8.20 shows a patient with BRVO with a circinate area of lipid deposition encircling clear serous fluid. Laser burns have been placed in a grid fashion within the distribution of the vein, preferentially at the site of leaking aneurysms noted on angiography. Figure 8.21 shows resolution of the serous and lipid exudation in the same patient several months later.

Argon or krypton laser treatment is placed in a "grid" over the region of the leaking retinal vessels but not in the foveal avascular zone or peripheral to the major vascular arcades. Collateralized and surviving vessels ought to be identified by fluorescein angiography and avoided during treatment.

In Fig. 8.22, note the retinal thickening, retinal vascular prominence and tortuosity, scattered hemorrhages, and perifoveal serous as well as trace lipid exudation associated with BRVO. Figure 8.23 is the fluorescein angiogram from the same patient showing chronic leakage in the distribution of the vein as well as in the perifoveal area. Figure 8.24 shows the same patient following laser photocoagulation treatment using krypton red near the perifoveal area and argon green more peripherally in the distribution of the BRVO. The same patient is shown in Fig. 8.25, several

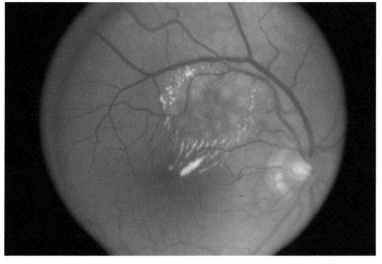

FIG. 8.20

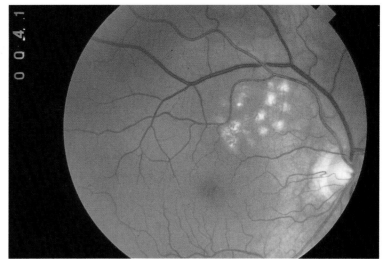

FIG. 8.21

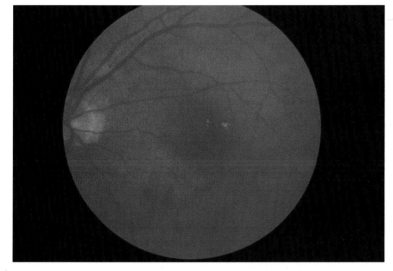

FIG. 8.22

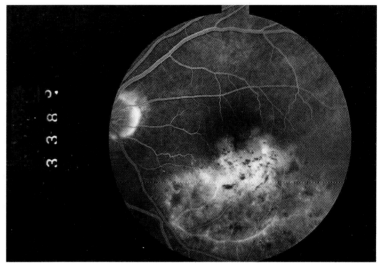

FIG. 8.23

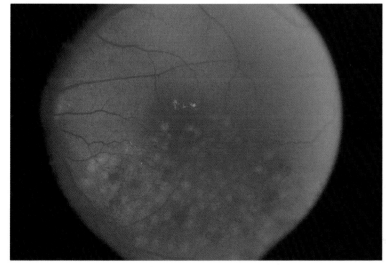

FIG. 8.24

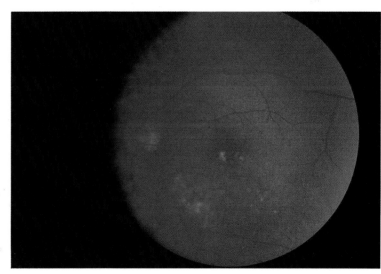

FIG. 8.25

months following treatment. Note the atrophy at the site of the photocoagulation burns and resolution of the hemorrhage and exudation. Figure 8.26 is the fluorescein angiogram from the same patient in the postoperative phase. No persistent leakage is seen.

The mechanism leading to resolution of the edema following laser treatment is unknown. The same factors implicit in the laser response to diffuse diabetic macular edema may play a role. In the BRVO study, contraindications to argon laser treatment included the presence of hemorrhage in the fovea or area to be treated and severe capillary nonperfusion. Roseman and Olk have successfully used krypton red laser for patients with extensive intraretinal hemorrhage or media opacity. We advocate the use of argon green laser for portions of the macula greater than ⅔ DD from the foveal center and krypton red laser closer than ½ DD to the edge of the foveal avascular zone. Figure 8.27 demonstrates the use of krypton red laser in juxtafoveal and argon green laser in macular treatment for macular edema in BRVO.

Retinal and Disk Neovascularization The risk of neovascular complications in BRVO is directly related to the degree of associated capillary nonperfusion. Causes of acute capillary closure in BRVO may reflect endothelial ischemia, retinal edema from infarction which lowers the critical closing pressure of these vessels, or localized intravascular coagulation. Decreased arteriolar perfusion (autoregulatory or arteriosclerotic) may also enhance progressive capillary closure. Since only a portion of the retina is involved in BRVO, this region is relatively hypoxic, creating presumably an angiogenic stimulus for growth of new vessels. If this stimulus is "subthreshold" for neovascularization, only endothelial proliferation such as collaterals and microaneurysms may be observed. However, a larger stimulus might cause retinal neovascularization, most commonly at the borders of the ischemic quadrant. Figure 8.28 shows ischemic retina superior to the disk associated with a huge area of preretinal neovascularization. Figure 8.29 shows the intensity and distribution of the krypton laser photocoagulation burns in

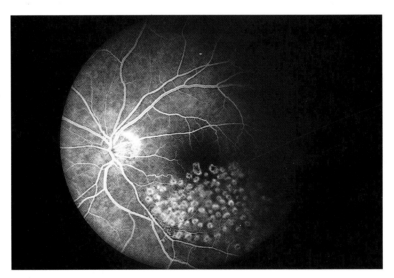

FIG. 8.26

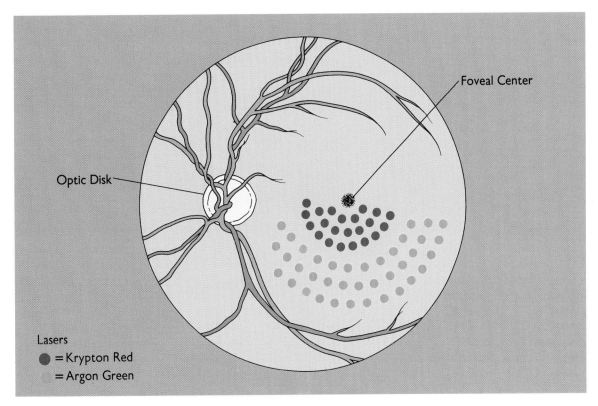

FIG. 8.27

Optic Disk

Foveal Center

Lasers
● = Krypton Red
○ = Argon Green

Branch Retinal Vein Occlusion: Retinal and Disk Neovascularization

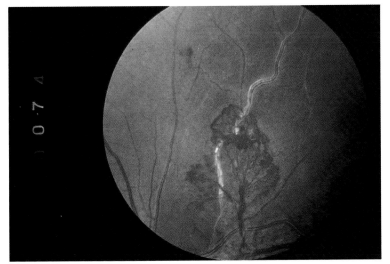

FIG. 8.28

FIG. 8.29

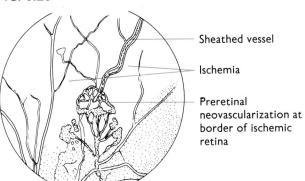

Sheathed vessel

Ischemia

Preretinal neovascularization at border of ischemic retina

the same patient. In Fig. 8.30, note the marked regression of the neovascularization several months following laser treatment.

Disk neovascularization or, very rarely, anterior segment neovascularization, also may evolve. The BRVO Study Group concluded that peripheral scatter argon laser photocoagulation may significantly reduce the complications of neovascularization by nearly a 2:1 ratio. The study recommended that only eyes with documented neovascularization be treated. Other studies have found that retinal neovascularization occurs 6 months or more after ischemic BRVO in 17%–34% of cases. The retina is involved more often than the disk. A classification scheme, or "ischemic index," has been suggested to identify those patients at risk for neovascularization based on a 30° fluorescein angiographic sweep within the region of affected retinal vasculature.

Argon laser scatter photocoagulation is indicated to treat cases of neovascularization. Moderately intense, 200–500-μm burns are placed one burn width apart, covering the entire involved segment 2 DD from the fovea to the periphery. Eyes with extensive intraretinal hemorrhage should be observed until clear or may be considered for treatment with krypton red laser. Figure 8.31 shows fibrovascular proliferation and vitreous traction along the course of the superior temporal arcade. In Fig. 8.32, note the distribution and intensity of the krypton laser burns immediately following treatment in the same patient.

A combination of factors may explain why photocoagulation stabilizes neovascularization in BRVO, including direct coagulation of leaking microaneurysms and foci of neovascularization with selective destruction and consequent reduction of a certain volume of tissue. This may allow the surviving tissue to be adequately oxygenated, or facilitate drainage of angiogenic factors into the choroidal circulation.

Macular BRVOs do not cause neovascularization but often cause subtle macular edema and vision loss best diagnosed by fluorescein angiography. Treatment guidelines for grid laser application are based on vision, chronicity, presence and location of collaterals, and degree of lipid exudation.

PERIPHERAL RETINAL VASCULAR OCCLUSIVE DISEASE

Peripheral retinal vascular occlusive disease may lead to retinal neovascularization and, rarely, disk neovascularization. Numerous entities make up the spectrum of this disease: sickle cell retinopathy, idiopathic peripheral occlusive disease (Eales' disease), granulomatous diseases such as sarcoidosis, blood dyscrasias, familial exudative vitreoretinopathy, retinopathy of prematurity, incontinentia pigmenti, and intermediate uveitis. The general principles for laser photocoagulation in these diseases relate to the location and extent of associated ischemia. If there is concomitant inflammation such as vitritis or a phlebitis, it is prudent to use antiinflammatory medications prior to, or in conjunction with, photocoagulation in order to control and eliminate the neovascularization. Findings in the management of sickle cell retinopathy and Eales' disease (idiopathic peripheral neovascularization) typify peripheral retinal vascular occlusive disease.

Sickle Cell Retinopathy

Visual loss can occur from the neovascular and hemorrhagic sequelae of proliferative sickle cell retinopathy. Fluorescein angiography has been instrumental in demonstrating that occlusion begins in small retinal arterioles, usually at bifurcations and often in the temporal periphery. Goldberg has classified five stages in proliferative sickle cell retinopathy: peripheral arterial occlusion, arteriovenous anastomoses, neovascularization, vitreous hemorrhage, and finally retinal detachment.

Vitreous attachments to the sea fans and proliferative tissue can cause vitreous hemorrhage, retinal tears, and even retinal detachments. Twenty to sixty percent of proliferative lesions autoinfarct, leading to a relatively low overall rate of blindness (12%–14%). However, the peripheral retina in these patients is ischemic and thinned, increasing the risk of tear formation even if the vascular lesions involute by themselves. This complicates any decision regarding the indications for laser treatment. Large elevated neovascular lesions ought to be treated, since they are at a higher risk of vitreous hemorrhage than flat, smaller lesions. Previous vitreous hemorrhage, retinal tears, associated diabetes, or bilateral involvement are indications for treatment, at least in one eye.

Small flat sea fans can be photocoagulated directly, using a hemoglobin-absorbing wavelength (argon green or dye yellow). A large spot size (200–500 μm) with long exposure (0.5 s) and moderate intensity should be used to limit complications. Often a lower-power intensity is needed in these patients due to the darker fundus pigmentation.

Previously, larger sea fans were closed by the feeder vessel technique. Advocates of this technique used moderate-to-high intensity burns of argon laser with a large spot size (500 μm) and long duration (0.2–0.5 s) to treat the feeding arteriole in the flat retina. After the arterial blood supply was segmented, the venules were then treated directly. Figure 8.33 shows a patient with sickle cell retinopathy with

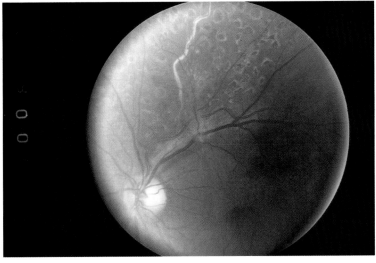

FIG. 8.30

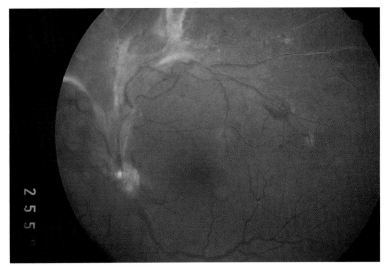

FIG. 8.31

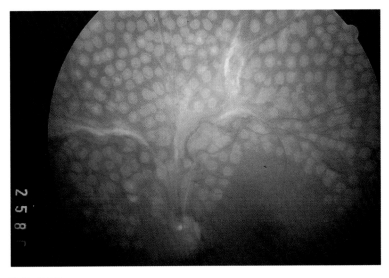

FIG. 8.32

Sickle Cell Retinopathy

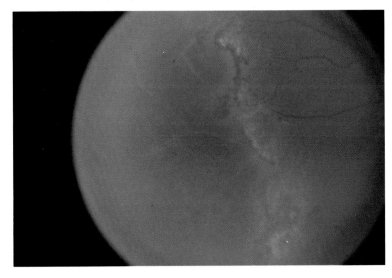

FIG. 8.33

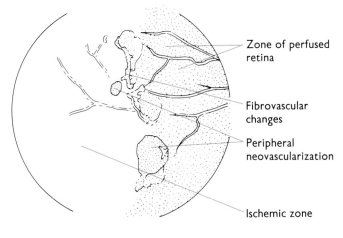

Zone of perfused retina

Fibrovascular changes

Peripheral neovascularization

Ischemic zone

peripheral neovascularization at the junction between perfused and nonperfused peripheral retina. A fluorescein angiogram on the same patient in Fig. 8.34 reveals hyperfluorescence of the neovascularization, which is partially obscured by preretinal hemorrhage. Figure 8.35 shows the same patient following photocoagulation treatment. Direct treatment of the feeder arterioles and draining venules resulted in an infarction of the preretinal neovascularization. The fluorescein angiogram of the same patient (Fig. 8.36) delineates the nonperfusion induced by the laser treatment. Although 95% of lesions could be effectively closed by this technique, potentially serious complications can occur. These include "blow out" vitreous hemorrhage or the creation of a nidus for future development of choroidal neovascularization, peripheral choridal ischemia, and retinal tears. Direct treatment of these lesions should be avoided.

A far safer and comparably effective technique is peripheral scatter photocoagulation. Figure 8.37 shows regression of neovascularization in the midperipheral retina following laser photocoagulation treatment by the grid or ablative technique. These vessels will respond to such treatment with less associated vitreoretinal traction and risk of retinal breaks. Occasionally, the vessels will have some residual perfusion compared with the more infarcted vessels from direct treatment. The large, elevated sea fans, however, do not respond to this method as well as less-severe proliferative sickle retinopathy. Burns are placed with light to moderate intensity at least 1–2 DD anterior and posterior to the lesion and at least one clock hour to either side, separated by one burn width. It is controversial whether to treat infarcted tissue peripheral to neovascular lesions or only to treat the region of "relative" hypoxia around and posterior to the sea fans. The efficacy of scatter photocoagulation may be related to destruction of the hypoxic retina with suppression of presumed "angiogenic factor" release (Glaser) or to allowing better oxygenation of the inner retina with stabilization of neovascularization, as in diabetes.

Although speculative, krypton red laser may be a useful adjunct in eyes where there is overlying vitreal hemorrhage, causing less absorption by hemoglobin and therefore less peripheral thermal vitreal contraction.

Eales' Disease

Eales' disease is an idiopathic bilateral vasoocclusive periphlebitis occurring mostly in males. It may cause severe vision loss secondary to capillary nonperfusion, retinal neovascularization with extensive fibrovascular proliferation, vitreous hemorrhage, vitreoretinal traction, and neovascular glaucoma. It is a diagnosis of exclusion once simulating disorders such as sickle cell retinopathy, diabetes, branch vein occlusion, lupus erythematosis, sarcoidosis, and other granulomatous, metabolic, and hematologic diseases have been ruled out. It is differentiated from peripheral uveitis with secondary neovascularization by the lack of vitreal inflammation.

Laser treatment has been successful in reversing the progression of neovascularization seen clinically and angiographically and in preventing eventual vitreous hemorrhage and retinal detachment. In patients with neovascularization, photocoagulation should be placed in a scatter pattern in the nonperfused retina, adjacent to areas seen to be leaking on angiography. The technique is similar to that used for proliferative sickle cell retinopathy. Neovascular tissue should not be treated directly.

ARTERIOLAR MACROANEURYSMS

Acquired retinal macroaneurysms are relatively common lesions usually seen in hypertensive patients in their sixth decade. They are slightly more common in women. The development of macroaneurysms is chiefly thought to be due to arterial wall damage caused by atherosclerotic thrombi, emboli, or venous stasis. Vision is threatened when the aneurysm, usually located in the posterior pole, leaks proteinaceous and lipid-rich exudate along with blood into the surrounding retina. This may occur slowly or suddenly (e.g., after a Valsalva maneuver). Serous detachments, circinate maculopathy, and hemorrhage (subretinal, subhyaloid, and vitreal) may occur. Some macroaneurysms close spontaneously through a process of thrombosis and sclerosis.

Laser photocoagulation is indicated when detachment or yellowish exudate persists or progressively accumulates in the macula. Moderate hemoglobin-absorbing laser photocoagulation (argon green or dye yellow) is applied directly to the aneurysm, using a large spot size (250–500 μm, larger than the lesion itself) and a long duration setting. It is not necessary to treat so heavily as to infarct the lesion completely; achievement of only a mild grayish color is all that is needed. Presumably, thermal absorption causes healing by accelerating the cicatricial change in the wall of the aneurysm, eliminating its permeability and bleeding tendencies. Following spontaneous or laser-induced resolution of the aneurysm, a fibrous shell that varies from a barely visible to opaque structure evolves.

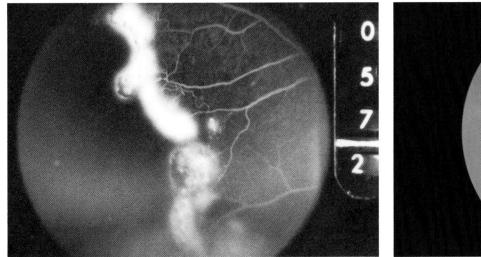

FIG. 8.34

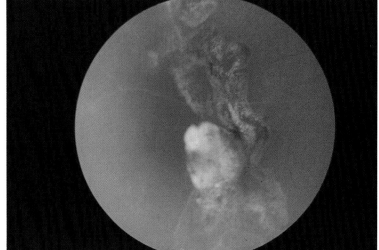

FIG. 8.35

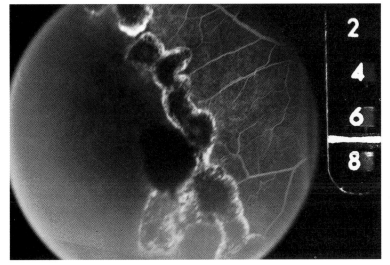

FIG. 8.36

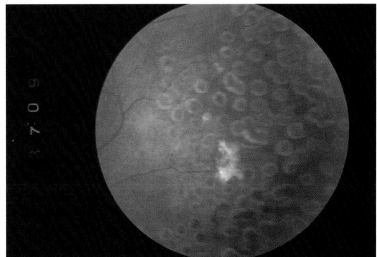

FIG. 8.37

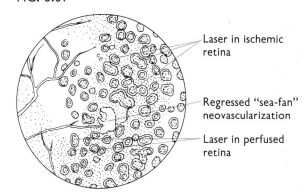

Laser in ischemic retina

Regressed "sea-fan" neovascularization

Laser in perfused retina

In Fig. 8.38 note the nodular arteriolar swelling surrounded by serous and lipid deposition in a circinate ring converging toward the macula. The fluorescein angiogram on the same patient in Fig. 8.39 demonstrates the marked hyperfluorescence of the macroaneurysm (light bulb phenomenon). Figure 8.40 shows the same patient several weeks following laser treatment. Some retinal pigment epithelial hyperplasia has been induced by treatment at the site of the aneurysm. There has been gradual resolution of the serous and lipid exudation. Figure 8.41 shows the same patient several months after treatment. There is continued resolution of the exudation and a cicatricial change in the wall of the aneurysm.

Risks of the procedure include incomplete closure, bleeding, and distal arterial obstruction with visual field loss. Postoperative oozing of blood and transiently increased lipid precipitation into the macula as the serous subretinal fluid resolves is not uncommon.

RETINAL TELANGIECTASIA

Retinal telangiectasia may be a nonhereditary congenital or acquired retinal vascular anomaly. Primarily, retinal capillaries (and, rarely, major retinal vessels) become irregularly dilated and incompetent with associated exudative leakage. Figure 8.42 demonstrates a case of congenital telangiectasia. Note the prominent aneurysms in the macular region surrounded by intraretinal serous edema and an irregular circinate or stellate ring. Figure 8.43 shows the same patient after laser photocoagulation treatment. Under fluorescein guidance, only a few burns were applied directly to the leaking aneurysms.

Massive yellow exudative retinal detachment in infancy or childhood (usually in one eye of a male patient) comprises Coats' syndrome; less widespread leakage and more focal involvement occur in adults with Leber's miliary aneurysms. Children with Coats' syndrome should have rapid ablative photocoagulation applied directly to destroy telan-

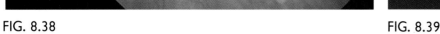

Arteriolar Macroaneurysm

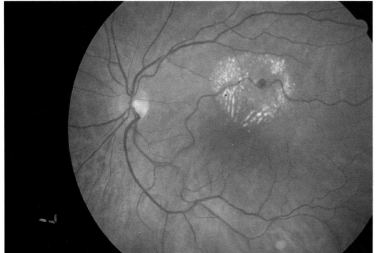

FIG. 8.38

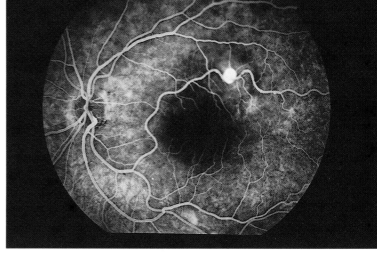

FIG. 8.39

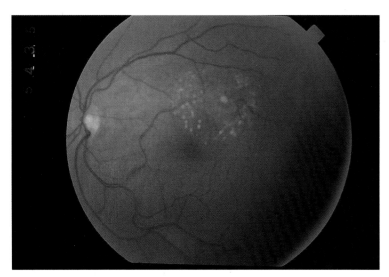

FIG. 8.40

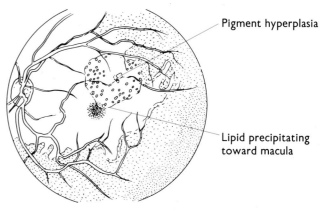

Pigment hyperplasia

Lipid precipitating toward macula

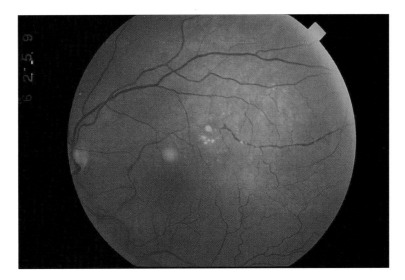

FIG. 8.41

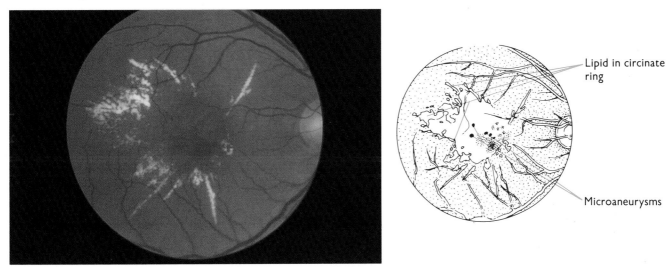

Lipid in circinate ring

Microaneurysms

FIG. 8.42

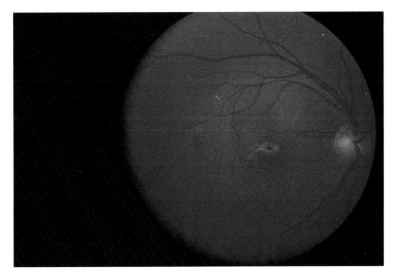

FIG. 8.43

giectatic vessels in order to preserve visual function and prevent rubeotic glaucoma. General anesthesia is often used. If subretinal exudate prevents adequate thermal laser energy absorption, cryotherapy may be indicated.

Treatment of adults with Leber's miliary aneurysms is dictated by progression of the disease, which causes widespread retinal exudation and detachment or macular edema. Patients with accumulation of yellowish macular exudate or macular edema associated with visual loss ought to be considered for focal or grid laser treatment to the telangiectatic areas. Figure 8.44 illustrates a case of congenital telangiectasia. Note the peripheral exudative detachment secondary to retinal telangiectatic vascular change. Figure 8.45 shows the same patient with a simultaneous macular exudative response from chronic lipid that has seeped under the retina and settled in the posterior pole. Photocoagulation was performed on the peripheral retina; the results are shown in Fig. 8.46. Figure 8.47 shows the macula in the same patient two years later. Dramatic resolution of the serous and lipid exudation and some patchy residual pigment epithelial hyperplasia and atrophy are seen.

Idiopathic juxtafoveal telangiectasia, which is often bilateral and limited to the perifoveal area, generally begins in the temporal half of the fovea. It is characterized by minimal intraretinal serous exudation, superficially glistening crystalline dots, and, in some cases, retinal pigment epithelial hyperplasia, retinal–choroidal anastomoses, and disciform scarring. Laser photocoagulation treatment may be indicated for a patient who has developed an extrafoveal neovascularized membrane in this disease (see section on treatment of subretinal neovascularization). Focal laser in a grid pattern may also be used to treat outside the foveal avascular zone in those cases with extensive macular leakage and associated visual decline.

Figure 8.48 shows grayish thickening in the perifoveal area in a patient with idiopathic juxtafoveal telangiectasia. The early phase fluorescein angiogram in Fig. 8.49 reveals dilated perifoveal capillaries and a few aneurysmal changes. Lipid deposition and nonperfusion are absent in this eye; this is characteristic of this disorder. Figure 8.50 shows the late stage angiogram, revealing intraretinal leakage and perifoveal cystoid edema. Perifoveal laser photocoagulation

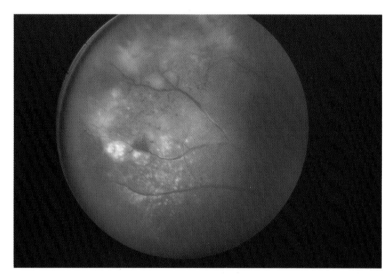

FIG. 8.44

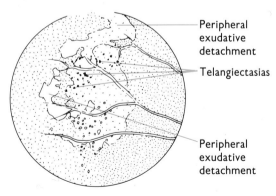

Peripheral exudative detachment

Telangiectasias

Peripheral exudative detachment

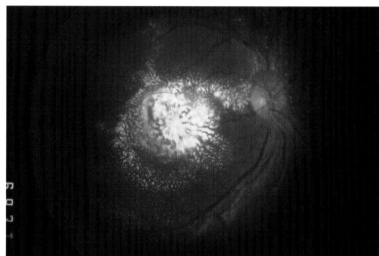

FIG. 8.45

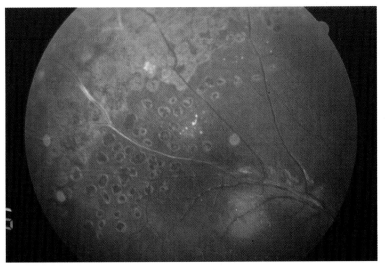

FIG. 8.46

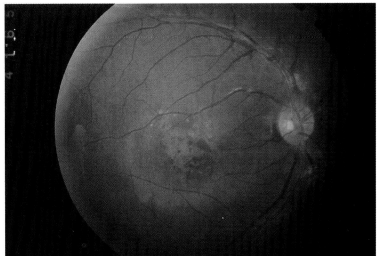

FIG. 8.47

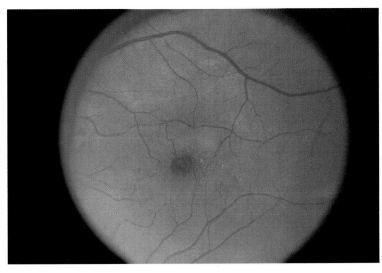

FIG. 8.48

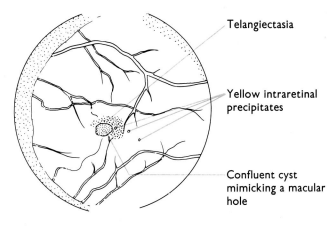

Telangiectasia

Yellow intraretinal
precipitates

Confluent cyst
mimicking a macular
hole

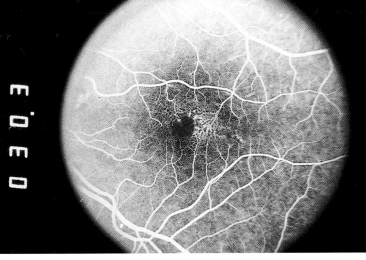

FIG. 8.49

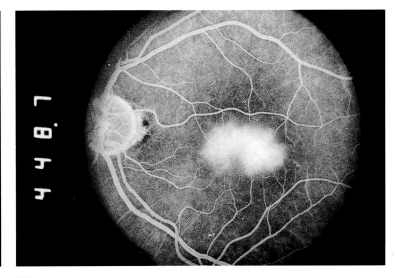

FIG. 8.50

has been performed in Fig. 8.51. Note the flattening of the retina in the perifoveal area. In Fig. 8.52, a fluorescein angiogram of the same patient after treatment reveals marked improvement of the perifoveal leakage, particularly inferiorly.

A careful clinical and fluorescein angiographic examination is needed in all cases of retinal telangiectasia to rule out simulating diseases, including diabetic retinopathy, venous occlusion, and radiation retinopathy.

ANGIOMATOSIS RETINAE

Capillary hemangiomas of the disk and retina can grow toward the inner (endophytic) or outer (exophytic) retinal layers. They have a predilection for the juxtapapillary area and may cause serous detachments of the retina and circinate maculopathy, probably due to fenestrated endothelium in the tumor capillaries. Peripheral angiomas leak lipid-rich exudates that also may accumulate in the macula. These lesions, due to their capillary nature and the associated development of arteriovenous fistulas and exudation, are capable of reactive proliferation and continued growth into adulthood.

Photocoagulation with a hemoglobin-absorbing wavelength (argon green or dye yellow) is most effective when these lesions are small in size and identified in their early stages of development. They often can be recognized in the temporal periphery as small red-gray lesions without abnormal efferent or afferent vessels and later as a cluster of capillaries with dilated feeder vessels. Large spot sizes (250–

500 μm) of long duration (0.5 s) and moderate intensity are used. Larger lesions generally cannot be treated with photocoagulation alone.

Figure 8.53 shows a capillary hemangioma on the nasal side of the disk with associated preretinal gliosis. The corresponding fluorescein angiogram in Figure 8.54 shows hyperfluorescence of the tumor on the disk. The color photograph in Fig. 8.55 taken after direct argon green laser treatment shows complete involution of the hemangioma. Retinal striae are still present. Figure 8.56 is a fluorescein angiogram confirming involution of the lesion.

Exophytic juxtapapillary hemangiomas are difficult to treat because of their frequent papillomacular bundle location, and because laser is often ineffective in arresting the exudation derived from the outer portion of the tumor that protrudes into the subretinal space. Lesions larger than 1–2 DD are harder to obliterate because they are associated with excessive subretinal exudate and a predilection for vitreoretinal proliferation on their surfaces.

RETINAL BREAKS

Laser photocoagulation is commonly applied around retinal breaks to prevent or limit the extension of retinal detachment. Three-mirror contact lenses with and without scleral depression enable peripheral visualization for treatment. Several wavelengths may be used to produce an adequate chorioretinal adhesion: argon green, krypton red, or dye yellow. Selection depends on the transmission characteris-

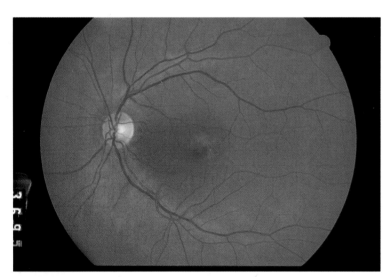

FIG. 8.51

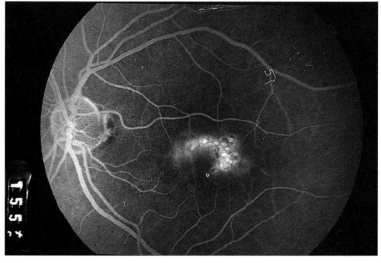

FIG. 8.52

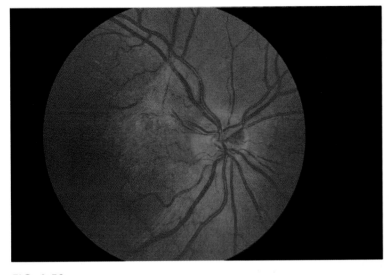

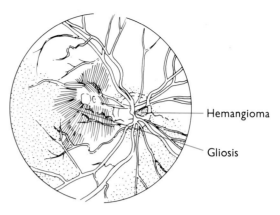

Hemangioma

Gliosis

FIG. 8.53

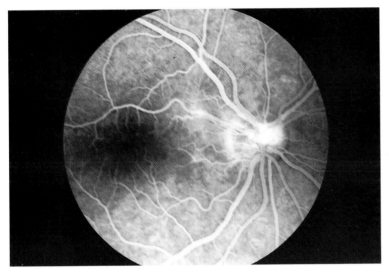

FIG. 8.54

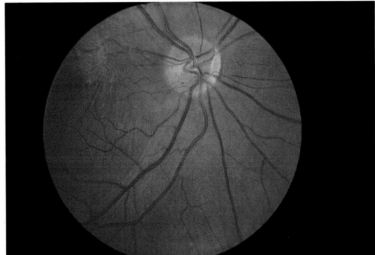

FIG. 8.55

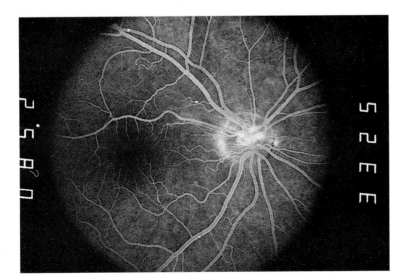

FIG. 8.56

tics of the ocular media and the pigmentary variations of a particular patient's eye.

Indications for laser treatment of retinal breaks are given in Fig. 8.57. Asymptomatic round holes (without vitreoretinal traction) and lattice degeneration with atrophic holes do not need treatment unless there is a history of retinal detachment. This is particularly true for eyes that are not very myopic (less than 3.00 diopters).

A double or triple row of nonconfluent laser burns of moderate-to-heavy intensity (200–500 μm) and 0.1–0.5-s duration are placed around the break. A tractional retinal break associated with a retinal branch vein occlusion is demonstrated in Fig. 8.58. Laser photocoagulation has been used in a double row barrage to surround the break, which developed secondary to the ischemic vasculopathy. After treatment, the patient is advised to rest, avoid overexertion, and refrain from reading for 7–10 days. Followup visits are usually scheduled at 1 and 2 weeks, at which time pigmentary changes corresponding to an adequate chorioretinal adhesion should be observed.

Laser treatment also may be used to reinforce a scleral buckle, especially if there is residual vitreoretinal traction following surgery. Laser treatment without surgery may be appropriate in the management of an inferior retinal break associated with minimal traction and a localized inferior retinal detachment. Two to three rows of laser burns are placed in the region of the attached retina surrounding the elevated retina to "wall-off" future spread. Endophotocoagulation techniques are used routinely during vitreoretinal surgery to seal breaks and to perform panretinal photocoagulation. If needed, laser can also be applied through an intraocular gas bubble postoperatively.

RETINAL PIGMENT EPITHELIAL–CHOROIDAL DISEASES

AGE-RELATED MACULAR DEGENERATION

The most important cause of irreversible legal blindness in patients over the age of 60 in the United States is age-related macular degeneration (AMD), particularly the exudative form. The 10% minority of the group with "wet" degeneration accounts for 90% of the patients with severe vision loss to 20/200 or worse.

Subretinal neovascularization (SRN) with subfoveal disciform scarring is the principal mechanism of severe vision loss in these patients. Eccentric SRN (at least 1,000 μm from the foveal center) and peripapillary SRN usually have a relatively good visual prognosis, but associated exudative detachments may cause RPE atrophy with subsequent vision loss without actual subfoveal invasion. Documented progression of clinical signs extending to or directly affecting the fovea is an indication for treatment. Most often, SRN tends to originate in the juxtafoveal area. Many of these cases are treatable; 75% will lead to legal blindness if left alone. Figure 8.59 shows a grayish-red subretinal neovascular membrane temporal to the fovea and drusen in the nasal macula. This is a case of age-related macular degeneration. Figure 8.60 is the corresponding fluorescein angiogram, showing lacy hyperfluorescence of the SRN. The late phase angiogram, showing diffuse subretinal hyperfluorescence, is seen in Fig. 8.61. In Fig. 8.62, the post-laser photograph reveals obliteration of the SRN and formation of a grayish-yellow scar.

In 1982, the Macular Photocoagulation Study (MPS) group showed definitively that argon laser photocoagula-

Retinal Breaks

INDICATIONS FOR LASER TREATMENT OF RETINAL BREAKS	
CONDITION OF EYE	INDICATIONS FOR TREATMENT
Phakic	Symptomatic horseshoe tears Symptomatic large or superior operculated holes (controversial) Asymptomatic horseshoe tears (large, superior, or in pathologic myopes)
Aphakic	Symptomatic horseshoe tears Symptomatic operculated holes Asymptomatic large or superior horseshoe tears
Fellow eye (Retinal detachment in other eye)	Symptomatic horseshoe tears Symptomatic operculated holes Asymptomatic horseshoe tears Asymptomatic large or superior operculated holes Lattice degeneration with round holes

FIG. 8.57

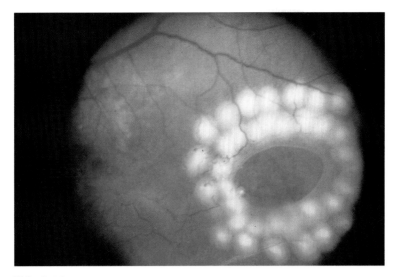

FIG. 8.58

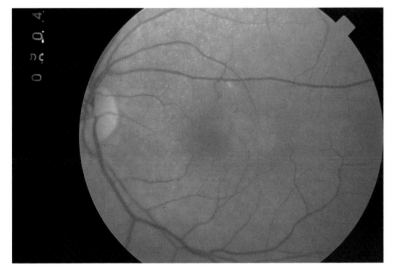

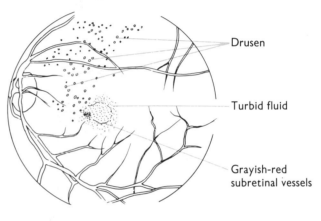

Drusen

Turbid fluid

Grayish-red
subretinal vessels

FIG. 8.59

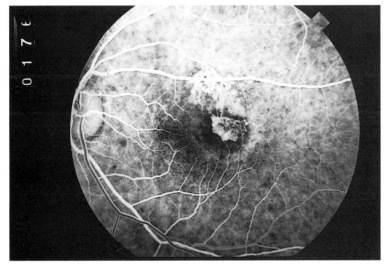

FIG. 8.60

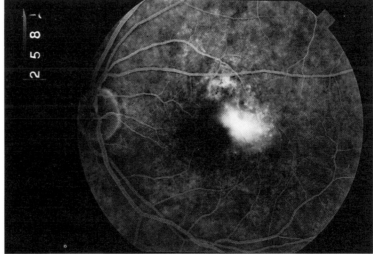

FIG. 8.61

tion is beneficial in treating extrafoveal SRN in AMD. After 18 months, 60% of the untreated eyes with SRN located 200 μm or more from the center of the FAZ lost 6 or more lines of visual acuity, compared with only 25% of treated eyes. After 3 years, a 24% difference in risk of severe vision loss still existed in patients who received treatment. It is important to note that the MPS and similar studies have had strict eligibility requirements, which included only well-defined SRN complexes that were eccentric to the center of the FAZ by at least 200 μm.

Preoperative Management for Subretinal Neovascularization

Before treating a patient with SRN, several issues need to be addressed. First, a high-quality preoperative fluorescein angiogram should be projected and magnified as an anatomic guide for the treating ophthalmologist. One taken within 72 hours illustrating the SRN is preferable. This may also help in illustrating the visual implications to the patient and family.

Next, a frank discussion concerning the potential benefits, risks, limitations, alternatives, and complications of laser treatment should follow. As part of the informed consent, the patient and family should fully understand that it may not be possible to restore vision to its original status before exudative changes occurred. Laser photocoagulation may be 100% technically and anatomically "successful," yet result in either no improvement or actually a decline in vision. Causes of decreased vision after laser treatment include the presence of permanent paracentral scotomas (hampering reading vision), inner sensory retinal thermal damage with retinal surface contraction, or progression of the underlying macular disease itself. Risks of photocoagulation in the FAZ and inadvertent treatment to an area of eccentric fixation must be considered. Lastly, the moderately high recurrence rate of SRN after laser treatment should be explained. The patient who understands the serious nature of his problem will be more inclined to return for careful postoperative surveillance, including fluorescein angiography.

The pupil should be well dilated with cycloplegic and sympathomimetic drops. Foveal fixation, using a different laser color than that to be used during treatment, should be reevaluated while sitting at the laser. The aiming beam is set at a small spot size (50–100 μm) at low intensity with minimal background illumination of the fundus by the split lamp beam through the contact lens. A tranquilizer can be given to the overanxious patient. If ocular immobility is not adequate, a retrobulbar anesthetic injection may be given. Maximal immobilization of the head and face as well as the eye to be treated should be obtained. It is important to reassure the patient and make him as comfortable as possible to avoid a Valsalva reaction. The surgeon should be alert to the possibility of micronystagmoid movements and Bell's phenomenon, which could rotate the FAZ toward the laser beam path particularly when inferior juxtafoveal SRN is being treated. Even with retrobulbar block, the intact superior oblique muscle can rotate the eye downward, bringing the fovea dangerously close to the laser beam path when SRN superior to the fovea is being treated.

The treatment areas should then be centered in the illuminated fundus to ensure high degrees of accuracy of axial focusing of the aiming and therapeutic beams and to widen the geographic area in the fundus available for treatment in the event of head or eye movement. Topical corneal anesthetic (proparacaine) is applied and a contact lens placed on the cornea. The Yannuzzi Macular Photocoagulation lens (Fig. 8.63) is suitable here; it has a wide flange extending beyond the limbus to provide lens stability and ocular immobility. Intraocular pressure can be uniformly increased without corneal distortion because of the steep posterior curve design of the lens. This is a valuable technique for slowing down choroidal circulation to minimize the possibility of choroidal hemorrhage during treatment and to control the spread of hemorrhage should it occur.

Laser Selection

Absorption characteristics of the commonly used laser wavelengths are given in Fig. 8.64. Although data proving the efficacy of photocoagulation for SRN came from studies

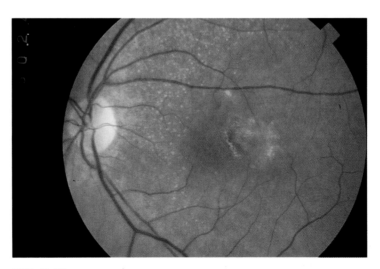

FIG. 8.62

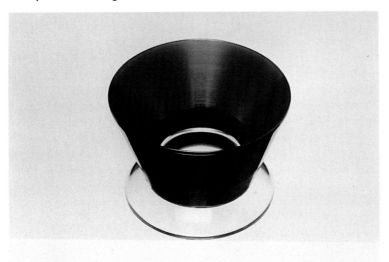

FIG. 8.63

Age-Related Macular Degeneration: Laser Selection

COMPARISON OF COMMONLY USED LASER WAVELENGTHS

	WAVELENGTH			
CHARACTERISTICS*	ARGON BLUE-GREEN (488 nm)	ARGON GREEN (514 nm)	DYE YELLOW (577 nm)	KRYPTON RED (647 nm)
Hemoglobulin absorption	80%	78%	98%	5%
Macular xanthophyll absorption	59%	11%	0%	0%
Melanin (RPE)† absorption	50%	45%	40%	35%
Transmission through ocular media‡	29%	35%	47%	50%

**All percentages given are approximations.*
†Depends on light versus dark fundi.
‡Depends on age.

FIG. 8.64

where argon blue-green laser (ABGL) was used, the blue wavelength (488 nm) of the argon biochromatic laser currently is not used by most retinal specialists for several reasons: (1) it is scattered greatly by ocular media, requiring three times as much energy at the cornea to produce equal retinal burns compared with argon green laser; (2) it is highly absorbed by xanthophyll, causing inner sensory retinal damage near the fovea and whitish opacification obscuring further laser treatment; and (3) it may be cataractogenic since it is absorbed by yellow xanthochrome pigments in the aging lens.

Argon green laser (AGL) (514 nm) is only minimally absorbed by xanthophyll. It is absorbed by hemoglobin, which can cause damage to the inner retinal layers and vessels, and it is especially hazardous to use in the event of significant subretinal blood due to absorption and spread of thermal damage. It is useful in treating (1) hypopigmented eyes, (2) SRN that originates from an atrophic scar or is associated with RPE atrophy, (3) "recurrent SRN" adjacent to an atrophic laser burn, (4) SRN that is associated with red choroidal vessels, (5) SRN that originates from idiopathic juxtafoveal retinal telangiectasia, and (6) SRN that has eroded through Bruch's membrane and the RPE and is underneath the sensory retina.

Krypton red laser (KRL) (647 nm) is not absorbed by xanthophyll but is absorbed by melanin (35%) in the RPE and choroid. This feature makes treatment of a lightly pigmented membrane in a hypopigmented eye difficult. Thermal damage to the inner retina is minimized and, whenever possible, it is our first choice among wavelengths. It is particularly desirable when there is (1) juxtafoveal SRN, (2) blood overlying SRN or between the fovea and the edge of the SRN, (3) a turbid detachment of the sensory retina or RPE associated with SRN, (4) preexisting preretinal membrane disease, (5) a nuclear sclerotic cataract, and (6) a hazy vitreous body.

Dye yellow laser (DYL) (577 nm) appears ideal as a hemoglobin-absorbing wavelength. It is transmitted well by the nuclear sclerotic cataract, and is not absorbed by xanthophyll in the perifoveal area. It is a highly efficient wavelength to use since it is minimally scattered by the ocular media and maximally absorbed by the hemoglobin-containing vasculature. The limiting factor regarding this particular wavelength has been, until recently, the technological unreliability of the dye laser systems. However, currently available dye laser systems are now of adequate power and stability to provide this monochromatic wavelength.

We prefer photocoagulation systems with dual wavelength capabilities such as the AGL and KRL or dye laser systems that contain adequate power in the yellow (577 nm) and red (640 nm) wavelengths. In the same patient, for example, a hemoglobin-absorbing wavelength (AGL or DYL) would be used to treat SRN associated with atrophic regions of the retina, while a non-hemoglobin-absorbing wavelength (KRL) or the dye (640 nm) would be used in the pigmented portions of the retina.

Laser Settings

The KRL is set at 0.5-s duration with a 200–500 μm spot size and a level of energy (150–400 mW) predetermined by the clinician based on the biologic nature of the fundus and the clarity of the ocular media. If the aiming beam is sharply focused, one can assume efficient ocular transmission of laser energy with minimal scatter. Test burns are hazardous and unreliable and the clinician should become familiar with the degree of aiming beam intensity required to induce a therapeutic response in a given patient. Parfocal (columnar) laser systems may be superior to "defocused" (conical) laser systems since the power density at the target tissue remains the same with alterations in focus. It is important to note that if the operator reduces the spot size, he must also decrease the power since a reduction of one-half the spot size will increase the power density four times at the target tissue.

Photocoagulation

A mild degree of pressure is placed on the contact lens to slow down the choroidal circulation if possible and to stabilize the eye. If the preoperative fluorescein angiogram shows a discrete source of neovascularization within the SRN ("feeder vessel"), treatment is directed first to this area. AGL is very effective here. The tendency for bleeding is minimized with this approach since it reduces perfusion to the rest of the SRN.

Next, the foveal side of the SRN is treated. The burns are allowed to extend over the edge of the membrane into the surrounding relatively normal RPE by approximately 100–200 μm (less if the SRN is juxtafoveal). A moderately intense grayish-white confluent burn of the SRN, surrounded by a softer yellowish color change at the uninvolved margins, is desired. Chalk-white burns like those employed by the MPS probably cause unnecessary thermal damage, but, as of yet, there is no evidence to indicate which approach is ideal or which wavelength is superior. As the photocoagulation burn spreads beyond the SRN into the surrounding RPE, a silhouette beneath the retina of the SRN is usually seen.

Post-Laser Management

After photocoagulation of the SRN, pressure on the contact lens is released slowly. If the membrane becomes darker, active perfusion is occurring and additional laser treatment is performed. Once pressure is released, a few minutes of observation is advised to check for slow "oozing" from the treatment site. Upon completion of the treatment session, a color photograph of the macula should be taken. Avoidance of exertional activities and non-aspirin analgesics are suggested. Follow-up normally should be done at 1,2,4,6, and 12 weeks.

Subretinal fluid should dissipate by the first week and subretinal blood and lipid should resolve over the first two or more weeks. Special attention should be directed to the edges of the treatment area. A variable degree of pigment granularity or an atrophic corona should be seen surrounding the obliterated SRN. This region also should be flat; thickening or elevation at the edge of the treatment area may be indicative of residual SRN. Fluorescein angiograms are recommended at weeks 2 and 6, even if the patient is asymptomatic and there is minimal clinical suspicion of residual disease. This is important because most recurrences occur during the first two months following treatment. Visual acuity should stabilize or improve by the second postoperative week and there should be a reduction in metamorphopsia.

Overall visual outcome will depend on additional variables, including associated RPE detachments, RPE rips, sensory retinal detachments, residual subretinal blood and lipid, CME, cystic foveal degeneration, perifoveal RPE atrophy, and confluent drusen. Functional visual success depends on patient adaptation to the scotomas from SRN and treatment scars and patient motivation in coping with partial central visual acuity loss, eccentric viewing, and visual aids. The patient should also be given an Amsler grid or Yannuzzi card to monitor vision in both eyes on a weekly basis.

Complications of laser treatment for SRN include choroidal hemorrhage, RPE rips, choroidal ischemia, and choroidal folds. Paracentral scotomas are common but macular pucker and inadvertent foveal burns fortunately are rare.

Recurrent Subretinal Neovascularization

Recurrence rates for SRN after laser treatment vary from 39% to nearly 60%. All recurrences must be recognized and treated promptly before they extend subfoveally. In one study, two factors were significantly related to higher recurrence rates: (1) juxtafoveal SRN and (2) light-colored SRN. Recurrent neovascularization can be separated into residual SRN and true recurrences. Residual SRN is any part of the new vessel membrane that survives up to 2 weeks following laser treatment. True recurrences can be marginal (associated with the edge of the photocoagulation burn) or independent. Most recurrences are associated with thickening or pigmentary elevations at the edge of the burn or exudative manifestations of the retina (serous, hemor-

rhagic, or CME). Central atrophic areas of the laser burn are generally devoid of SRN and a recurrence will usually proliferate away from the center of the scar.

Fluorescein angiography in the post-laser period is especially challenging. Normal fluorescence at the margin of a laser burn due to intact choriocapillaris causes a "brushfire" of pseudohyperfluorescence, in contrast to the lack of fluorescence of the laser scar. Late staining of the sclera within the laser scar occurs but does not intensify or spread as much as in recurrent SRN. "Lacy" hyperfluorescence is rarely seen in recurrent SRN; rather, "fuzzy" hyperfluorescence associated with shallow exudative detachments is the rule, but to a lesser degree than in primary SRN since fusion of the retina to the RPE by laser limits the pooling of fluorescein dye.

Guidelines for retreatment include the presence of (1) new or persistent areas of hyperfluorescence on the angiogram that do not correspond to RPE atrophy at the edge of the scar and (2) RPE thickening if associated with exudative changes, even if no hyperfluorescence is seen on the angiogram.

RETINAL PIGMENT EPITHELIAL DETACHMENTS

Laser treatment of serous RPE detachments is controversial since vision has rarely improved despite successful flattening after laser. Since up to 67% of serous RPE detachments are associated with SRN, it is imperative to identify the extent of the SRN angiographically and to treat the membrane specifically. If the RPE detachment has a meniscus of blood, a fringe of subretinal lipid, or choroidal folds, SRN is extremely likely. Figures 8.65 to 8.68 demonstrate such a case. Figure 8.65 shows an extremely turbid pigment epithelial detachment in the temporal macula fringed with

Retinal Pigment Epithelial Detachments

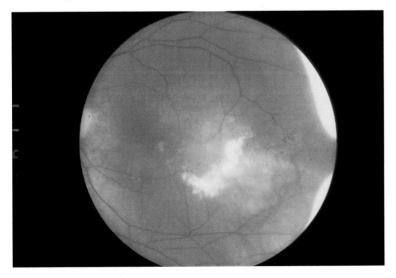

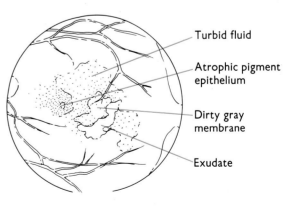

Turbid fluid

Atrophic pigment epithelium

Dirty gray membrane

Exudate

FIG. 8.65

lipid exudation. There is also an overlying sensory retinal detachment. The fluorescein angiogram in Fig. 8.66 reveals a ring of visible vessels in the temporal macula surrounded by an area of occult neovascularization. The pigment epithelial detachment extends nasally to involve the center of the macula. There is a focal area of hyperfluorescence in this region, corresponding to an atrophic change in the pigment epithelium. Figure 8.67 is the post-laser photograph showing atrophy at the site of treatment with obliteration of the SRN and resolution of the detachments. Figure 8.68 is the post-laser angiogram revealing infarction of the SRN and no evidence of persistent leakage.

Turbid subretinal fluid or blood may, however, obscure clinically or angiographically associated SRN, which is likely to be present at the margin of the RPE detachment, often at a concave notch. However, it should be noted that exudative drusen may cause a scalloped margin of the RPE detachment without actual SRN present.

Figure 8.69 shows a huge exudative pigment epithelial detachment of the macula associated with AMD. There is peripapillary thickening of the pigment epithelium and a focal area of hemorrhage in the papillomacular bundle as well. In Fig. 8.70, the fluorescein angiogram shows homogeneous hyperfluorescence in the sub-pigment epithelial space. There is a silhouette of actively proliferating vessels in the nasal macula, originating from the occult neovascularization present in the peripapillary region. The posttreatment color photograph in Fig. 8.71 shows obliteration of the neovascularization and resolution of the detachment. The corresponding angiogram in Fig. 8.72 reveals no persistent actively proliferating neovascular hyperfluorescence. There is a discrete ring of hyperfluorescence surrounding the perifoveal region corresponding to the border of the old detachment.

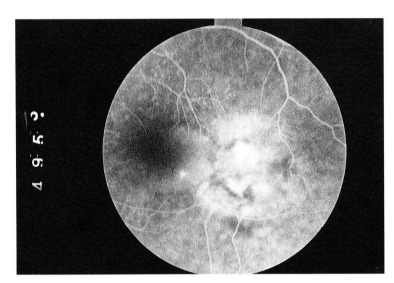

FIG. 8.66

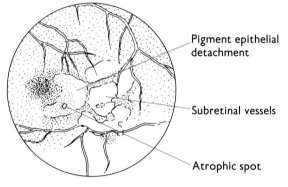

Pigment epithelial detachment

Subretinal vessels

Atrophic spot

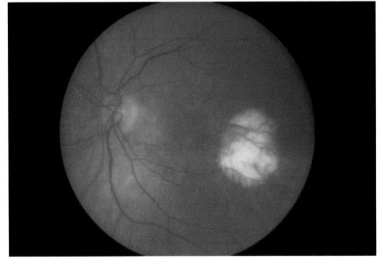

FIG. 8.67

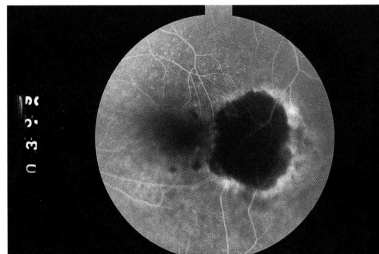

FIG. 8.68

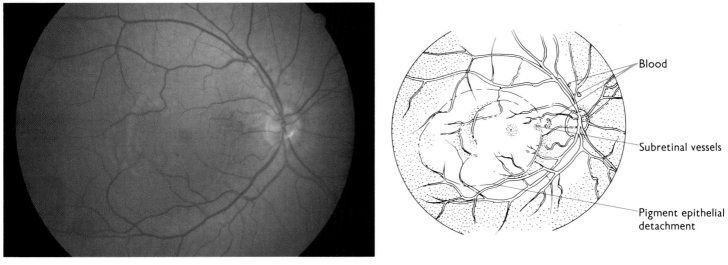

FIG. 8.69

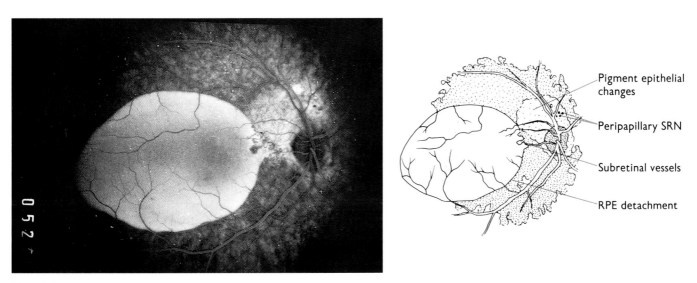

FIG. 8.70

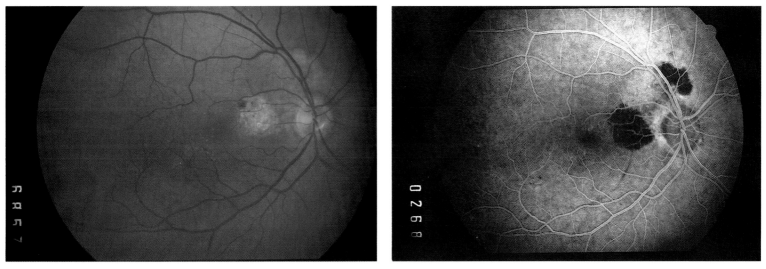

FIG. 8.71

FIG. 8.72

Retinal pigment epithelial rips also must be differentiated from SRN. They are red-orange, atrophic, and flat where the RPE is absent but thickened where the edge is coiled. They are tractionally associated with SRN and occur at the edge of the RPE detachment but do not represent SRN and should not be treated.

Several methods of laser photocoagulation treatment for RPE detachments have been proposed, including (1) placement of a grid pattern over the entire RPE detachment, (2) confluent obliteration of the RPE detachment, and (3) focal coagulation of any associated neovascular membrane at or near the edge of the RPE detachment. Although most RPE detachments will flatten when treated with a grid, clinical experience has shown that visual outcome is often poor; thus this technique has largely been abandoned. Confluent laser photocoagulation of the RPE detachment, sparing the fovea, is aimed at obliterating presumed occult SRN. This method can be effective, but large areas of retinal tissue are sacrificed. In Fig. 8.73, note the massive exudative detachment of the macula fringed with heavy lipid exudation. The fluorescein angiogram shown in Fig. 8.74 reveals indistinct leakage consistent with occult neovascularization that extends from the temporal aspect of the disk to the fovea. Figure 8.75 is the immediate postphotocoagulation photograph showing the confluent, moderately intense treatment to the occult neovascularization, sparing the fovea. Figure 8.76, taken several months later, shows complete resolution of the serous and lipid exudation with obliteration of the neovascularization.

The best (though not always possible) approach is to attempt clinical and angiographic identification of an associated neovascularized membrane in order to perform focal photocoagulation only. Figures 8.77 to 8.80 demonstrate a hemorrhagic detachment secondary to AMD. Figure 8.77 shows subretinal hemorrhage in the center of the macula. There is a reddish discoloration in the supratemporal macula consistent with actively proliferating neovascularization as a source of the bleeding. The fluorescein angiogram shown in Fig. 8.78 reveals an indistinct area of hyperfluorescence at the site of the presumed neovascularization. The same patient is shown following photocoagulation treatment in Fig. 8.79. Note the moderately intense treat-

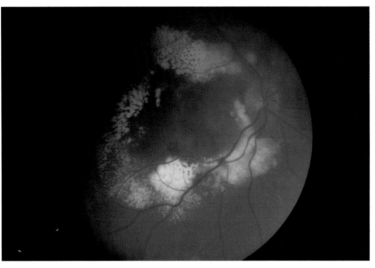

FIG. 8.73

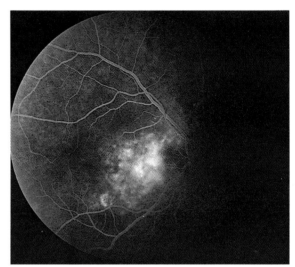

FIG. 8.74

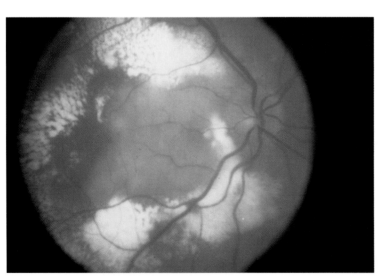

FIG. 8.75

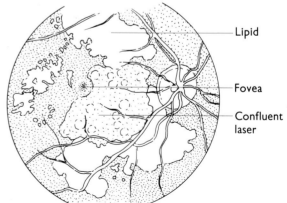

Lipid

Fovea

Confluent laser

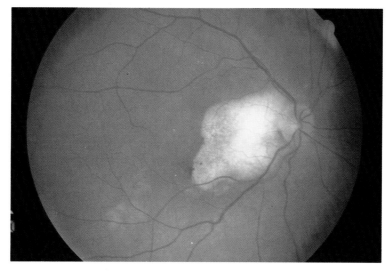

FIG. 8.76

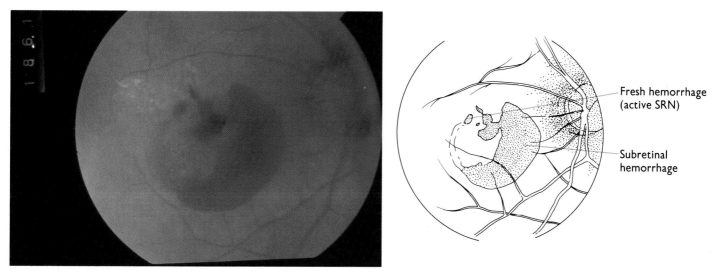

Fresh hemorrhage
(active SRN)

Subretinal
hemorrhage

FIG. 8.77

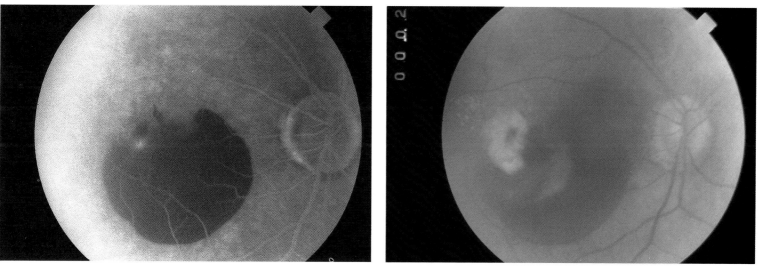

FIG. 8.78

FIG. 8.79

ment at the site of the presumed neovascularization. Figure 8.80 shows obliteration of the neovascularization, resolution of the hemorrhage, and some atrophy secondary to the antecedent hemorrhagic detachment. In our experience, RPE detachments will flatten if associated SRN is obliterated, and this usually allows vision to improve. However, many RPE detachments are partly serous and partly "organized" (referring to a region of homogeneous pooling of fluorescein dye adjacent to a darker, more variable, region of fluorescence), making localization of a discrete neovascular membrane difficult. The MPS is currently investigating the laser treatment of RPE detachments. Figure 8.81 provides a guide to clinical and angiographic diagnosis of RPE detachments.

Any disturbance of the RPE–Bruch's membrane complex, including trauma, tumors, inflammation, and even laser-induced chorioretinal scars themselves, may predispose to SRN. Laser treatment in these circumstances may be judiciously aimed at direct coagulation of extrafoveal SRN rather than the primary lesion itself.

OTHER DISEASES ASSOCIATED WITH SUBRETINAL NEOVASCULARIZATION

Subretinal neovascularization is a common histopathologic manifestation associated with numerous other macular diseases, such as pathologic myopia, angioid streaks, presumed ocular histoplasmosis syndrome (POHS), choroidal rupture, inflammatory disorders, and optic nerve head drusen. SRN may be suspected by a myriad of clinical manifestations, including the presence of hemorrhage, lipid, discoloration, pigment ring, CME, choroidal folds, and RPE detachment,

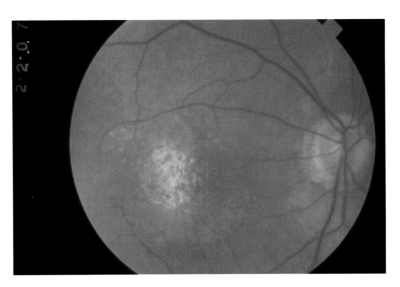

FIG. 8.80

FLUORESCEIN ANGIOGRAPHIC FEATURES OF RETINAL PIGMENT EPITHELIUM DETACHMENT AND SUBRETINAL NEOVASCULARIZATION

TYPE OF DETACHMENT OR NEOVASCULARIZATION	FLUORESCEIN ANGIOGRAPHIC FEATURES		
	CLINICAL	EARLY	LATE
RPE detachment (uncomplicated)	Circumscribed well-demarcated serous elevation of RPE.	Homogeneous progressive increase in fluorescence underneath RPE detachment. Some fluorescence may be masked by xanthophyll and perifoveal RPE pigment.	Increased intensity without increased area of hyperfluorescence as pooling occurs in sub-RPE space (margins remain sharp).
Focal RPE atrophy ("window defect")	Thinned, depigmented area of RPE detachment.	Focal choroidal transmitted hyperfluorescence ("hot spot").	Essentially unchanged but more intense fluorescence than overall RPE detachment.
RPE avascular leak (central serous type)	No discernible lesions on RPE detachment.	Focal hyperfluorescence at level of RPE ("hot spot").	Increase in area and intensity of hyperfluorescence as dye leaks into subsensory retinal space but does not fill it.
RPE rip	Flat reddish-orange disturbance at margin of RPE detachment. Retracted RPE edge sharp or coiled and concave. SRN located on side of retracting RPE.	Hyperfluorescence of large choroidal vessels followed by choriocapillaris deep to the edge of the RPE tear ("hot spot").	Pooling into overlying sensory retinal detachment. Scleral staining.
Prominent choroidal vessel ("pseudo SRN")	Significant choriocapillaris and RPE atrophy. Large choroidal vessel visible.	Hyperfluorescence of medium and large choroidal vessels without leak.	Outline of these vessels emptied of fluorescein dye against background of scleral staining ("silhouette sign").
SRN	Thickened, pigmented or discolored RPE. Subretinal fluid, lipid, blood.	Early hyperfluorescence as a "hot spot" under and at the level of the RPE detachment. Hypofluorescence by blood.	Diffuse leakage under and above RPE. May see silhouette of vessels in late stages when dye leaves choroidal circulation. Leakage often fills sensory detachment.
"Occult" SRN (organized RPE detachment)	Thickened or slightly elevated and granular-appearing RPE.	Irregular slow filling of RPE detachment.	Gradual increase in sub-RPE fluorescence, but not as intense as pure serous elevation.

FIG. 8.81

with or without distinct fluorescein angiographic leakage. Occult SRN may not hyperfluoresce by virtue of blocking subretinal blood, pigment, or turbid fluid.

The MPS study has provided guidelines for treating patients with AMD, POHS, and idiopathic SRN. Figure 8.82 shows a fluorescein angiogram of idiopathic SRN demonstrating actively proliferating vessels in the nasal macula. Figure 8.83 shows the moderate intensity of the confluent treatment. Figure 8.84 illustrates obliteration of the neovascularization with a resultant atrophic scar. Results were more encouraging with respect to laser treatment for SRN in the POHS group than the AMD group. A 78% reduction in risk of severe visual loss after 3 years could be attributed to treatment. Figure 8.85 shows the pigmentary disturbances in the infrajuxtafoveal area and in the temporal macula in a case of POHS. The fluorescein angiogram in Fig.

8.86 shows actively proliferating neovascularization at the site of the two pigment epithelial hyperplastic changes. There is also some vascular hyperfluorescence overlying the atrophic scar in the infranasal macula. In Fig. 8.87, photocoagulation treatment has caused regression of the neovascularization at the three leakage sites. Figure 8.88 confirms angiographically the obliteration of the SRN. Other diseases of the macula associated with SRN have not been studied in clinical trials.

Pathologic myopia and other hypopigmented conditions, such as angioid streaks, in the fundus with SRN present a challenge to the clinician. Examination, photography, and fluorescein angiography are more difficult and the lack of pigmentation makes evaluation of the extent of the SRN difficult. It is difficult to locate the FAZ and the patient's point of fixation as well as the retinal and choroidal vascular land-

Other Diseases Associated With Subretinal Neovascularization

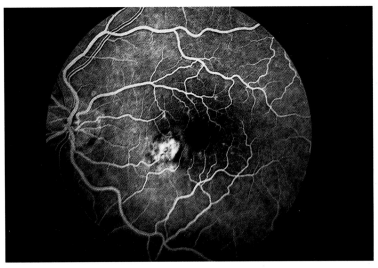

FIG. 8.82

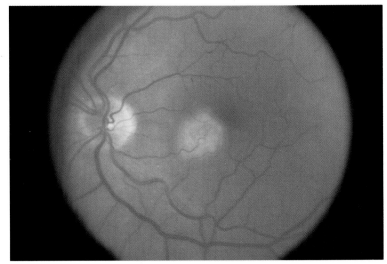

FIG. 8.83

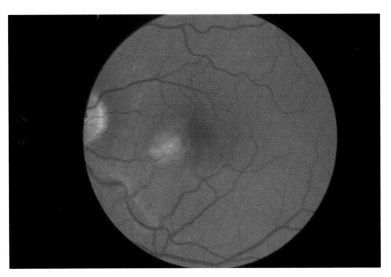

FIG. 8.84

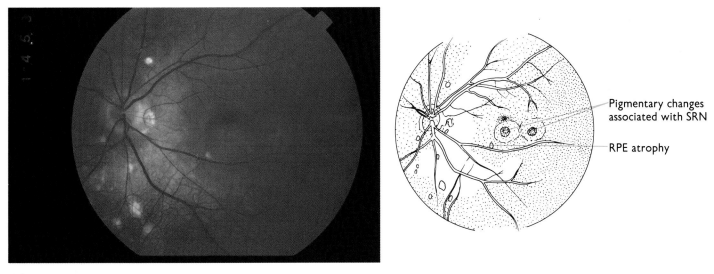

Pigmentary changes
associated with SRN

RPE atrophy

FIG. 8.85

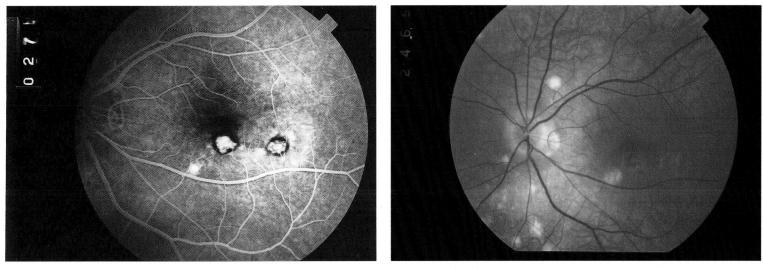

FIG. 8.86

FIG. 8.87

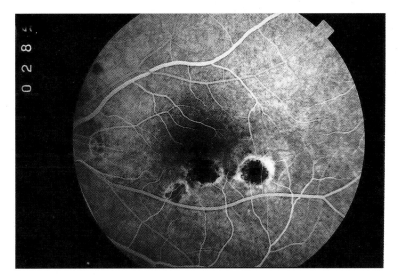

FIG. 8.88

marks when treating a pathologic myope. Figure 8.89 demonstrates a case of pathologic myopia, revealing chorioretinal atrophy and several lacquer cracks. A vertical crack in the temporal macula has become neovascularized, fringed with pigment epithelial hyperplasia. The fluorescein angiogram in Fig. 8.90 shows vascular hyperfluorescence at a foveal area of the lacquer crack in the temporal macula. The postphotocoagulation color photograph in Fig. 8.91 reveals obliteration of the neovascularization with an atrophic laser scar. Figure 8.92 shows the corresponding angiogram confirming the clinical impression. Five months later, the atrophic laser scar has enlarged (Fig. 8.93). This is a characteristic of pathologic myopia.

Eyes with angioid streaks also have widespread atrophy, diffuse SRN, and fragile occult vessels, which are subject to hemorrhage and recurrence. Figures 8.94–8.96 illustrate a case of SRN associated with angioid streaks in a patient with pseudoxanthoma elasticum. Figure 8.94 reveals a cicatricial change from previous laser treatment in the superior macula. There is also an exudative detachment with a pigmentary disturbance near the fovea. The fluorescein angiogram in Fig. 8.95 reveals obliteration of the choroid at the site of

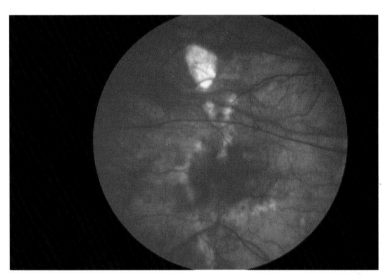

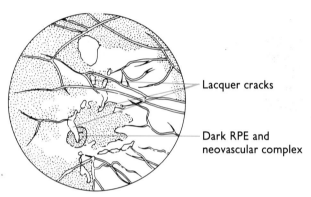

Lacquer cracks

Dark RPE and
neovascular complex

FIG. 8.89

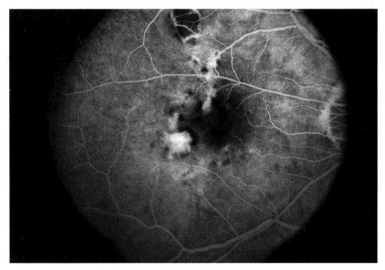

FIG. 8.90

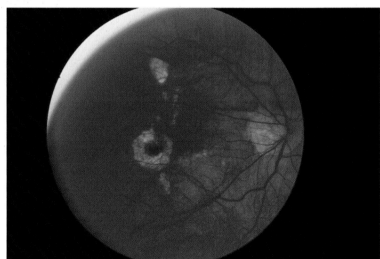

FIG. 8.91

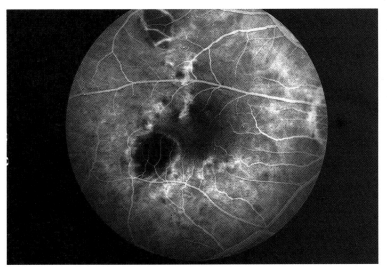

FIG. 8.92

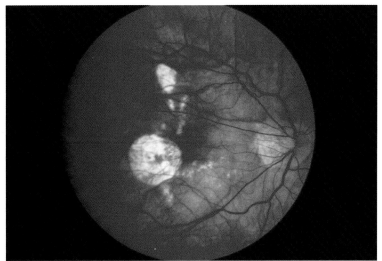

FIG. 8.93

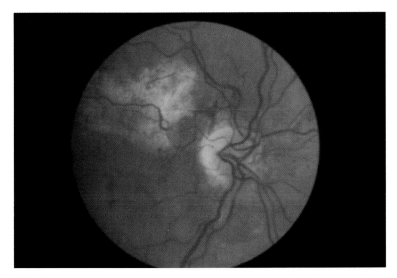

FIG. 8.94

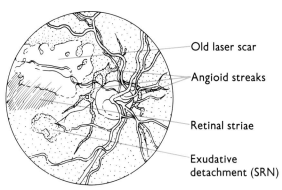

Old laser scar

Angioid streaks

Retinal striae

Exudative detachment (SRN)

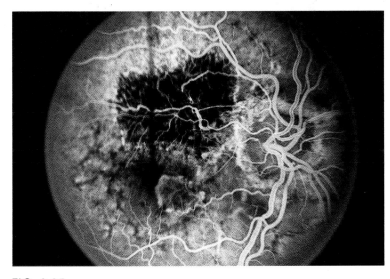

FIG. 8.95

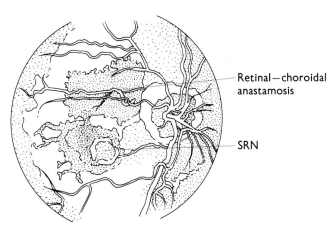

Retinal—choroidal anastamosis

SRN

previous laser treatment. There is also a retinal choroidal anastamosis and contraction of the surface of the retina in that area. An active ring of neovascularization is present just nasal to the fovea. The post-laser photograph in Fig. 8.96 shows obliteration of the SRN.

Juxtafoveal and Subfoveal Subretinal Neovascularization

The efficacy and safety of treatment have not been proven for SRN closer than 200 μm to the center of the FAZ (juxtafoveal), for perifoveal or subfoveal SRN, for RPE detachments with or without SRN, and for indistinct or "occult" SRN. The MPS group concluded that KRL treatment was effective in reducing severe vision loss in juxtafoveal SRN and in cases of extrafoveal membranes associated with blood or pigment extending closer than 200 μm to the foveal center in POHS patients. Most experienced clinicians treat juxtafoveal SRN if the neovascular membrane is well defined angiographically. Treatment of subfoveal SRN to limit the size of scotomas is controversial, and is probably indicated only in the situation where a disciform scar exists in one eye and the other eye develops a subfoveal membrane with severe visual acuity loss that the clinician suspects is largely due to exudation.

Inflammatory retinal–choroidal diseases can also be associated with SRN. In serpiginous choroidopathy, photocoagulation *is* indicated for the rare occurrence of extrafoveal SRN located at the margin of an active or inactive scar and is aimed at eradicating the vascular membrane only. In Fig. 8.97, note the peripapillary hyperplastic change. There is an area of secondary neovascularization in the macula, associated with a grayish subretinal discoloration, a ring of subretinal hemorrhage, and a shallow overlying detachment. Figure 8.98 is the fluorescein angiogram of the actively proliferating neovascularization on the temporal side of the scar. Figure 8.99 was taken following krypton red laser treatment of the same patient. Note the moderately intense confluent burns at the site of the neovascularization. In Fig. 8.100, the post-laser photograph reveals obliteration of the neovascularization and resolution of the detachment. The corresponding fluorescein angiogram at this stage shows infarction of the SRN and no significant subretinal vascular leakage (Fig. 8.101). Systemic steroids are a useful adjunct in almost all acute exacerbations of this disease.

Prophylactic photocoagulation of inactive toxoplasmosis scars is not indicated because not all scars become active. Scars associated with SRN can be treated effectively after careful clinical and angiographic localization of the extra-

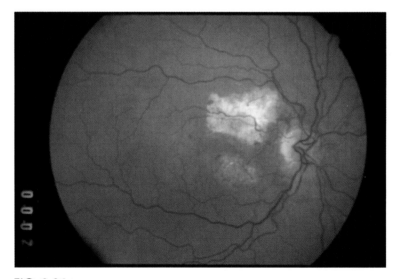

FIG. 8.96

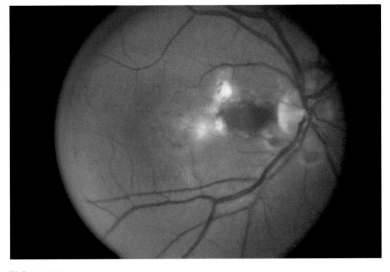

FIG. 8.97

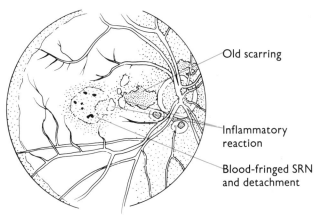

Old scarring

Inflammatory
reaction

Blood-fringed SRN
and detachment

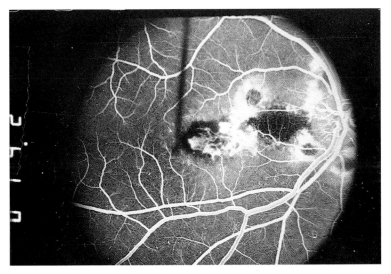

FIG. 8.98

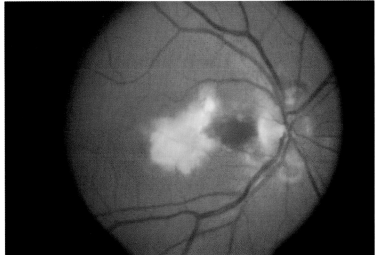

FIG. 8.99

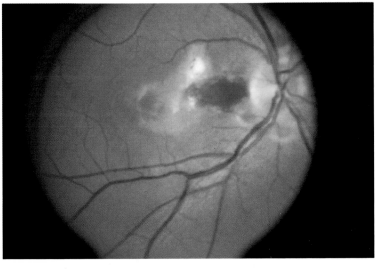

FIG. 8.100

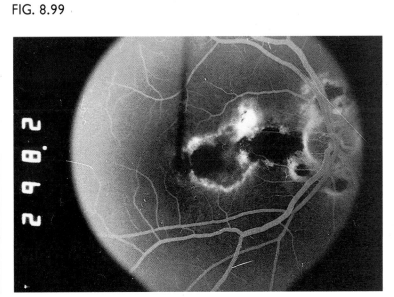

FIG. 8.101

foveal neovascularization. In Fig. 8.102, note the SRN associated with the retinal folds radiating toward the active foveal side of the toxoplasmosis scar. The fluorescein angiogram in Fig. 8.103 reveals diffuse leakage of the SRN and staining of the scar. Figure 8.104, taken after laser treatment, shows obliteration of the SRN and a juxtafoveal atrophic corona.

The precise mechanism of closure of SRN with laser is not known but is believed to be due to one or more of the following: (1) thermal infarction, (2) reversal or alteration in proposed angiogenic mediating factors present in the RPE or choriocapillaris (via RPE hyperplasia and choriocapillaris atrophy), (3) production of drainage sites for the exudative debris in the macula, (4) reconstitution of Bruch's membrane and the RPE, thereby reestablishing the outer BRB, and (5) relaxation of scleral rigidity, perhaps leading to less venous choroidal obstruction and less accumulation of sub-RPE debris.

CENTRAL SEROUS CHORIORETINOPATHY

Central serous chorioretinopathy (CSC) is a syndrome that causes transient episodes of serous detachment of the retina; there is a predilection for mildly hyperopic men between the ages of 30 and 50 who characteristically exhibit "Type-A" behavioral patterns. It tends to be bilateral and recurrent. It is most commonly seen in whites in New York and Hispanics in southern Florida, and is thought to be most prevalent in Asians and rare in blacks.

The precise pathophysiologic etiology for macular detachment is probably located at the level of the RPE. The defect leading to focal breakdown of the outer BRB may be due to a number of mechanisms: (1) a nonvascular physical disruption in continuity, (2) a focal area of inflammation or ischemia, (3) a localized immunologic or biochemical reaction, (4) a physiologic breakdown in the junctional complexes or diffusion barriers (zonula occludens and zonula adherens), or (5) other unknown factors.

Variants of CSC include multiple localized detachments of the RPE with bullous retinal detachment, CSC with atrophic RPE tracts and peripheral retinal detachments, and CSC associated with subretinal yellow precipitates, presumably fibrin.

Since CSC is generally a self-limited disease and there are no clinical trials that have established definitively the efficacy and safety of laser treatment, indications for treatment can only be based on clinical judgments. It is known that laser treatment does shorten the duration of the detachment, which is likely related to the ultimate visual outcome.

However, this concept is still unproven. It is also known that the disease tends to be chronic–recurrent acute in some patients with ultimate perifoveal pigment epithelial atrophy, cystic–macular degeneration, and irreversible and profound loss of vision. However, there is also some risk to laser photocoagulation treatment, particularly when the laser applications are applied very close to the fovea.

With these considerations in mind, the following is recommended. Laser treatment should be considered in a patient who has a persistent and progressive detachment and associated visual decline after a period of 3–4 months when there is a remote pigment epithelial leak at least 1 DD from the center of the fovea. When the detachment is associated with a more proximal pigment epithelial leak, it is recommended that more time (5–6 months) be allowed for a spontaneous resolution. If a patient has had a poor result from a relatively short detachment of the macula in one eye, there is a rationale for earlier photocoagulation treatment in the fellow eye. Finally, patients with variants of CSC with multiple pigment epithelial detachments, with a bullous sensory detachment, or with widespread pigment epithelial disease and multiple recurrent leaks should be managed with earlier laser photocoagulation intervention. These patients generally have a poorer visual prognosis.

The principle complications associated with laser treatment are inadvertent damage to the fovea, a persistent scotoma at the site of photocoagulation treatment, and a thermal reaction that may become associated with the development of subretinal neovascularization. All patients receiving juxtafoveal laser treatment for CSC must be informed that they may experience a recognizable corresponding permanent scotoma. Treatment, if possible, should not be placed closer to the fovea than the perifoveal capillary net. A recent fluorescein angiogram demonstrating the exact location of the RPE leaks is placed on a viewer. Stereoscopic contact lens examination is used to identify the sites to be treated and the associated serous detachment.

Either argon green, dye yellow, or krypton red wavelengths can be employed effectively. Krypton is recommended for juxtafoveal and papillomacular bundle treatment. A spot size that is slightly larger than the pinpoint leak (usually 200 μm or larger) is used with minimum intensity (100–150 mW) and a long duration (0.5 s), focused at the level of the RPE to obtain a slow and mild burn that turns the RPE a faint grayish color.

A case of CSC is shown in Figs. 8.105–8.108. In Fig. 8.105, note the serous detachment of the macula, with an oval depigmentary change of the RPE just nasal to the fovea. The fluorescein angiogram of the same patient (Fig.

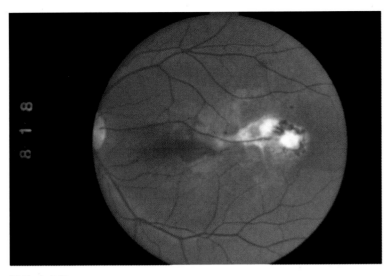
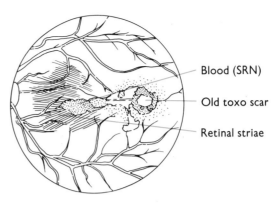

Blood (SRN)
Old toxo scar
Retinal striae

FIG. 8.102

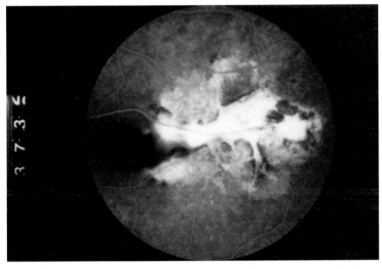

FIG. 8.103

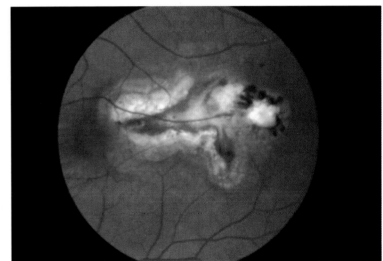

FIG. 8.104

Central Serous Chorioretinopathy

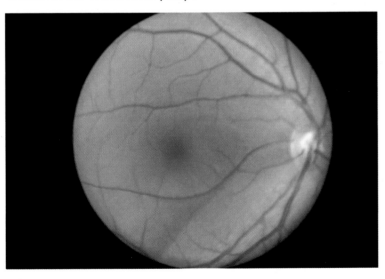
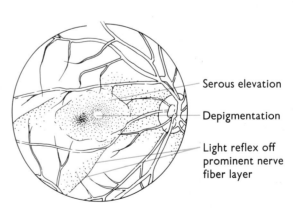

Serous elevation
Depigmentation
Light reflex off prominent nerve fiber layer

FIG. 8.105

8.106) shows a focal "smokestack" leak into the subsensory retinal space. Figure 8.107 shows the clinical appearance after krypton red photocoagulation, demonstrating flattening of the macula and a grayish discoloration at the level of the RPE. The fluorescein angiogram taken after treatment shows the "window defect" but no active leak (Fig. 8.108).

It takes approximately 2–6 weeks for the neurosensory detachment to resolve following photocoagulation of the leak. The duration will be dependent on the chronicity of the detachment, usually indicated by the degree of turbidity of the subretinal fluid. An additional 4–6 weeks is needed for full visual recovery potential in most patients. An atrophic or granular pigment spot will commonly mark the site of the laser treatment.

MISCELLANEOUS
TUMORS
Choroidal (Cavernous) Hemangioma
Cavernous hemangiomas of the choroid usually occur as orange-red, round, solitary tumors. They are often detected in early adulthood and are most commonly found in the posterior pole. Symptoms begin when serous leakage occurs from the edge of the tumor into the macular area. Cystic degeneration of the retina overlying the growth, along with extensive metaplasia of the RPE, are common findings.

Guided by fluorescein angiography, moderately intense photocoagulation using large spot sizes and long duration times should be directed to the portion of the lesion where the greatest leakage of fluorescein dye occurs. Re-treatments may be needed. Collapse of the cystic retina and resolution of leakage, rather than obliteration or shrinkage of

the tumor (which usually does not occur), determine success. The goal of treatment is to stimulate the RPE and reconstitute the outer BRB.

Choroidal Melanoma
Photocoagulation is rarely used for eradicating choroidal melanomas due to their large size at diagnosis and the danger that penetration of the laser beam (even with krypton red) may not carry through the complete thickness of the tumor, leaving residual viable cells and increased inflammation.

Choroidal Osteoma (Osseous Choristoma)
A choroidal osteoma (osseous choristoma) is a yellowish-orange lesion usually seen in the vicinity of the optic nerve head in the posterior pole and often associated with a sensory retinal elevation. Laser treatment is ineffective in penetrating deeply enough into the bony growth to efficiently cause involution. Rarely, SRN is associated at the edge of the osteoma and may be treated directly by laser.

SUBRETINAL PARASITES
Nematodes may cause retinal and RPE damage due to their motility and toxic excretions.

Photocoagulation may be used to attempt thermal destruction of the organism if it is visible clinically and can be identified and localized to a region away from the macula. This is a difficult undertaking. An interesting case of ophthalmomyiasis is shown in Figs. 8.109–8.113. Figure 8.109 shows a patient with pigmentary and atrophic changes in the macula. The fluorescein angiogram in Fig. 8.110 shows the atrophic tracks secondary to the migratory behavior of the nematode. Figure 8.111 shows the nema-

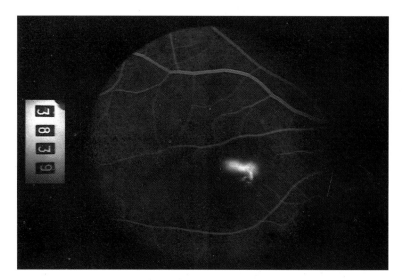

FIG. 8.106

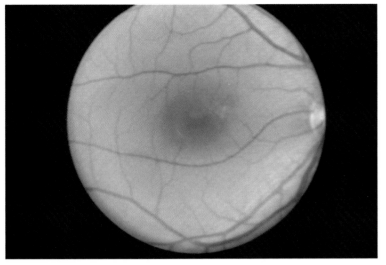

FIG. 8.107

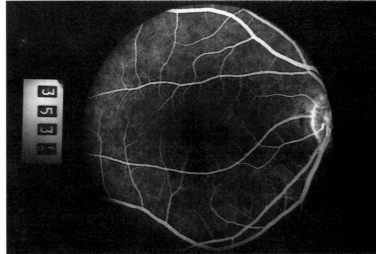

FIG. 8.108

Subretinal Parasites

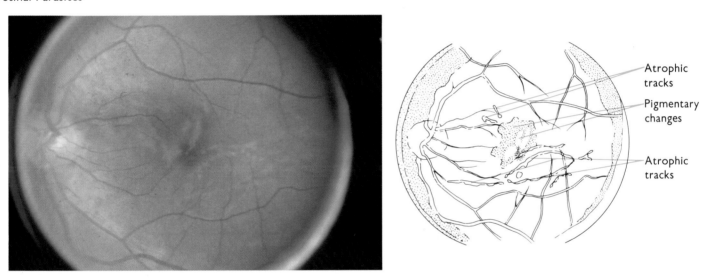

FIG. 8.109

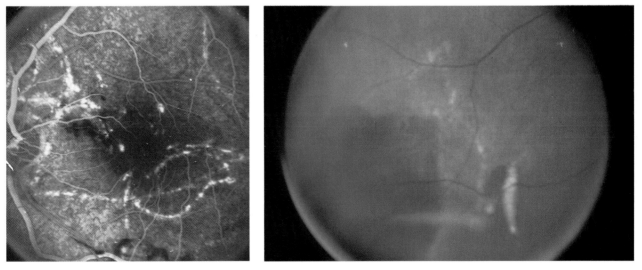

FIG. 8.110

FIG. 8.111

tode located underneath the retina. Figure 8.112 shows successful photocoagulation of the nematode. In Fig. 8.113, there has been a cicatricial retinal response at the site of photodestruction of the nematode. Often, the worm escapes from clinical view when the first shots are fired by the laser, making this a time-consuming and frustrating management consideration.

INFLAMMATIONS

In serpiginous choroidopathy, photocoagulation to "wall off" centrifugal progression of lesions into the fovea is usually unsuccessful. "Skip lesions" may occur and normal tissue itself would be sacrificed by the laser.

In toxoplasmosis, photocoagulation of active whitish retinal lesions, although tempting, is unpredictable. Thermal absorption of different wavelengths by inflamed vitreous and retinal tissue is variable. If the photocoagulation is minimally absorbed, the organism may not be eradicated; if it is maximally absorbed (often by the adjacent pigmented scar, in part) damage to normal surrounding retinal tissue and macular pucker may result.

Indications for various retinal diseases, along with current laser photocoagulation techniques, have been discussed. Ophthalmologists should familiarize themselves with color fundus photographs and the fluorescein angiogram that best demonstrate the disease entity, and carefully evaluate the region of proposed treatment by contact lens examination. Informed consent covering the potential risks, benefits, limitations, alternatives, and possible complications of laser intervention is mandatory. Clinical trials have demonstrated the effectiveness of certain wavelengths, but more clinical experience is needed to definitively prove which wavelengths are superior in any given situation.

Picture credits for this chapter are as follows: Figs. 8.38–8.41 courtesy of Harold Weissman, MD; Fig. 8.81 previously published in Judson PH, Yannuzzi LA: Subretinal neovascularization: Diagnosis and Treatment, in L'Esperance FA (ed): Ophthalmic Lasers. St. Louis, C.V. Mosby, 1989, vol 2, p. 543; Figs. 8.109–8.113 courtesy of Connie Fitzgerald, MD.

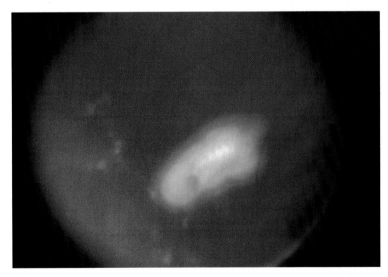

FIG. 8.112

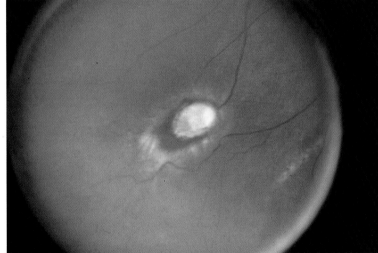

FIG. 8.113

SUGGESTED READING

CHAPTER 1   **CATARACT SURGERY AND INTRAOCULAR LENS IMPLANTATION**

Apple DJ, Reiddy JJ, Googe JM, et al: A comparison of ciliary sulcus and capsular bag fixation of posterior chamber lenses. *Am Intra-Ocular Impl Soc J* 1985;11:44–63.

Caldwell DR (ed): *Cataracts,* New Orleans Academy of Ophthalmology (trans). New York, Raven Press, 1988.

Clayman HM, Jaffe NS, Galin MA: *Intraocular Lens Implantation. Techniques and Complications.* St Louis, CV Mosby Co, 1983.

Emery JM, McIntyre DJ: *Extracapsular Cataract Surgery.* St Louis, CV Mosby Co, 1983.

Jaffe NS, Galin MA, Hirschman H, Clayman HM: *Pseudophakos,* St Louis, CV Mosby Co, 1978.

Jaffe NS, Jaffe MS, Jaffe GF: *Cataract Surgery and Its Complications,* ed 5. St Louis, CV Mosby Co, 1989.

Maloney WF, Grindle L: *Textbook of Phacoemulsification.* Fallbrook, Calif, Lasenda Publishers, 1988.

Maumenee AE, Stark WJ, Isente I (eds): *Cataract Surgery and Visual Rehabilitation.* Amsterdam, Kugler Publications, 1985.

Stark WJ, Terry AC, Maumenee AE (eds): *Anterior Segment Surgery.* Baltimore, Williams and Wilkins, 1987.

Tarkkanen A (ed): Pathology of intraocular lens implantation. *Acta Ophthalmol* 1985;(suppl 170).

CHAPTER 2   **TECHNIQUES IN CORNEAL TRANSPLANTATION**

Barraquer J, Routtlan J: *Microsurgery of the Cornea, An Atlas and Textbook.* Barcelona, Ediciones Scribasa, 1982.

Bruner WA, Stark WA, Maumenee AE: *Manual of Corneal Surgery.* New York, Churchill Livingstone, 1987.

Casey TA, Mayer DJ: *Corneal Grafting, Principles and Practice.* London, WB Saunders Co, 1984.

Leibowitz HM: *Corneal Disorders, Clinical Diagnosis and Management.* Philadelphia, WB Saunders Co, 1984.

Troutman RC: *Microsurgery of the Anterior Segment of the Eye: The Cornea: Optics and Surgery.* St. Louis, CV Mosby Co, 1977, vol. 2.

CHAPTER 3   **SURGERY FOR GLAUCOMA AND RELATED CONDITIONS**

Anderson DR: Trabeculotomy compared to goniotomy for glaucoma in children. *Ophthalmology* 1983;90:805–806.

Burian HA: A case of Marfan's syndrome with bilateral glaucoma: With description of a new type of operation for developmental glaucoma. *Am J Ophthalmol* 1970;50:1187–1192.

Cairns JE: Trabeculectomy, preliminary report of a new method. *Am J Ophthalmol,* 1968;66:673–679.

Epstein DL: *Chandler and Grant's Glaucoma,* ed 3. Philadelphia, Lea & Febiger, 1986.

Hoskins HD Jr, Shaffer N, Hetherington J: Goniotomy versus trabeculotomy. *J Ped Ophthalmol Strabismus* 1984;21:153–158.

King JH Jr, Wadsworth JAC: *An Atlas of Ophthalmic Surgery,* ed 3. Philadelphia, JB Lippincott, 1981.

Kolker AE, Hetherington J Jr: *Becker-Shaffer's Diagnosis and Therapy of the Glaucomas,* ed 5. St. Louis, CV Mosby, 1988.

Luntz MH: The advantages of trabeculectomy over goniotomy. *J Ped Ophthalmol Strabismus* 1984;21:150–152.

Marion JR, Shields MB: Thermal sclerostomy and posterior lip sclerectomy: A comparative study. *Ophthalmic Surg* 1978;9:67–75.

Olander KW, Zimmerman TJ, Mandelkorn RM: Non-perforating trabeculectomy: Results in phakic and aphakic patients with glaucoma. *Invest Ophthalmol Vis Sci* 1980;suppl:141.

Scheie HG: Retraction of scleral wound edges—as a fistulizing procedure for glaucoma. *Am J Ophthalmol* 1958;45:220–229.

Shaffer RN, Hoskins HD: Goniotomy in the treatment of isolated trabeculodysgenesis (Primary congenital [infantile] developmental glaucoma). *Trans Ophthalmol Soc UK* 1983;103:581–585.

Shields MB: *A Study Guide for Glaucoma,* ed 2. Baltimore, Williams and Wilkins, 1987.

Spaeth GL: A prospective, controlled study to compare the Scheie procedure with Watson's trabeculectomy. *Ophthalmic Surg* 1980;11:688–694.

Spaeth GL, Joseph NH, Fernades E: Trabeculectomy: A re-evaluation after three years and a comparison with Scheie's procedure. *Ophthalmic Surg* 19756:27–38.

CHAPTER 4 SURGERY OF THE RETINA AND VITREOUS

Benson WB: *Retinal Detachment Diagnosis and Management.* Philadelphia, JB Lippincott, 1988, pp 113–155.

Blankenship GW: Management of postvitrectomy diabetic vitreous hemorrhage, in Blankenship GW, Stirpe M, Gonvers M, Binders S (eds): *Basic and Advanced Vitreous Surgery.* Padua, Liviana, 1986, pp 295–300.

Byer NE: A clinical definition of lattice degeneration of the retina and its variations. *Mod Probl Ophthalmol* 1975;15:58–67.

Chang S, Lincoff H, Ozmert E, et al: Management of moderate PVR, in Freeman HM, Tolentino FI (eds): *Proliferative Vitreoretinopathy (PVR).* New York, Springer-Verlag, 1988, pp 54–59.

Charles S: *Vitreous Microsurgery,* ed 2. Baltimore, Williams & Wilkins, 1987, pp 89–92.

Coleman, DJ: Early vitrectomy in the management of the severely traumatized eye. *Am J Ophthalmol* 1982;93:543.

Elner SG, Elner VM, Diaz-Rohena R, et al: Anterior PVR: II. Clinicopathologic, light microscopic, and ultrastructual findings, in Freeman HM, Tolentino FI (eds): *Proliferative Vitreoretinopathy (PVR).* New York, Springer-Verlag, 1988, pp 34–45.

Flynn HW, Blumenkranz MS, Parel JM, et al: Cannulated subretinal fluid aspirator for vitreoretinal surgery. *Am J Ophthalmol* 1987;103:106–108.

Freeman HM, Elner SG, Tolentino FI, et al: Anterior proliferative vitreoretinopathy (PVR): I. Clinical findings and management, in Freeman HM, Tolentino FI (eds): *Proliferative Vitreoretinopathy.* New York, Springer-Verlag, 1988, pp 22–33.

Freeman HM, Humphrey WT, Schepens CL, et al: Transillumination and choroidal diathermy in the drainage of subretinal fluid, in Pruett RC, Regan CDJ (eds), *Retina Congress.* 1974, pp 391–396.

Glaser BM, Cardin A, Biscoe B: Proliferative vitreoretinopathy. The mechanism of development of vitreoretinal traction. *Ophthalmology* 1987;94:327–332.

Hannekan AM, Michels RG: Surgical treatment of PVR, in Freeman HM, Tolentino FI (eds): *Proliferative Vitreoretinopathy (PVR).* New York, Springer-Verlag, 1988, pp 60–69.

Hilton GW, Grizzard WS: Pneumatic retinopexy: A two-step outpatient operation without conjunctival incision. *Ophthalmology* 1986;94:307–314.

Lewis H, Aaberg TA: Anterior proliferative vitreoretinopathy. *Am J Ophthalmol* 1988;00:277–284.

Lincoff H, Coleman J, Kreissig I, et al: The perfluorocarbon gases in the treatment of retinal detachment. *Ophthalmology* 1983;90:546–552.

Machemer R, McCuen BW, de Juan E: Relaxing retinotomies and retinectomies. *Am J Ophthalmol* 1986;102:7–12.

McCuen BW II, de Juan E Jr, Machemer R: Management of severe (grade D) PVR with mechanical fixation of the retina, in Freeman HM, Tolentino FI (eds): *Proliferative Vitreoretinopathy (PVR)*. New York, Springer-Verlag, 1988, pp 70–75.

McDonald HR, Abrams GW, Irvine AE, et al: The management of subretinal gas following attempted pneumatic retinal reattachment. *Ophthalmology* 1987;94:319–326.

McPherson A: Prophylactic treatment of retinal detachment, in Brockhurst RJ, Boruchoff SA, Hutchinson TB, Lessell S (eds): *Controversy in ophthalmology*. New York, WB Saunders, 1977, pp 517–538.

Morse PH, Scheie HG: Prophylactic cryoretinopexy of retinal breaks. *Arch Ophthalmol* 1974;92:204.

Nussbaum JJ, Freeman HM: Peripheral retinal breaks and degeneration, in Fraunfelder FT, Roy FH (eds): *Current Ocular Therapy 2*. Philadelphia, WB Saunders, 1985, pp 471–473.

Pruett RC: The fishmouth phenomenon: 1. Clinical characteristics and surgical options. *Arch Ophthalmol* 1977;95:1782–1787.

Ryan SJ: The pathophysiology of proliferative vitreoretinopathy in management. *Am J Ophthalmol* 1985;100:188–193.

Schepens CL: Retinal detachment and allied diseases. Philadelphia, WB Saunders, 1983, pp 374–435.

Tasman W, Shields JA: *Disorders of the Peripheral Fundus*. Hagerstown, Harper & Row, 1980, pp 7–11.

Tolentino FI, Refojo MF, Schepens CL: A hydrophilic acrylate implant for scleral buckling: Technique and clinical experience. *Retina* 1981;12:281–286.

Trese MT, Cox MS: The role of vitreoretinal surgery in ocular trauma, in Spoor TC, Nesi FA (eds): *Management of Ocular, Orbital and Adnexal Trauma*, 1988, pp 29–135.

Zivojnovic R: *Silicone Oil in Vitreoretinal Surgery*. Dordrecht, Martinus Nijhoff, 1987, pp 45–72.

CHAPTER 5   TECHNIQUES IN STRABISMUS SURGERY

Calhoun JH, Nelson LB, Harley RD: *Atlas of Pediatric Ophthalmic Surgery*. Philadelphia, WB Saunders Co, 1987.

Helveston EM: *Atlas of Strabismus Surgery*. St. Louis, CV Mosby Co, 1985.

Helveston EM, Eris FD: Superior oblique tuck for superior oblique palsy. *Aust J Ophthalmol* 1983;11:215–220.

Parks MM: *Atlas of Strabismus Surgery*. Philadelphia, Harper and Row, 1983.

Parks MM: Fornix incision for horizontal rectus muscle surgery. *Am J Ophthalmol* 1968;65:907–915.

Parks MM: The overacting inferior oblique muscle. *Am J Ophthalmol* 1974;77:787–797.

Steger DR, Parks MM: Inferior oblique weakening procedures. *Arch Ophthalmol* 1973;90:15–16.

Swan KC, Talbott: Recession under Tenon's capsule. *Arch Ophthalmol* 1954;51:32–41.

VanNoorden GK: The limbal approach to surgery of the rectus muscles. *Arch Ophthalmol* 1968;80:94–97.

CHAPTER 7   REFRACTIVE SURGERY

Arrowsmith PN, Marks RG: Evaluating the predictability of radial keratotomy. *Ophthalmology* 1985;92:331–338.

Arrowsmith PN, Marks RG: Visual, refractive, and keratometric results of radial keratotomy: Two year follow up. *Arch Ophthalmol* 1987;105:76–80.

Barraquer JT: *Queratomikosis y Queratofaguia*. Colombia Institute Barraqer de America, 1980, pp 34,35,379.

Hoffer KJ, Darin JJ, Pettit TH, et al: UCLA clinical trial of radial keratotomy. *Ophthalmology* 1981;88:729–736.

Kremer FV, Marks RG: Radial keratotomy: Prospective evaluation of safety and efficacy. *Ophthalmic Surg* 1983;14:925–930.

Maxwell WA, Nordan LT: Optical and wound complications of keratomileusis, in Cavanaugh D (ed), *The Cornea.* New York, Raven Press, 1988.

McDonald MB, Kaufman HE, Aquavella JV, et al: The nationwide study of epikeratophakia for aphakia in adults. *Am J Ophthalmol* 1987;103(2):358.

McDonald MB, Kaufman HE, Aquavella JV, et al: The nationwide study of epikeratophakia for myopia. *Am J Ophthalmol* 1987;103(2):358.

McDonald MB, Koenig SB, Safir A, et al: Onlyha lamellar keratoplasty for the treatment of keratoconus. *Br J Ophthalmol* 1983;67:615.

Nordan LT: *Current Status of Refractive Surgery.* San Diego, Steinway Instrument Co, 1983.

Nordan LT: Quantifiable astigmatism correction: Concepts and suggestions. *J Cataract Refract Surg* 1986;12(Sept).

Nordan LT, Fallor M: Myopic keratomileusis: 74 consecutive cases with one year follow up. *J Refract Surg* 1986;1(May/June).

Nordan LT, Maxwell WA: Keratomileusis, in Schwab I (ed): *Refractive Keratoplasty.* New York, Churchill Livingstone, 1987.

Nordan LT, Maxwell, WA: Myopic keratomileusis: Early experience. *J Refract Surg* 1985;1(July/Aug).

Sawelson HR, Marks RG: Two year results of radial keratotomy. *Arch Ophthalmol* 1985;103:505–510.

Sawelson HR, Marks RG: Three year results of radial keratotomy. *Arch Ophthalmol* 1987;105:81–85.

Srinivasan R, Sutcliff E: Dynamics of the ultraviolet laser ablation of corneal tissue. *Am J Ophthalmol* 103(no 3, pt 2):470–471.

Waring GO, Lynn MJ, Gelender H, et al: Results of the prospective evaluation of radial keratotomy (PERK) study 1 year after surgery. *Ophthalmology* 1985;92:177–198.

CHAPTER 8   LASER SURGERY OF CHORIORETINAL DISEASES
Diabetes Mellitus

Blankenship GW: Diabetic macular edema and argon laser photocoagulation: A prospective randomized study. *Ophthalmology* 1979;86:69–75.

Bresnick GH: Diabetic macular edema: A review. *Ophthalmology* 1986;93:989–997.

Diabetic Retinopathy Study Research Group: Photocoagulation treatment of proliferative diabetic retinopathy. Clinical applications of Diabetic Retinopathy Study (DRS) findings, DRS report 8. *Ophthalmology* 1981; 88:585–600.

Early Treatment Diabetic Retinopathy Study Group: Photocoagulation for diabetic macular edema: Early Treatment, DRS report 1. *Arch Ophthalmol* 1985;103;1796–1806.

Ferris FL, Podgor MJ, Davis MD: The Diabetic Retinopathy Study Research Group: Macular edema in DRS patients. DRS report 12. *Ophthalmology* 1987;94:754–760.

Klein R: The epidemiology of diabetic retinopathy: Findings from the Wisconsin Epidemiologic Study of Diabetic Retinopathy. *Int Ophthalmol Clin* 1987;27(winter):230–237.

MacDonald HR, Schatz H: Macular edema following panretinal photocoagulation. *Retina* 1985;5:5–10.

Olk RJ: Modified grid argon (blue green) laser photocoagulation for diffuse diabetic macular edema. *Ophthalmology* 1986;93:938–948.

Patz A, Fine SL: Observations in diabetic macular edema, in *Symposium on Retinal Diseases. Transactions of the New Orleans Academy of Ophthalmology.* St. Louis, CV Mosby, 1977, p 112.

Venous Occlusive Disease

Branch Vein Occlusion Study Group: Argon laser photocoagulation for macular edema in branch retinal vein occlusion. *Am J Ophthalmol* 1984;98:3.

Branch Vein Occlusion Study Group: Argon laser scatter photocoagulation for prevention of neovascularization and vitreous hemorrhage in branch vein occlusion. A randomized trial. *Arch Ophthalmol* 1986;104:34–41.

Hayreh SS, Rojas P, Podhajsky P, et al: Ocular neovascularization with retinal vascular occlusion: III. Incidence of ocular neovascularization with retinal vein occlusion. *Ophthalmology* 1983;90:488–506.

Magargal LE, Brown GC, Augsberger JJ, et al: Efficacy of panretinal photocoagulation in preventing neovascular glaucoma following ischemic central retinal vein occlusion. *Ophthalmology* 1982;89:780–784.

Magargal LE, Brown GC, Augsberger JJ, et al: Neovascular glaucoma following central retinal vein occlusion. *Ophthalmology* 1981;88:1095–1101.

Roseman RL, Olk RJ: Krypton red laser photocoagulation for branch retinal vein occlusion. *Ophthalmology* 1987;94:1120–1125.

Sickle Cell Retinopathy

Goldberg MF: Retinal neovascularization in sickle cell retinopathy. *Trans Am Acad Ophthalmol Otolaryngol* 1977;83:409.

Goldberg MF, Jampol LM: Treatment of neovascularization, vitreous hemorrhage and retinal detachment in sickle cell retinopathy, in *Symposium in Medical and Surgical Diseases of the Retina and Vitreous. Transactions of the New Orleans Academy of Ophthalmology.* St. Louis, CV Mosby, 1983, pp 53–81.

Redman KRV, Jampol LM, Goldberg MF: Scatter retinal photocoagulation for proliferative sickle cell retinopathy. *Am J Ophthalmol* 1982;93:594.

Macroaneurysms

Cleary PE, Kohner EM, Hamilton AM, et al: Retinal macroaneurysms. *Br J Ophthalmol* 1975;59:355.

Gass JDM: *Stereoscopic Atlas of Macular Diseases: Diagnosis and Treatment,* ed 3. St. Louis, CV Mosby, 1987, vol 1, pp 362–367.

Palestine AG, Robertson DM, Goldstein BG: Macroaneurysms of the retinal arteries. *Am J Ophthalmol* 1982;93:164.

Eales' Disease

Gass JDM: *Stereoscopic Atlas of Macular Diseases: Diagnosis and Treatment,* ed 3. St. Louis, CV Mosby, 1987, vol 1, pp 410–411.

Renie WA, Murphy RP, Anderson KC, et al: The evaluation of patients with Eales' disease. *Retina* 1983;3:243.

Telangiectasias

Gass JDM, Oyakawa RT: Idiopathic juxtafoveal telangiectasia. *Arch Ophthalmol* 1982;100:769.

Ridley ME, Shields JA, Brown GC, et al: Coat's disease: Evaluation and management. *Ophthalmology* 1982;89:1381.

Angiomatosis Retinae

Annesley WH Jr, Leonard BC, Shields JA, et al: Fifteen year review of treated cases of retinal angiomatosis. *Trans Am Acad Ophthalmol Otolaryngol* 1977;83:OP446.

Gass JDM, Braunstein R: Sessile and exophytic capillary hemangiomas of the juxtapapillary retina and optic nerve head. *Arch Ophthalmol* 1980;98:1790.

Retinal Breaks

Byer NE: Prognosis of asymptomatic retinal breaks. *Arch Ophthalmol* 1974;92:108–210.

Davis MD: The natural history of retinal breaks. *Arch Ophthalmol* 1974;92:183–194.

Davis MD, Segal PP, MacCormack A: The natural course followed by the fellow eye in patients with rhegmatogenous retinal detachment, in Pruett RC, Regan CDJ (eds): *Retina Congress.* New York, Appleton-Century-Crofts, 1972, pp 643–660.

Subretinal Neovascularization

Braunstein RA, Gass JDM: Serous detachments of the retinal pigment epithelium in patients with sensile macular disease. *Am J Ophthalmol* 1979;88:612–620.

Gass JDM: Pathogenesis of macular detachment and degeneration. *Ophthalmol Forum* 1984;2:8–17.

Macular Photocoagulation Study Group: Argon laser photocoagulation for neovascular maculopathy. Three year results from randomized clinical trials. *Arch Ophthalmol* 1986;104:694–705.

Macular Photocoagulation Study Group: Argon laser photocoagulation for senile macular degeneration. Results of a randomized trial. *Arch Ophthalmol* 1982;100:912–918.

Macular Photocoagulation Study Group: Recurrent choroidal neovascularization after argon laser photocoagulation for neovascular maculopathy. *Arch Ophthalmol* 1986;104:503–512.

The Moorfields Macular Study Group: Retinal pigment epithelial detachments in the elderly: A controlled trial of argon laser photocoagulation. *Br J Ophthalmol* 1982;66:1–16.

Poliner LS, Olk RJ, Burgess D, et al: Natural history of retinal pigment epithelial detachments in age-related macular degeneration. *Ophthalmology* 1986;93:543–551.

Shakin JL, Yannuzzi LA, Shakin EP, et al: Krypton red laser photocoagulation for subretinal neovascularization. *Ophthalmology* 1985;92:1364–1370.

Sorenson JA, Yannuzzi LA, Shakin JL: Recurrent subretinal neovascularization. *Ophthalmology* 1984;92:1059–1074.

Yannuzzi LA: Krypton red laser photocoagulation for subretinal neovascularization. *Retina* 1982;2:29–46.

Central Serous Chorioretinopathy

Mazzuca DE, Benson WE: Central serous retinopathy. *Surv Ophthalmol* 1986;31:170–174.

Slusher MM: Krypton red laser photocoagulation in selected cases of central serous chorioretinopathy. *Retina* 1986;6:81–84.

Yannuzzi LA: Type-A behavior and central serous chorioretinopathy. *Retina* 1987;7(2):11–130.

Yannuzzi LA, Shakin JL, Fisher YL, et al: Peripheral retinal detachments and retinal pigment atrophic tracts secondary to central serous pigment epitheliopathy. *Ophthalmology* 1984;91:1554–1572.

Choriodal Hemangioma

Gass JDM: *Stereoscopic Atlas of Macular Diseases: Diagnosis and Treatment,* ed 3. St. Louis, CV Mosby, 1987, vol 1, pp 172–176.

Sanborn GE, Augsberger JJ, Shields JA: Treatment of circumscribed choroidal hemangiomas. *Ophthalmology* 1982;89:1374.

INDEX